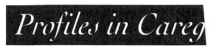 *Profiles in Careg*

The Unexpected Career

DATE DUE

Carol S. Aneshensel
Department of Community Health Sciences
School of Public Health
University of California
Los Angeles, California

Leonard I. Pearlin
Human Development and Aging Program
Department of Psychiatry
Center for Social and Behavioral Sciences
University of California
San Francisco, California
and
Department of Sociology
University of Maryland
College Park, Maryland

Joseph T. Mullan
Department of Psychiatry
University of California
San Francisco, California

Steven H. Zarit
Department of Human Development and Family Studies
Pennsylvania State University
University Park, Pennsylvania

Carol J. Whitlatch
Department of Psychiatry
University of California
San Francisco, California
and
The Margaret Blenkner Research Center
The Benjamin Rose Institute
Cleveland, Ohio

Profiles in Caregiving

The Unexpected Career

Carol S. Aneshensel

Leonard I. Pearlin

Joseph T. Mullan

Steven H. Zarit

Carol J. Whitlatch

Academic Press

San Diego   New York   Boston   London   Sydney   Tokyo   Toronto

Front cover photograph: The types of primary stressors that sometimes generate intrapsychic strains are illustrated by this caregiver as he moves his wife, gets her settled, and attends to her needs (see photograph 11, page 134).

Academic Press, Inc.
A Division of Harcourt Brace & Company
525 B Street, Suite 1900, San Diego, California 92101-4495

United Kingdom Edition published by
Academic Press Limited
24-28 Oval Road, London NW1 7DX

Library of Congress Cataloging-in-Publication Data

Profiles in caregiving : the unexpected career / by Carol S.
  Aneshensel . . . [et al.].
          p.   cm.
  Includes bibliographical references and index.
  ISBN 0-12-059540-0 (alk. paper)
   1. Alzheimer's disease--Patients--Care.   2. Caregivers.   3. Senile
dementia--Patients--Care.   I. Aneshensel, Carol S.
  RC523.P76   1995
  362.1'9897683--dc20   95-3498
                                                           CIP

PRINTED IN THE UNITED STATES OF AMERICA
95 96 97 98 99 00 MM 9 8 7 6 5 4 3 2 1

To Carel Joyce, the one who cares for our family, C. S. A.

Contents

Chapter 5   *The Natural History of Care-Related Stress*

Chapter 6   *Stress Proliferation*

Chapter 7   *The Containment of Care-Related Stressors*

Chapter 8   *The Transition to Institutional Care*

Chapter 9   *Adaptation Following Institutionalization*

Chapter 10   *The Timing and Settings of Patient Death*

Chapter 13   *Implications for Public Policy and Society*

Chapter 14   *A Review and Overview of Caregiving Careers*

Preface

This book is the end product of a lengthy process of sifting and sorting through a vast volume of information collected from people caring for close relatives with Alzheimer's Disease. In the course of this process, countless decisions were made concerning the data that should be emphasized, the statistical strategies best suited to our analytic goals, and the styles of presentation that would most clearly describe our findings. It is easy to imagine that a very different book might have been written had we made a few of these decisions differently. However, we can attest that our choices were made with careful consideration and that they are consistent with the purposes that guided the substance and direction of the work.

Among these purposes was the desire to highlight the long-term and varied course of caregiving to someone suffering from dementia. These caregivers provide an outstanding case study of a group that, for the most part, succeeds in maintaining its equilibrium while being engaged in a challenging mission that typically spans many years. To capture the transitions and changing conditions that caregivers experience during the extended trajectories of their activities, we formulated the construct of caregiving careers. This construct, in turn, was instrumental in determining how we approached the analysis of the data and, in fact, how we organized this book.

We also sought to create a book that would appeal to the interests of multiple audiences, each very different from the others. Included among the audiences we hope to reach are caregivers such as those who participated in this study. Unfortunately, these caregivers are found everywhere, a consequence of the aging of the population. Some of the unavoidable technical and procedural parts of this book might not be easy going for many in the lay audience of caregivers, but we have attempted to make the substance of each chapter accessible to all readers.

A second audience that is important to us is made up of our academic colleagues whose research is concerned with stress and well-being. Although in some respects caregivers are a special group, they nonetheless provide a clear and stunning lesson for scholars interested in stress and its consequences in other populations. In particular, much can be found between these covers that helps to illuminate processes of chronic psychosocial stress. The hardships and demands faced by caregivers are not in the form of eruptive events that quickly become part of one's past. Indeed, they are persistent conditions that can come to shape the organization of experiences across a significant portion of the life course. Despite the uniqueness of the caregivers described here, what we are able to learn about them has general applicability to other groups facing enduring hardship.

Still another audience this book addresses is clinicians, program planners, and others whose work entails ameliorative interventions in the lives of caregivers. In the course of interviewing the participants in our study, we were occasionally asked what difference the research would make, how it might lighten the burdens of caregiving. We ardently hope that it will make a difference, but we recognize that the knowledge we have gained will not by itself directly make caregivers' lives easier. If this research is to make a difference, it will be because it has informed the actions of the front-line professionals who work with caregivers, who create intervention programs, and who advocate public policies. This is an audience that remained very salient in our awareness throughout the writing of this book.

Because of the vast body of data that passed through our scrutiny and the diverse audiences which we seek to reach, this was far from an easy book to assemble. But it was as rewarding as it was difficult. In large measure, the rewards came from our own opportunities for learning. The very process of selecting, analyzing, organizing, and presenting the information repeatedly forced us to reconsider our own thinking and assumptions. A kind of dialectic was set in motion, where our findings led to a refinement of our theoretical and conceptual orientations and these refinements, in turn, resulted in new perspectives on our findings. There was nothing routine about the work; on the contrary, each day seemed to bring its own challenges and discoveries.

The work presented in this volume is the result of the collective efforts of a large number of people in several institutions. It is a pleasure to acknowledge their contributions formally. First of all, this research was made possible by a MERIT award made to Dr. Pearlin by the National Institute of Mental Health (MH-42122). Our special thanks go to Drs. Enid Light and Barry Lebowitz of the NIMH Mental Disorders of Aging Research Branch for their encouragement, support, and guidance. Also among the early supporters of the study are Dr. William Jaqust, Director of the Northern California Alzheimer's Center, and David Lindeman, formerly the Administrative Director of the Center. Both gave us critical intellectual and practical assistance in laying the groundwork for the study and generously served as our co-investigators during the early phases of the work.

An enormous effort was required to implement the fieldwork for this inquiry. Our large-scale sample of caregivers was largely recruited through the good offices and generous help of the executive directors of two Alzheimer's Disease and Related Disorders Associations. One is William Fisher of the San Francisco Bay Area Chapter and the other is Peter Braun of the Greater Los Angeles Chapter. We cannot overstate our gratitude for the facilitation of the research by these individuals and their organizations.

Several members of both the San Francisco and the Los Angeles research teams are veterans of each step of the study and it is impossible in this brief space to give a fair account of all of their contributions. We note but a few. In San Francisco, Anita O'Connor was responsible for the quality of the interviewing and is herself an interviewer nonpareil. Jane Karp monitored the scheduling of interviews and maintained the data management system, including the computer storage of all of the information drawn from the interviews. Shirley Yuen and Kali Zivitz examined virtually every page of every interview for errors and completeness and were instrumental in the complex computerized "cleaning" of the data. With Ellen Grund, they also helped to generate compilations of data and tabular presentations of results.

In Los Angeles, sample recruitment and data collection activities were organized and supervised by staff of the UCLA Survey Research Center. Roberleigh Schuler worked as the principal statistical analyst for this project and the meticulousness and sophistication of her work is evident throughout this volume. She also undertook the onerous task of proofreading text, tables, and figures against original output.

Had we known in advance the amount of work entailed in the sheer preparation of materials for this monograph, aside from the conduct of the research itself, we might never have embarked on this journey. Having undertaken it, however, we are grateful to those who helped bring us safely back to port. As all experienced scholars know, contemporary research is conducted in the context of a bewildering web of bureaucratic requirements. Protecting us from hopeless entanglement in this web were our two peerless administrative assistants, Liz Merry in Los Angeles and Les Gundel in San Francisco. They enabled us to keep most of our energies focused upon the research itself.

Several individuals have been through the text of this book with a fine-toothed comb. Dr. Allen LeBlanc reviewed and critiqued the entire manuscript, turning a researcher's eye to its conceptual and empirical content. We are particularly grateful to Dannah Grancell for transforming our drafts into a coherent text by imposing a uniformity of style and technique, a task of more than ordinary difficulty because of the multiple authors. Ms. Grancell prepared the bibliography, completing and verifying it against the citations in the text. Derrick Hindery prepared all of the graphics, helping to convert numbers into images reflective of the substance of the findings. Finally, Alicia Padilla conducted the word processing for the manuscript, repeatedly revising each chapter without losing her good humor or patience.

Barbara Barer is responsible for two features of the book that help to illustrate how some of the quantitative findings we present are abstracted from the daily lives of individual caregivers. The vignettes and statements of caregivers that are interspersed throughout this monograph are one such feature; these materials emerged from qualitative interviews she conducted. Ms. Barer is as sensitive a photographer as she is an interviewer and her pictures poignantly bring to life some of the activities and emotional currents that are difficult to capture by words alone.

Finally, a unique reward came from studying caregivers, a very special group.

It is difficult to imagine a population more cooperative or more encouraging than this one. We feel privileged to have been taught by them.

Carol S. Aneshensel
Los Angeles
Leonard I. Pearlin
San Francisco

For a copy of the interviews conducted for this work, please address inquiries to: Academic Publishing Service, 308 Westwood Plaza, Room 2414AU, Los Angeles, California 90024, (310) 825-2831. Please make reference to *Compendium for Profiles in Caregiving* in your request.

Chapter 1

Setting the Stage

Introduction
The Aging of the Population and the Need for Family Care
The Late-Life Dementias
The Epidemiology of Late-Life Dementia
Precursory Commentary

Introduction

As the American population continues to age, the number of older persons with health impairments and associated dependencies grows. Consequently, the ranks of family caregivers whose assistance enables their elderly relatives to live in the community (i.e., outside of nursing homes) increases as well. This book describes the experiences of a select group of these caregivers, who assist elderly relatives afflicted with Alzheimer's disease (AD) or a related dementia. It is based upon a longitudinal survey of a demographically diverse sample of 555 principal caregivers living in San Francisco or Los Angeles. At the time of the first interviews in 1988, all of the cognitively impaired persons resided at home, usually with their caregivers. Over the next 3 years, we watched as the caregivers traveled a course encompassing an extended and varied set of experiences: active in-home caregiving, the decision to institutionalize one's parent or spouse, the transition to a nursing home, the provision of supplemental care within a nursing home, death of the dementia patient, grief and bereavement, and finally, the social and psychological reorganization of their lives in the aftermath of caregiving.

The wives, husbands, and children who were taking care of relatives suffering from dementia have been, in a real sense, our active partners in this research endeavor. Later in this book, we describe in detail these caregivers and how they were brought into the study. For now, we wish only to point out the splendid and exceptional quality of their participation. With extraordinary enthusiasm, forbearance, and support, they bountifully and openly shared with us their lives, experiences, feelings, and thoughts as caregivers. It is difficult to imagine a research project receiving more encouragement and involvement from the people it was studying than this one fortuned. To be sure, as the study progressed, some grew impatient with us and our questions, and some were disappointed that the study could offer no immediate relief for them and others in similar situations. Yet the vast majority worked with us to the conclusion of the interview process, providing us the opportunity to observe them as they contended with the hardships and frustrations of protecting the welfare of their impaired relatives. Some fared better than others in this struggle, and much of this volume is dedicated to identifying the conditions contributing to such differences.

One of the reasons this study has enjoyed the interest and loyalty of so many of its participants resides in the nature of caregiving itself and its effect on the organization of people's lives. The degenerative and irreversible course of AD and other late-life dementias typically results in family caregivers becoming increasingly engulfed by the needs of impaired relatives. The time and energies of caregivers come to be consumed by this single enveloping role. Absorption into caregiving, of course, is often at the expense of the activities and relationships across which their lives had previously been spread. Understandably, these overwhelming circumstances may also result in isolation, a sense of being invisible in the larger society, and a conviction that no one "out there" understands or cares about their plight (Skaff & Pearlin, 1992). This picture describes the typical context into which researchers wanting to learn about caregiving and about the people who provide it were welcomed. We were undoubtedly seen by many caregivers both as a rare opportunity to express their views about issues of paramount importance and as a possible vehicle for communicating their stories to the outside world. We do not wish to ennoble people who provide, or have provided, care to close relatives with AD or similar disorders. There is no reason to believe that there are fewer characterological frailties in this population than in any other. Yet, all of them have stepped forward to take on a role that few, if any, sought or desired. At a historical time and in a society in which people are presumably driven by motives of self-gratification, caregivers as a group outstandingly embody many of the best humanitarian values.

> We've been married for 50 years. I owe it to her. She'd do the same for me.

For most of us, it is relatively easy to assist others when their needs are limited and transient; it is a different matter when the help others need is both continuous and progressively expanding. The latter condition tests our mettle; to pass the test requires resolute commitment to a difficult and frustrating role. For many people then, caregiving is an expression of extreme altruism, where one's own well-being is sacrificed for the benefit of another. As observers who have had the opportunity to watch each caregiver over a critical segment of his or her life course, we frequently have been struck by the generosity of spirit and action displayed by this group. As emphasized previously, they have also been open-handed collaborators in this study, leaving us with a keen sense of responsibility for reconstructing the important thematic narratives of their lives as caregivers.

It is one thing to feel a responsibility to relate meaningfully the narratives of caregivers; it is another to find the best way to accomplish this complicated task. The difficulty, in part, exists because caregiving often involves not one story or narrative, but several, each evolving over time. In some respects, the course of caregiving is similar to a theatrical drama. In a theatrical drama, there are shifts in scenes with the significance of events and exchanges that occur in early scenes revealed only as the play moves forward to its finale, and the meaning of the ending revealed only against the backdrop of the beginning. Similarly, in order to make sense out of the twists and turns in the unfolding drama of caregiving, the audience ideally needs to watch carefully from beginning to end. Our own effort does not reach this ideal. We entered the theater only after everyone was already acting out their roles, some for very short times and others for longer periods, and we left before all of the actors had finished their parts. Nevertheless, the material we present in this book is drawn from 3 years of sitting in the audience and observing different story lines being played out.

The parallels between the theater and caregiving should not be exaggerated. Unlike the drama of the theater, caregiving to a loved one being transformed by dementia virtually never has a happy ending. There are no happy beginnings either. The mystifying and frightening emergence of cognitive and behavioral impairments can only leave caregivers hoping for the best, but fearing the worst. Unlike the drama of the theater, too, much must be ad-libbed, for there is no script guiding the drama of caregiving; on the contrary, the actors are frequently surprised by unanticipated incidents and scenarios. Although most learn early that future scenes are bleak, it is difficult for caregivers to foresee with clarity either the exigencies that eventually will appear or the timing of their appearance.

Probably the most striking difference between caregiving and theatrical dramas is that there are as many narratives as there are actors playing the role of caregiver. In some important respects, the story of each caregiver is different from that of all others. Many factors converge and combine in the caregiving situation: personal and family histories; material, physical, and social resources; aspirations and values; the needs and capabilities of the impaired relatives; and so forth, ad infinitum. At some level, the particular mix of these kinds of conditions results in each actor playing out the caregiver role in a fashion that is unique.

Given that in some ways any one caregiver is different from all other caregivers, it would seem that we could easily become immersed in the details that distinguish each and every one of the 555 individuals whom we have observed. The volume of detail, moreover, is particularly great by virtue of our having interviewed each individual on multiple occasions. One of the tasks we faced, therefore, was finding the appropriate level at which to organize and present our observations. Ideally, our methods should neither be so global and abstract that we lose touch with the texture of caregiving experiences and some of their nuances, nor so microscopic and concrete that circumstances shared within socially defined groups of individuals are obscured.

The desired ground between these two extremes is less elusive than might at first appear to be the case. It is reached, by and large, by the kinds of questions we pose in this book and the kinds of information we mobilize in looking for answers. Thus, as will be seen in several chapters, one of our major interests is the level of emotional distress that caregivers exhibit: Some will be very high on our measures of distress, some virtually free of distress, and others will be somewhere in between. It is our goal, however, not merely to describe these kinds of differences, but to explain them as well. For this purpose, we seek to determine if the variations in distress are associated with a host of conditions: the social and economic characteristics of caregivers; features of the caregiving situations, such as whether the caregivers are the spouses or adult children of relatives impaired by dementia; the level of exposure to a variety of stressors; and access to various personal, social, and material resources. The psychosocial conditions and experiences we have chosen to consider in this regard are not those that are idiosyncratic elements of the lives of individual caregivers. Instead, these attributes are likely to be differentially distributed among subgroups of caregivers. Our analytic job, therefore, is to identify and explain both the themes common to the lives of all caregivers and those that tend to be found primarily within specific subgroups.

It is a far more challenging and complicated task to explain the variations in well-being among caregivers than to establish that such variations exist. The former task is difficult because there is not simply one factor contributing to well-being, but multiple factors with configurations that change as caregiving continues over time or moves to another set of circumstances. Of course, this is to be expected: All of us inhabit a multifaceted world, and caregivers to relatives with dementia are certainly no exception. As researchers, it is our job to sift and sort data in order to identify those factors that adversely impact the lives of caregivers and those that enable people to avoid or limit the harmful effects of caring for someone with dementia.

We are aided in this analytic task by organizing much of our inquiry around a dominant question: Given that caregiving has the inherent capacity to evoke stress, what processes generate successful adaptation as opposed to generally maladaptive outcomes? Our attempts to answer this question are oriented toward two phenomena, each of which is explicated in the following chapters. The first we refer to as *stress proliferation:* the encroachment of care-related stress into areas of life previously insulated from hardship. Stress proliferation points up that persistent stressors within important life domains tend to generate other stressors. The second phenomenon entails the regulation or control of the impact of numerous care-related stressors, largely through various material and psychosocial resources, which we refer to as *stress containment.* It will be shown that both circumstances, the extent of stress proliferation and the degree of stress containment, help to explain why the well-being of some people is put at extreme risk by caregiving, whereas other people seemingly are able to survive with little apparent damage to themselves.

Obviously, it is much simpler to state the purposes of our analyses than to describe the many decisions and the intricate procedures involved in actually conducting them. Consequently, one of the obstacles we faced in writing this book was to communicate information with sufficient clarity so as to allow the reader to make critical judgments about not only the appropriateness of our analytic strategies, but the conclusions we have drawn from them as well. For several reasons, this challenge is occasionally difficult to meet: we frequently weigh and evaluate relatively large numbers of variables simultaneously; in keeping with the longitudinal design of the study and alterations in the lives of caregivers, we gear much of our analyses to understanding the dynamics of change; and we use several modes of multivariate analyses, choosing statistical techniques yielding the most accurate assessment. In dealing with these complexities, we seek to provide sufficient technical detail for the reader to grasp which procedures or techniques are being used, why they were chosen, and what the results mean. Where possible, we attempt to limit the presentation of information that might unnecessarily divert the attention of the reader from the substantive issues under consideration. Ideally, we would like to avoid leading our readers through all of the distracting twists and turns of analytic problem solving that we have traversed. We should also regretfully acknowledge in this introduction that at various points we come up short of this ideal.

The Aging of the Population and the Need for Family Care

We have speculated about some of the reasons caregivers were willing to invest considerable time and energy in this study. But what about those of us who are the researchers in this enterprise, what is it that drives our interests in this work? To some extent, the answer to this query is embedded in the pages of this book. However, superimposed over the mixed interests and motives of the research team is the consensual conviction that caregivers to impaired family members represent a vitally important group in our society. The significance of this group, moreover, can only become more relevant as the vast social and demographic changes that are underway in the United States and in many other countries continue on their present course. We refer specifically to the aging of populations, commonly known as the "graying of society."

As a result of advances in public health and medical technology, people are likely to live appreciably longer than their parental generation. Consequently, the population has aged markedly over the past century and will continue to do so well into the next century. At the present time, there are approximately 32 million people aged 65 years and older, which is about 12.6% of the total population (U.S. Bureau of the Census, 1992). This group is projected to number 79 million, or 20.6% of the population, by the middle of the next century (U.S. Bureau of the Census, 1992). Furthermore, the elderly population itself is aging (U.S. Department of Health and Human Services, 1992; Zedlewski, Barnes, Burt, McBride, & Meyer, 1990). The "oldest old," those aged 85 years and older, are the fastest growing segment of the population and are expected to double in their present size by the year 2020 (U.S. Bureau of the Census, 1992).

These demographic trends portend concomitant increases in the number of elderly persons with chronic disease, disability, and dependency upon others for assistance with activities of daily living (ADLs). Although functional loss and disability are not necessary consequences of the aging process, both tend to increase with age as a result of underlying chronic disease (Manton, 1989). A product of the demographic aging of the population, especially the rapid growth of the most highly disabled segment of the elderly population (i.e., those aged 85 years and older) is that the elderly population is becoming increasingly more disabled over time despite biomedical and public health interventions (Kunkel & Applebaum, 1992; Manton, 1989; Rogers, Rogers, & Belanger, 1989). Concretely, the need for assistance with one or more ADLs, such as personal needs (e.g., dressing, eating, and hygiene), outside mobility, housework, meal preparation, and finances, is under 3% for those less than 65 years of age, but increases progressively with age from 9.3% for ages 65 through 69 years, to 10.9% for ages 70 through 74 years, 18.9% for ages 75 through 79 years, 23.6% for ages 80 through 84 years, and 45.4% for those 85 years or older (U.S. Bureau of the Census, 1990). It should be emphasized that the vast majority of the elderly (82%) do not have limitations with regard to ADLs (Zedlewski et al., 1990). Nonetheless, there is a large population of elderly requiring long-term assistance, and this segment of society has been, and will continue, increasing in both absolute number and as a percentage of the population.

Most of the impaired elderly reside in the community, including the majority of persons with severe dementia and almost all of those with mild dementia syndromes (Day, 1985; Doty, 1986). The preponderance of the disabled elderly are able to do this only because they receive needed care from their families. In fact, various researchers have found that over three-quarters of the help received by the impaired elderly is provided by family members (Abel, 1987; Day, 1985; Doty, 1986). The family, therefore, plays a pivotal role in averting institutionalization.

Previous research, though, has documented incontrovertibly that family care is not cost free (Abel, 1987). According to Day (1985), the cash value of services performed by families far exceeds the combined cost of government and professional services to both the elderly who live in the community and those who live in institutions. Caregivers also incur "invisible" expenses, including home modifications, rented equipment, special foods, higher heating bills, and the "opportunity costs" of caregivers who forego paid employment. This type of family support is estimated to be the equivalent of full-time work in about one-third of households providing elder care (Day, 1985).

The social psychological costs incurred by family caregivers are more difficult to tabulate. Day (1985) provided vivid description of the stakes entailed in family caregiving:

> *The strain on caregivers must be considered in any cost calculation. If the burden of caring for a disabled elderly relative becomes too great and the goodwill and personal reserves of the caregiver are exhausted, serious consequences for both the elderly dependent and the family emerge. The caregiver's own health may be impaired, institutionalization may be sought, older dependents may be abused or neglected, and families may break down under conflicting loyalties to their own interests and needs of an older relative. Thus, the health and quality of life of those who provide care is tied — and therefore of equal importance in policy terms — to the health and quality of life of the aging who receive support. (p. 14)*

This passage introduces a theme to which we shall return, namely that the needs and interests of care recipients may be very different from those of caregivers, differences that pit the well-being of one against that of the other.

The Late-Life Dementias

The aging of the population, the increase in dependency with age, and the scope of care provided by the family are especially consequential in the case of late-life dementias. Although dementia has been described since antiquity, it has generally been regarded as part of the normal aging process. Over the past 30 years, however, researchers have identified specific disorders that cause dementia. Although these disorders become more frequent at advanced ages, they do not appear to be inherent to the aging process, rather these disorders are the result of specific pathological processes. Nonetheless, dementing illnesses are among the most feared and devastating disorders of late life.

It is necessary to have some understanding of the nature of dementia to grasp the challenges faced by caregivers to persons afflicted with these disorders. Detailed clinical descriptions of dementia, its etiology, and its course, however, are beyond the scope of this book. Instead, we present a thumbnail sketch. For a comprehensive discussion of the dementing illnesses, we recommend *Dementia: A Clinical Approach* (Cummings & Benson, 1992). An excellent nontechnical introduction to dementia and its consequences for the family may be found in *The 36-Hour Day* (Mace & Rabins, 1991). *The Diagnostic and Statistical Manual IV (DSM-IV)* of the American Psychiatric Association (1994) defines dementia as a disorder involving impairments in memory, intelligence, judgment, and neuropsychology, which are sufficient to inhibit carrying out social activities or work. Individuals with dementia have evidence of other intellectual and personality changes as well. Although symptoms vary according to the specific underlying disease, progressive memory and intellectual impairments are the core of the syndrome.

> She said that she sometimes felt "fuzzy brained," that she couldn't find words. I didn't really pay any attention.

Several disorders are grouped together under the label of dementia, or senile dementia, because they share the same cluster of symptoms. Indeed, over 50 different disorders have been identified as leading to dementia-like symptoms (Cummings, 1987). Among the irreversible diseases and most frequent causes of dementia are AD and multi-infarct dementia (MID). Potentially treatable causes of dementia symptoms include metabolic disorders, infections, severe depression, and other psychiatric disorders. These problems may be the primary source of symptoms or may exist simultaneously with an irreversible dementia in older persons.

AD accounts for a majority of cases of dementia in the United States and Europe (Anthony & Aboraya, 1992; Kokmen, Beard, Offord, & Kurkland, 1989; Mortimer, 1988; Mortimer & Hutton, 1985; Sulkava, et al., 1985). AD leads to progressive deterioration in memory, intellectual ability, behavior, and personality. It is characterized by an insidious onset and gradual, steady deterioration. Impairments in memory and new learning typically are noticed first, but visual, spatial, and language problems also may be present early in the disease. The person gradually loses the ability to perform ADLs, starting with complex activities, such as managing finances, and progressing to basic activities, such as dressing and bathing. Personality changes may occur as well, including increased apathy, dependency, anger, aggressiveness, and sometimes, inappropriate sexual behavior. The rate of this progression varies. Severe disability and death may occur within a few years of onset. More typically, however, deterioration is gradual, and patients survive from 10 to as long as 20 years after diagnosis. Death is often brought about by other illnesses or by complications of AD, such as loss of the ability to swallow or increased susceptibility to infections.

The search for the cause of AD has been the subject of intensive research. Theories have focused on genetic influences, neurochemical deficits, neurotoxic effects, and the role of head trauma. Much of the recent research has investigated possible genetic causes and their possible link to beta amyloid, a protein that accumulates in abnormal structures called *plaques* in the brains of AD patients. Unfortunately, the cause of AD has proved to be elusive.

As mentioned above, numerous other conditions besides AD produce the cluster of symptoms known as dementia. After AD, the most frequent type of dementia is MID, which involves the occurrence of multiple small strokes, or infarcts, and produces widespread damage in both hemispheres of the brain.[1] Several additional types of vascular disorders may lead to dementia, such as lacunar states and Binswanger's disease. Other diseases associated with dementia include frontal lobe disorders such as Pick's disease, and a recently described syndrome called dementia of the frontal lobe type (DFT). Another frequent cause is Parkinson's disease, which affects subcortical regions of the brain, producing motor symptoms like rigidity and tremor that are characteristic of the disease. Most Parkinson's patients, however, have some intellectual impairment due, at least in part, to slow thought processes and motor impairment that interfere with performance of some cognitive tasks. Other common causes of dementia include Huntington's disease, progressive supranuclear palsy, Wilson's disease, hydrocephalus, human immunodeficiency virus (HIV),[2] encephalopathy, slow virus dementias (e.g., Creutzfeld-Jakob's disease), and toxic and metabolic dementias (see Cummings & Benson, 1992, for additional sources of dementia).

Depending upon the location and extent of brain damage, specific symptoms vary somewhat across the numerous disorders that cause dementia. There is, however, considerable overlap in the functional and behavioral problems associated with these diseases, especially as they progress over time. As a result, families face similar challenges in providing care to dementia patients regardless of the underlying illness. Thus, the specific cause of dementia typically is less relevant to understanding caregiver stress than the cognitive and behavioral impairments encountered as a result of the underlying disease.

A variety of dementias are represented in our sample, just as in the population at large. However, because our sample is composed of a large majority of patients suffering from AD, we make no attempt to distinguish care recipients by their diagnoses.

The Epidemiology of Late-Life Dementia

Estimates of the prevalence of dementia vary from one study to another. This is mainly due to the absence of clear markers identifying the underlying disease, such as AD, for which definitive diagnosis depends upon postmortem examination. At present, diagnosis is based on evidence from several domains, not from a single test or indicator. Epidemiological studies that estimate prevalence, however, usually have relied on brief evaluations that assess cognitive tasks such as orientation, information, and memory. Although reliable for identifying obvious cases of dementia, these procedures are less accurate when symptoms are mild; diagnoses of less severe cases require more comprehensive examinations. Consequently, epidemiological surveys typically distinguish moderate and severe dementia from mild dementia. Diagnosis of mild dementia is usually made on less firm criteria (Mowry & Burvill, 1988) and as a result may include people whose impairment is due to other causes and is not progressively degenerative (Johansson, Zarit, & Berg, 1992). Because of these limitations, there is a general consensus on the prevalence of moderate and severe dementia, but estimates of mild dementia vary considerably (Mowry & Burvill, 1988).

Most studies from North America and Europe report rates of moderate and severe dementia somewhere between 4% and 7% of the population over the age of 65 (Anthony & Aboraya, 1992; Cummings & Benson, 1992; Kay & Berg-mann, 1980; Mortimer, 1988). One recent study, though, estimated the prevalence of AD alone at 10% for this age group (Evans et al., 1989).[3] Estimates of mild dementia have fluctuated widely, from a low of 3% to a high of 64% (Mowry & Burvill, 1988). The typical range, however, is 10–15%.

Although estimates of prevalence may differ, it is clear that rates of dementia increase sharply with age. In general, prevalence rates before age 65 years are very low, but rise dramatically thereafter (Jorm, Kortem, & Henderson, 1987; Kokmen et al., 1989; Regier et al., 1988). The most rigorous demonstration of this pattern may be found in a study of a representative, nationwide sample in Finland, which used health interviews, cognitive testing, and medical records in a comprehensive assessment (Sulkava et al., 1985). Rates of moderate and severe dementia numbered 2.6% for the population under age 65 years, 4.2% for those aged 65 through 74 years, 10.7% for those aged 75 through 84 years, and 17.3% for those over 85 years. The few available longitudinal studies confirm this pattern of increasing risk of dementia with age (Berg, Nilsson, & Svanborg, 1988; Johansson et al., 1992; Nilsson & Persson, 1984).

Precursory Commentary

From our discussions, it should thus be clear that (1) as longevity is extended and the number of older people increases, there is a commensurate increase in the number of people suffering from dementia; and (2) people who suffer from dementia, regardless of its type, are likely to require high levels of caregiving. The findings of several early studies, moreover, have established that the people who provide this care are overwhelmingly likely to be either spouses or adult children of the impaired elder (Brody, 1985; Cantor, 1983; Johnson & Catalano, 1983; Shanas, 1979). Taken together, the studies show beyond any doubt that a substantial proportion of Americans are committed to the care of their impaired parents, husbands, and wives, and institutionalization, as we further document in chapter 8, is not a choice of first resort. In general, family care of frail or demented elders stands as a powerful contradiction of any notion that the impaired aged are abandoned by families preoccupied with the pursuit of their own life agendas.

It may be assumed with confidence that the society at large benefits from the willingness and ability of families to care for their members who are unable to care for themselves. Were it otherwise, impaired elders would be institutionalized sooner and in larger numbers than is currently the case. This, in turn, would impose a far greater economic burden on society to provide long-term care to elders. Although family caregiving may help to contain costs to the society and its citizens as a whole, it often results in serious costs concentrated in the caregiving families. The breadth and magnitude of these costs cannot be calculated solely in economic terms. A large body of research has established that there are also profound costs to caregivers associated with disruption of their normal activities and social relationships, and with injury to their mental and physical health (see Baumgarten, 1989; Schulz, Visintainer, & Williamson, 1990; Wright, Clipp, & George, 1993, for comprehensive reviews). A major purpose of this book is to identify and probe these kinds of costs as they accrue across the entire trajectory of caregiving, including the postcaregiving period.

From the vantage point of certain theoretical perspectives, the lessons that may be learned from caregivers, as important as they are in their own right, extend far beyond the boundaries of caregiving. In particular, caregiving represents an unusual opportunity to scrutinize the processes surrounding long-term hardships. As we elaborate in chapter 2, caregiving to cognitively impaired relatives is likely to be an enduring situation, one capable of giving rise to a variety of chronic stressors. Although there is reason to believe that chronic stressors, more than those that are eventful, may be particularly damaging to an individual's well-being, surprisingly little study has been directed towards them, possibly because the observation of their unfolding consequences requires multi-year inquiries such as this one. At any rate, in addition to caregivers being a demographically growing population deserving scrutiny for their own sake, they are also a group from which a great deal may be learned concerning chronic stressors and the impact stressors have on people's health and well-being.

In addition to persisting over time, chronic stressors may multiply and inten-sify or, under certain conditions of change, diminish or recombine with other stressors. One of the opportunities provided by the study of caregivers is to observe such changes and their effects. As a result of intense chronic stressors in caregivers' lives, many caregivers transfer the care of their relatives from the home and community to long-term care facilities. Because dementia is most likely to afflict older people, many caregivers also experience the death of their impaired relatives. These kinds of transitions, as we refer to them, may yield a close-up picture of how constellations of stressors rooted in the circumstances of people's lives undergo change as situations change. Thus, the study of caregivers is also a study of the close connections between the changing situational contexts in which people are located and their changing exposure to stressors.

We may briefly assert, too, that the more we learn about the processes in-volved in caregiving, the wider are the possibilities for informed interventions. Although much of this volume is aimed at discovery, we believe that what we succeed in learning is of equal importance to the clinical worker as to the basic researcher. The most general point that we wish to argue is that the long-term study of caregivers may appeal to multiple intellectual and practical interests and agendas.

A final note concerns the organization of the book. The first several chapters are devoted to the groundwork on which the study stands. Thus, chapter 2 develops the theoretical orientations that serve as the guidelines for the inquiry. The perspectives primarily involved include the *stress process* and *caregiving careers,* the latter being the framework within which we examine the develop-mental trajectory of caregiving over time. Chapter 3 describes the sample, includ-ing the methods by which it was recruited and its composition. Additionally, this chapter outlines the multifaceted design of the inquiry, particularly as it reflects the division of the sample over time into three distinct subsamples of caregivers: those continuing to provide home care, those who have placed their relatives in long-term care facilities, and those who have become bereaved.

The ensuing chapters closely reflect our notion of caregiving careers, which rests on the subdivision of the sample outlined above. Thus, chapter 4 deals with the emergence of caregiving roles and describes the types of difficulties typically encountered by caregivers. Chapter 5 describes the ebb and flow of care-related stressors over time. Chapters 6 and 7 are at the heart of our theory about the stress process. Chapter 6 examines the proliferation of stressors that arise over time in the lives of caregivers as they provide in-home assistance. In chapter 7 we examine stress containment looking particularly at the contribution of social support and mastery in this respect. In chapter 8 we consider the transition to institutional care, identifying the conditions that hasten or inhibit placement. The institutional phase of caregiving and role restructuring are examined in chapter 9. The final phase of the caregiving career is analyzed in chapters 10 and 11, both of which examine an exigency ultimately experienced by all surviving caregivers: namely, the death of their relatives. Chapter 10 is a look at variability in the time of death, examining various reasons why some patients die earlier than others. Chapter 11 deals with the bereavement processes triggered by the death of an impaired relative and identifies the circumstances associated with the intensity and duration of bereavement.

The final three chapters consider some of the implications of what we have learned. Although we regard this study as falling more squarely in the realm of basic research than in applied, a powerful motivation driving our effort is the desire for our findings to be applied in a way that makes a difference to the lives of long-term caregivers. The application of these findings potentially occurs at two levels. One, addressed in chapter 12, concerns the use of this investigation in devising clinical and service interventions. We harbor no illusions that there is any intervention that can eliminate fully the hardships and anguish associated with caregiving. There is, nevertheless, much room for easing their effects. It is our hope that this study will inspire creative and efficacious interventions.

Public policy represents a second, though related, level at which we hope our study makes a difference. This is the subject of chapter 13. Public policy determines the allocation of societal resources, and in times of scarcity, these resources are likely to be devoted to ends that are clearly stated and that are closely entwined with widely shared values. Our best wish is that this book helps to make a strong case in behalf of family caregivers; there is no doubt in our minds that as a group, the actions of these caregivers bespeak much that is prized and esteemed in our society. Finally, chapter 14 is a brief overview of what we regard as some of the major substantive findings to emerge from this investigation.

In assembling the materials for this volume, we were struck by how easy it is to lose sight of the people whose experiences are captured in our empirical findings. To some degree, this loss is inevitable, because statistical compilations are most informative about average tendencies and experiences shared in common. Indeed, these techniques treat the unique experiences of a single individual as measurement error, a depersonalizing concept. Yet, the quantitative approach is necessary to address the core questions guiding this research as well as other investigations into caregiving. Nonetheless, numbers alone do an injustice to the spirit of participation that characterized the participants in this study and to the personal histories they shared with us.

We endeavor to correct this imbalance by telling the stories of four of the 555 caregivers who participated in this study: Frank, Constance, Rosemary, and Valerie. These narratives were recorded midway through our data collection, when we were searching for qualitative information to assist us in interpreting our quantitative findings. We introduce each caregiver early in the text and then trace their stories throughout the multiple stages of the caregiving career. Providing a platform for caregivers to speak in their own voices best conveys the substance of our findings.

Frank

Frank is almost 80 but seems years younger, his large build carried very erect, his step sprightly and robust. He's personable, a great talker, who also enjoys writing and spouting aphorisms, and an avid music lover. His home is furnished in a comfortable, "lived-in" look. His wife of many years, Beth, has recently died. He says of her,

We had a very good life together. She had many talents, especially a crackling sense of humor. Sharp as a razor. Great sensitivity. Was a frustrated ballerina, had an interest in fine china. We spent 5 weeks together in Italy and looked at china from one end of the country to the other.

I was so in love with Beth. That everything about her was so important to me. She never became like a stranger. It was singularly different with me. No children, no other support. All my love, dedication, poured on her, not spread out over others.

The person interviewing Frank observes that his main problem now is one of loneliness:

We shook hands when I left and he gallantly leaned down and kissed my hand and started to choke up. I heard him sobbing as I turned to go out the door.

The goal of the inquiry then is to describe the experiences of individuals as they go about providing care to relatives suffering from dementia. Caregivers are tracked as they clothe, feed, bathe, and protect their husbands, wives, mothers, and fathers, day in and day out, year in and year out. We describe how some survive and even thrive in harsh situations, while others lose ground. The circumstances under which caregivers are forced to turn to institutional care are identified, as are the personal, social, and economic resources that enable others to continue providing in-home care. Additionally, we follow caregivers as they ultimately lose their relatives to death and resume their lives without their spouses or parents. At each step of the way, we link the conditions the caregivers confront to changes in their mental health and emotional well-being. Finally, we ask ourselves, So what? What difference is made by what we have learned? Perhaps the payoff of this research will eventually be reflected in more effective help and planning for this burgeoning, but still largely invisible group.

Notes

[1]The terms *multi-infarct* and *vascular dementia* have replaced the older concept of arteriosclerosis dementia. Arteriosclerosis, per se, does not result in generalized intellectual decline and dementia. Rather, the decline associated with arteriosclerosis dementia is the result of specific pathological changes, such as small strokes (Funkenstein, 1988).

[2]Acquired immunodeficiency syndrome (AIDS) is most prevalent among relatively young adults, which distinguishes this type of dementia from late-life dementias.

[3]These findings appear to be study-specific. The population researched had exceptionally low rates of formal education (3 years of schooling on average) and included significant numbers of people for whom English was a second language. Both of these characteristics may interfere with performance on tests of cognitive ability. Additionally, the reported rates confound prevalence with incidence insofar as new cases identified 18 months after the baseline survey were added to those identified at baseline.

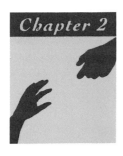

Caregiving Careers and Stress Processes

Many of the key decisions about the sort of study we wanted to conduct and the questions that needed to be asked were made far in advance of the initiation of our large-scale survey of caregivers. Nearly 2 years were spent conducting qualitative interviews, developing scales and measures, and, of paramount importance, crystallizing theoretical perspectives. These perspectives eventually guided our decisions about what data should be gathered, the way it should be analyzed, and the manner in which the results could best be arranged for presentation. This is not to say that everything about the research and organization of this book was by any means preconceived. On the contrary, the products of extemporaneous decisions and intuitive hunches are interspersed throughout the following pages. By and large, the crafting of the inquiry and the analyses of the data were closely shaped from the earliest stages of the project by two conceptual frameworks: caregiving careers and the stress process.

The notion of caregiving careers, which provides the structure for the organization of this book, stems directly from the sequence of experiences that normally characterizes the lives of caregivers. As indicated by the very term, the construct of *career* specifically directs attention to the orderly restructuring of responsibilities and activities that take place across time. Some of our thinking about caregiving careers is taken from studies of occupational life and its progression. However, in contrast to occupational careers that focus on achievement within opportunity structures, caregiving careers are driven not by personal ambitions, but by the pathogenesis of dementia and the functional dependencies it creates.

The stress process, the second conceptual perspective underlying this work, pertains to changes in the interrelated circumstances of life that affect people's well-being. One component of the process is made up of the clusters of psychosocial stressors that may form in people's lives and that vary over time in their intensity and configuration. Another element is represented by the various mechanisms that regulate the impact of such stressors on health and well-being. The thinking underlying the stress process, much of it developed from close to two decades of prior research and writing, was crucially instrumental in orienting the directions taken by this study. It is also the major analytic framework for understanding the experiences of caregivers at each stage of their caregiving careers.

Even with the theoretical perspectives of caregiving careers and the stress process shaping the presentation and analyses of the data, the application of theory to data is not as simple as applying a template to drawing paper. Instead, theory and data involve more of a dialectical exchange: Theory directs our attention to certain data and helps to make sense of our findings, whereas the data make us question and refine our theoretical perspectives. We would like to believe that our theoretical leanings have led us to a better understanding of caregivers, and we are quite certain that the caregivers have helped us to be more sensitive to our theoretical leanings and their potential for error.

The remainder of this chapter is devoted to a description of the two theoretical foundations and a discussion of their relevance to caregiving. We begin with a consideration of caregiving careers.

Caregiving as a Career

Our conceptualization of caregiving as a career emerged from our observations of a large sample of caregivers to family members suffering from dementia as they continued to provide care within the home, admitted their relatives to nursing homes, provided supplemental care within long-term care facilities, became bereaved, and carried on their lives after caregiving. In chapter 3 we chart the number of caregivers involved in each of these natural subdivisions over a period of time. For now, we wish only to call attention to the fact that with the passage of time, caregivers normatively experience considerable change.

Our description of caregiving as an evolving set of circumstances differs from the perspective implicit in most policy discussion wherein caregiving for the frail elderly often is equated with one particular set of circumstances: providing substantial assistance to a physically or mentally impaired person who lives outside of a formal institution, typically an older member of the immediate family. When we observe caregivers for an extended period of time, as we have done in this investigation, we see clearly that intensive in-home care usually does not stand alone in an individual's experience of providing care. Instead, caregiving may, and often does, reach across a rather prolonged trajectory that encompasses demands and situations that extend beyond this form of care. For example, at the beginning of care, demands may be quite limited in scope or intensity, readily incorporated into the routines of everyday home life (Matthews & Rosner, 1988). Later on in the caregiving process, long after an impaired person has been placed in a formal institution, a caregiver frequently continues to provide supplemental or "invisible" care (Wilson, 1989).

Thus, caregiving typically encompasses multiple stages. Three such stages are especially important: preparation for and acquisition of the caregiver role; enactment of care-related tasks and responsibilities within the home and possibly within a formal institution; and disengagement from caregiving, which often entails bereavement, recovery, and social reintegration. These three stages and the transitions from one to another comprise what we have come to recognize as a caregiving career (Pearlin, 1992; Pearlin & Aneshensel, 1994).

Caregiving should be viewed, then, not as a fixed set of experiences, but as a series of shifting configurations. The problematic conditions encountered early in the course of dementia give way to emergent challenges as the dementia follows its inevitable and irreversible degenerative course. Each stage of caregiving presents distinctive sources of stress; offers some strategies for addressing these difficulties, at the same time as it precludes alternative options; utilizes various personal, social, and economic coping resources, while depleting others; and shapes the choices available in ensuing stages. The career perspective highlights the stages of caregiving, drawing attention to commonalities in stress processes that extend across time, as well as to the unique dynamics inherent in each.

Some of the changes that occur in a caregiving career entail the yielding of one status and the acquisition of another, as when caregivers cease to be residential caregivers and become, instead, the relatives of an institutionally placed person. We borrow from life course literature the term *transitions*, which refers to movements from one status to another. In addition to transitional changes, caregivers are likely to experience other changes that occur within a status, such as providing more assistance with the activities of daily living (ADLs) when the progressive cognitive decline associated with dementia demands it.

As will be documented throughout this book, the conditions surrounding the lives of caregivers undergo constant shifts and realignments. The construct of career is particularly appropriate to describe this context of change because its imagery captures both the dynamic movement of caregivers from one status to another and the patterns of change they experience within status locations.

Occupational and Informal Careers

Careers are most often thought of in reference to the occupational sphere, especially as the work performed within formal organizations over a lengthy arc of the life course. The critical element distinguishing the concept of career from work is the presence of a *series* of related positions through which persons move in an ordered sequence: This sequence is usually arranged in a hierarchy of respect, responsibility, and reward (Wilensky, 1961). A career is formed not by a single job, but by a constellation of jobs held over time. Moreover, these jobs are not merely numerous, they are related to one another. The association among these jobs forms a developmental trajectory of progressive accomplishment, expertise, control, management, and complexity.

The construct of career has been applied to many roles outside of the institutional mainstream of occupation, just as we are applying it to caregiving. For example, Barley (1989) described the use of career in studying marginal or unconventional jobs such as the taxi-dancer (Cressey, 1932) and the professional thief (Sutherland, 1937). Other work in this classic tradition pertains to participation in deviant subcultures, such as marijuana users (Becker, 1953). The career motif also surfaces in studies that examine the course of illness, such as Goffman's (1961) description of the "moral career" of mental patients. More recent work has applied this concept to the management of chronic illness (Gerhardt, 1990).

We are not the first to associate the concept of career with caregiving. Brody (1985), for example, spoke of caregiving careers in reference to providing care to a succession of impaired elders, thus emphasizing serial engagement with multiple care recipients. From our perspective, however, career more heuristically refers to movement of an individual through a series of related stages as he or she helps a single care recipient. Also, we see the caregiving career as incorporating stages subsequent to in-home care, namely, institutional care, bereavement, and social readjustment.

In summary, the concept of career has a long and rich history of application beyond the formal workplace. In such far-reaching applications, the concept of career refers to any sphere of activity in which people move through a series of related and definable stages in a progressive fashion, moving in a definite direction or towards a recognizable endpoint or goal—the unfolding of a social role (Arthur, Hall, & Lawrence, 1989). It need not be institutionalized or enacted within a formal organization, but may instead be an informal social status, like family caregiver.

Characteristics of Careers and Caregiving

Some of the perspectives that have arisen from the study of occupational careers are useful in identifying similar features of caregiving. The concept of career encapsulates a set of characteristics: a temporal focus, usually of lengthy duration; change, especially growth or maturation; and a cumulative experience that merges into a holistic entity. We use the concept of career, then, as a shorthand notation for emphasizing the evolving character of caregiving.

This developmental attribute is implicit, for example, in models that describe multiple stages of caregiving. Given and Given (1991) referred to this sequence as the "natural course" of the caregiving experience. The stages they described, selection into the role, acquisition of care-related skills, provision of care, and cessation of care, parallel those that we use. The three stages identified by Wilson (1989) are alike as well: taking it up, deciding to become a caregiver; getting through it, enduring the unfolding sequence of problems entailed in providing care; and turning it over, relinquishing care and control to an institution. Similarly, Lewis (1987) differentiated three stages of caregiving: semi-care, entailing more of a sense of responsibility than instrumental tasks; part-time full care, characterized by increasingly heavy task demands; and full care, involving complete absorption in the task of caring. These descriptions reveal an essential characteristic shared by careers and caregiving: the evolution of role-related responsibilities across time.

In caregiving as in occupation, then, careers are neither suddenly nor quickly created, rather they emerge after being engaged in changing constellations of activities and functions. Moreover, as in occupation, caregiving careers are not built on repeating the same acts indefinitely, but on the restructuring of activities and responsibilities, sometimes gradually and other times precipitously. Finally, for both occupational and caregiving careers, it is possible to discern multiple transitions, each signaling movement from one stage to another.

The concept of career expands our view of caregiving because it orients our thinking towards the *entire* sequence of events leading up to the present time, as distinct from self-contained episodes. Although each caregiving stage or transition may be, and often is, examined in isolation, we believe the meaning and impact of one's current caregiving experience are shaped by what has passed before and by what is anticipated in the future. The caregiving career, therefore, is not static: In addition to the present, each phase embodies a history and foreshadows a future.

This situation is analogous to the world of occupations in that a worker's current position is inseparable from his or her cumulative work history. For example, the identical position may be a marker of status attainment and upward social mobility for a young person who is just starting out, but a sign of failure or stagnation for an older worker who has not ascended beyond the lower ranks of the occupational ladder. Thus, caregiving and occupational careers are isomorphic to the extent that they are both best understood as interrelated wholes viewed across their entire span of existence: from acquisition of role, through role enactment, to eventual disengagement from and termination of role.

Furthermore, occupational and caregiving careers parallel one another in the sense that for each, past events establish the various career paths that await the completion of the currently occupied position, closing some doors and opening others. Activities take place within the context of preceding events and establish boundaries for future events. For example, as we shall see in chapter 9, adaptation to institutional care is influenced by the nature of responses to care-related stressors during the earlier in-home phase of caregiving (Zarit & Whitlatch, 1992). Similarly, chapter 11 documents that adaptation to the death of the care recipient depends importantly upon how the caregiver has coped previously with the transformation of the patient from a self-sufficient, functional adult to a dependent (Mullan, 1992). Thus, the career perspective addresses not merely the interdependence of events over time, but also their cumulative impact.

The concept of career also helps to orient us to the fact that caregiving is closely bound by the biographies of caregivers. In the work force, an individual's history, including education, training, and experience, determines his or her occupational status. Similarly, in a caregiving career, for instance, the lifelong history of parent–child relationships influences who is drawn into the role of caregiver. Obligation is as potent a motivation for caregiving as affection insofar as some children take on caregiving responsibilities to reverse or overcome long-standing problems with parents (Townsend & Noelker, 1987). A critical contribution of the concept of career, therefore, is to orient us to not only what is transpiring currently, but also to events in the distant past that shape the context of contemporaneous elements of caregiving. Being drawn into the role, providing assistance at home, institutional placement, and bereavement each pose their own distinctive concerns for caregivers; yet, each is also joined to the other components to form a coherent entity.

Finally, the concept of career serves to focus attention upon social regularities in caregiving. It enables us to take the biographies of individuals and identify common threads among them. Individually experienced situations, circumstances, problems, and emotions are recast as the orderly unfolding of predictable care-related episodes, reactions, and consequences. The imagery of career focuses attention on experiences shared in common by individuals who are engaged in like activities with comparable intents and purposes. When an individual pursues a career, occupational or other, he or she walks down the same roads traversed by others following the same career; each individual encounters sets of experiences shared in common with many other individuals. These experiences arise not so much from individual choice or predisposition, or even personal sentiments, but from the nature of the job to be done—in our study's case, the caring for an impaired family member.

This emphasis on commonalities in care-related experience distinguishes the social, cultural, and economic contexts of individual action from the traits of individuals, such as intrapsychic coping mechanisms. For example, although the decision to admit a relative to a nursing home is experienced as intensely personal, it is shaped by external considerations like the availability of nursing home beds, the quality of nursing home facilities, and the family's socioeconomic resources. Each instance of family caregiving is unique in its specific attributes: in the historical bond between caregiver and care recipient, the current nature of family relations, the personalities of those whose lives have been touched and changed by the dementia, and so forth. These individualistic aspects of caregiving personalize the experiences shared in common by most, if not all, caregivers.

Yet they should not obscure the commonality in experience that affects incumbents of the caregiving role by virtue of the fact that they are role incumbents.

In summary, the concept of career evokes the image of a multistage trajectory spanning a lengthy interval of time and emphasizes the notion that each stage is understood best in relation to the totality of the career. The career perspective on caregiving, thus, stresses the linkages between current experience and that which has occurred previously, including the quality of family relationships prior to the emergence of the need for care. This accumulated experience sets the stage for future action, rendering some courses of action likely and foreclosing others. In this manner, the impact of caregiving is seen as extending beyond the actual provision of care, just as the nature of work influences the character of retirement. Finally, careers are enacted by multiple actors, a fact that focuses our attention on the social regularities of caregiving as distinct from the idiosyncratic experiences of individuals. This reorientation enables us to identify elements of caregiving that are inherent in role incumbency.

Points of Divergence

In using the term *caregiving career,* we do not mean that caregiving should be thought of as a job. Hence, it is useful to outline some fundamental differences between occupational and caregiving careers. In comparing the two, it becomes evident that the clarity and ambiguity of the timing of transitions differs between their spheres. Whereas people know precisely when they enter a job, entry into caregiving might be gradual and insidious, in some instances, becoming a fait accompli before one is fully aware of it. Once an incumbent of the caregiver role, people might have very little idea of how long they will be at a particular stage before entering a transition into another. Occupational careers, by contrast, often, but not always, follow a relatively well-defined time schedule through the ranks. One of the distinguishing features of caregiving transitions, therefore, is the relatively indeterminate character of their timing and duration.

Another major feature of caregiving careers, sharply differentiating them from occupational careers, is that family caregiver is an informal status, recognized only within the family or network core. Consequently, it lacks the rights, privileges, and prerogatives associated with formal statuses. Thus, a daughter caring for a parent suffering from dementia does not have any greater authority over the treatment of a parent than her siblings. In the eyes of the world, one is seen not as a caregiver, but primarily as a wife, husband, daughter, or son.

Moreover, an occupation exists as a durable position, independent of the individual who happens to occupy it. By contrast, of course, the caregiver role within the family exists because someone is ill and lasts only as long as the exigencies necessitating it. That is, the role ceases as soon as care is no longer required. No one stands in the wings awaiting their opportunity to take up the role, and most caregivers would be dismayed at the thought of their role continuing indefinitely as a fixture of their life course.

Finally, caregiving differs from other careers in that caregiving is unplanned.

It is for this reason that we think of it as "the unexpected career." There is a difference, indeed, between being "unknown" and being "unexpected." We assume that most people who become caregivers have had the opportunity to observe others in the same role, perhaps within the same kinship unit. Having been an observer of the role does not mean that one begins to plan and prepare for being an incumbent of the role. On the contrary, aversion to the caregiver role leads many of us to deny the strong possibility of ever becoming its incumbent. Despite the fact that caregiving to older impaired relatives is becoming a common contingency of the life course, people typically do not see themselves as caregivers when they project themselves into the future. In this respect, caregiving is far different from careers that require both clear decisions for entry and a lengthy period of preparation and training. Preparation for caregiving usually occurs after one is an incumbent of the role, which by itself may make adjustment to the role difficult.

In many respects, our conceptualization of a caregiving career corresponds more closely to female than male experience within the occupational sphere. Perhaps the similarity is not surprising because family caregivers are more likely to be women. As numerous observers of work life have noted, career paths differ by gender. The orderly male prototype of continuous labor force participation and progressive upward movement does not do justice to the "disorderly" experience of many women (cf. Wilensky, 1961). In particular, the latter model fails to incorporate the schism between occupational and family life that arises for women (Diamond, 1987). Larwood and Gutek (1987) identify several supplemental considerations for models of career that are relevant to women, including family obligations and restricted opportunity structures. These themes emerge as well with regard to gender and caregiving, especially to notions that women become caregivers more often than men for several reasons: women have been socialized into kin-keeping tasks and nurturing roles, women have more time available because they are less likely to be employed, and opportunity costs and external resources are lower for employed women than men given that women typically earn less than men (Montgomery, 1992; Walker, 1992). Caregiving careers may well impede the occupational attainments of women, sustaining the very gender stratification of the occupational sphere that channels women into caregiving.

Obviously, the analogy we construct between occupational and caregiving careers should not be taken too literally, but instead, as an image that illuminates critical aspects of caregiving that might otherwise be overlooked. Our purpose in drawing out the similarities and differences between caregiving and occupational careers has been to highlight some of the structural and experiential features of caregiving, particularly as they change over time. Change is the quintessential element of caregiving, and the construct of career sensitizes us to the continuities and discontinuities of the role and its effects as time passes. As we have indicated, the benchmarks of some of the changes reside in the transitions from one stage of the career to another. Indeed, the very organization of this book mirrors the major stages of the caregiving career. Although we have made reference to the stages and transitions, we have not yet described them. It is to this task that we now turn.

Stages and Transitions in Caregiving Careers

A typical caregiver's career comprises three stages: (1) *role acquisition*, the recognition of the need for the role and the assumption of its obligations and responsibilities; (2) *role enactment*, the performance of role-related tasks within the home and, for some, within the formal setting of a long-term care facility; and (3) *role disengagement*, the cessation of caregiving and the returning to other venues of life that typically follow the death of one's impaired relative. A stage is not necessarily a period of stability. As explained earlier in the chapter, all caregivers who are engaged at the same stage are not inevitably exposed to identical conditions; on the contrary, within each stage caregivers experience diverse circumstances. Moreover, the rapidity and direction of change and the timing and sequencing of transitions from one stage to another varies substantially among caregivers.

Thus, we regard the stages of caregiving as heuristic devices that help us both detect the threads connecting each part of caregiving to its other parts and identify conditions that move caregivers along their career trajectories at different rates and at different psychological and material costs to themselves. In Figure 2.1 we identify the three career stages, role acquisition, role enactment, and role disengagement. Three transitions—illness onset, nursing home admission, and death of the dementia patient—also play major roles in shaping the course of the caregiving career, especially with regard to the timing and sequencing of its component parts. In the following sections, we discuss each of the three major stages and then take up issues of sequencing and timing of transitions that help to define distinct career lines.

Pathways to Care: Role Acquisition

Despite the fact that many family members readily embrace the opportunity to care for loved ones in need, caregiving certainly presents itself as an unappealing line of work, a career to which few aspire. The tasks of care are physically exacting: lifting, dressing, cleaning, feeding, and so forth. The interpersonal demands, particularly in the presence of dementia, are taxing: confronting socially inappropriate or disruptive behavior, supervising the actions of an adult much as one would an infant, and forbearing in the face of frustration. Often, too, these activities are performed in isolation from others, depriving the caregiver of the ordinary social exchanges of adult life. In this regard, caregiving shares some of the disadvantages of the traditional role of housewife or homemaker: the work is unstructured and socially invisible; a high density of the tasks are boring, repetitive, and unskilled; and the role is enacted in social isolation (Gove & Geerken,

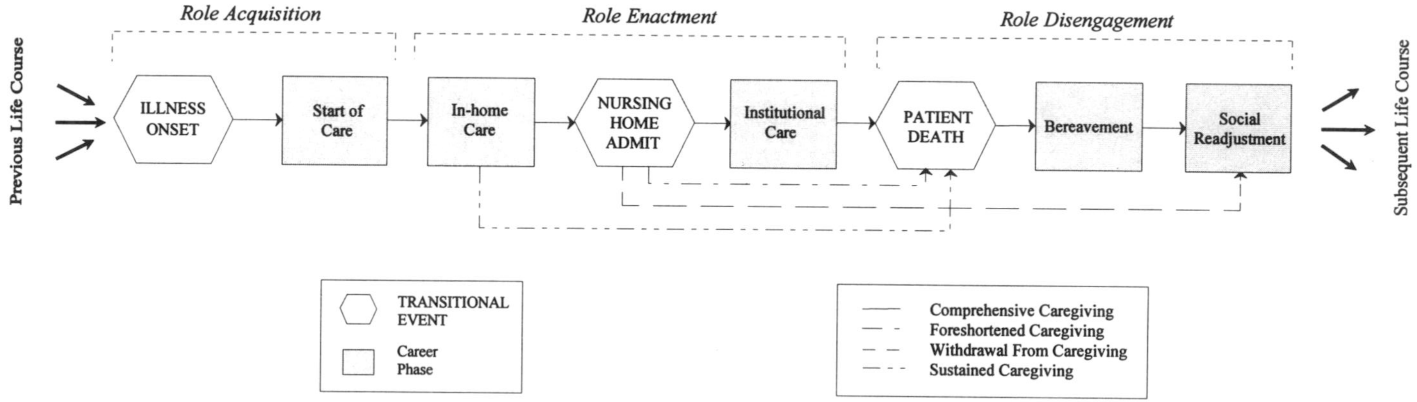

Previous Life Course

Role Acquisition

ILLNESS ONSET → Start of Care → In-home Care → NURSING HOME ADMIT

Role Enactment

Institutional Care → PATIENT DEATH → Bereavement → Social Readjustment

Role Disengagement

Subsequent Life Course

TRANSITIONAL EVENT

Career Phase

Comprehensive Caregiving
Foreshortened Caregiving
Withdrawal From Caregiving
Sustained Caregiving

Figure 2.1 Progression of caregiving careers.

1977; Gove & Tudor, 1973). Finally, though not least important, the very necessity to provide assistance stands as a constant reminder of the transformation and decline of a loved one.

Given the undesirable nature of the activities entailed in caregiving, why do so many step forward when the need for care arises within their families? There are multiple answers to this question: One provides care because one is supposed to, in order to fulfill an internalized norm of duty; there are no viable alternatives as no other person steps forward; institutional care is unavailable or unaffordable; one's parent or partner needs it; or one is convinced that if the shoe were on the other foot, the caregiver would be the beneficiary of the care recipient's solicitude. The intimacy and primacy of family relations might lead us to attribute caregiving solely to emotional attachment. However, personal affinity does not suffice to explain why some types of family members are more likely to become caregivers than others. As described previously, selection into the role depends upon the lifelong history and structural composition of relationships.

Constance

Constance lives in a semirural setting, set back from the main road. Her ranch-style house is comfortable, homey, and immaculate. She is a tall woman, trim, neatly groomed, with grey curly hair and bright blue eyes, a person who enjoys quiet afternoons, the garden, and crossword puzzles. Constance describes the tradition of caregiving in her family:

My mother's parents lived next door and my grandmother broke her hip at 88 and she lived to 97. In those days they stayed in bed. For nine years my mother was in charge of taking care of my grandmother in her home. I always promised myself that I'd do likewise when it would be my turn. It was never verbalized but through observation I saw it. I said it to myself, not to anyone else. I put it on myself that I'd take care of her.

My mother expected that she'd take care of herself!

This responsibility was taken on as a normal part of family obligation as distinct from a deep bond of affection.

She's my mother and for that reason we're close, but we don't have a lot in common with each other, other than our history. It's not that I enjoyed it or that we were that close or that I got that much out of the relationship. But she was my mother and it was a promise that I'd made to myself.

Although Constance institutionalized her mother only after it became a necessity, she wishes she could have continued to provide in-home care.

I feel that I've disappointed myself, that I didn't do what I hoped I would do. I can reason it all out, but I still wish that it was different. If she's begging me to take her home, I come home feeling down. If I could get her to realize that she has to be there, and she would accept it. My mother wants to be somewhere else. That is driven home to me daily.

In looking toward the future, she says of her children,

I sat them all down once and told them that I didn't want to live with any of them, to let them off the hook so that they wouldn't feel guilty. The boys laughed and said I was saying that because I knew how they keep house.

Although dementia may seem to afflict people at random, the absorption of individuals into caregiving careers is far from happenstance. Caregivers, at least primary caregivers to impaired elderly, are most likely to be female and to be drawn from the ranks of family rather than friends or acquaintances (Dwyer & Coward, 1992; Horowitz, 1985a, 1985b; Stoller, 1990). When an impaired person is married, care is almost invariably provided by the wife or husband—93.1% in our study—a testament to the bonds of affection, as well as to the power of norms concerning family obligations.

In cases of intergenerational caregiving, the selection of who will serve as caregiver is regulated not solely by the quality of the personal relationship between parent and child, but by powerful customs dictating the circumstances under which one is obligated to provide care and one is excused. Given and Given (1991) classified the factors leading to acquisition of the caregiving role as demographic imperatives, such as being an only child, normative obligations of reciprocity, and situational factors like having the fewest competing obligations to work and family. Occupancy of several other social roles—being employed, being married, and having children—tends to insulate grown children from parent care, as does geographical distance (Matthews & Rosner, 1988).

Given that informal care of impaired elders is economically and socially imperative, it may be reasoned that it is functionally beneficial for the selection of people into the role not to be haphazard or left to the capriciousness of individual proclivity. At any rate, the patterns of selection of people into the role clearly indicate that becoming a principal caregiver is not merely a matter of emotional affinity and convenience. More important, perhaps, are the institutional forces and their normative supports that sort and sift the possibilities and influence the choices of caregivers. These forces, moreover, may operate outside the awareness of those being affected by them, often leaving the people who ultimately become principal caregivers holding to the conviction that their entrance into the role is entirely the result of their own free choice, uninfluenced by extraneous circumstances. However incomplete it might be, this kind of understanding possibly further strengthens commitment to the role.

If the situation was reversed, she'd do the same thing for me.

The fact that caregiving is embedded within major societal institutions is easy to overlook in light of the intense emotional relations characterizing many families. Here, we see a strong parallel to occupational careers. It is the institutional climate of an occupation that gives work meaning, setting the context within which it contributes to collective ends and garners rewards. The imagery of career, therefore, serves to direct attention to the family as a social institution and to the social, economic, cultural, and political contexts within which families function.

The onset of family caregiving typically has an amorphous quality, not easily distinguished from the mutual exchange of assistance. The degenerative course of dementia gradually shifts preexisting patterns of aid increasingly towards the unilateral provision of aid to the impaired individual. The person providing this care, however, typically does not recognize the full extent of this transformation immediately. Consequently, many caregivers enter the role long before they apply this label to themselves.

Rosemary

Rosemary is a tall, thin, 82-year-old woman with short, white, tousled hair who herself suffered a stroke three years ago, which left her speech impaired. She wears glasses and a hearing aid, and uses a walking stick when she goes out—the result of two knee replacements; she has fallen several times, but without serious consequences. Rosemary describes the onset of her husband's dementia, a set of signs and symptoms she mistook for memory problems that could be remedied:

His judgment failed at least 20 years ago, during the early 1970s when he was in his late sixties. It got worse and worse and I don't think that I was very helpful. I kept suggesting that he try memory devices, and kept saying "Why don't you just try?" That didn't work and it simply made him mad and I can see why. At the time we were both very frustrated.

In 1975, when he was 70, he gave up his professional work, his writing, his studying, and giving lectures, etc., because he said "I no longer trust my judgment." He said that. I tried so hard telling him that he could overcome it, and I pooh-poohed this. I said, "Don't be silly, it's not true." He stuck to it mostly, and it's good that he did. When he did give a talk at a seminar, when he was talked into doing it, things were a mess, but by that time he didn't realize it. He thought everything went all right.

In 1980 a neurologist from Harvard, whom he'd known all his life, came to visit us for half a day. We had a good time, lots of conversation, laughing, but at the end of his visit he took me aside and said I should realize that something was very much the matter.

I didn't realize it because it had been going on so very gradually and I thought that he could overcome it if I could persuade him to. That was a shock to me.

> *Right away we went to UCSF and had a thorough examination and there was nothing found to be wrong with him other than the Alzheimer's disease.*
>
> *He went downhill pretty fast from then on.*

As we shall see in chapter 4, there are several major routes through which individuals come to be caregivers. Thus, a key feature differentiating caregiving career lines is the manner in which one enters the role. At one extreme, typified by Alzheimer's disease (AD), care responsibilities accrue insidiously, becoming discernible only in reflective retrospection; at the other extreme, caregiving responsibilities erupt with little warning, accelerating rapidly up a steep gradient (e.g., a debilitating stroke). As we have seen, a considerable transformation may take place in the preexisting relationship between the giver and the recipient of care before either party comes to recognize that the exchange of care has become largely unilateral. Alternately, one may be thrust into caregiving with little or no warning. The manner in which someone enters into caregiving, therefore, depends in part upon the nature of the impairment prompting the need for care. Yet there is considerable variation in how caregivers take up the role even with regard to the same illness. This variability reflects the importance of other contextual factors, such as characteristics of the patient, caregiver, patient–caregiver past and present relationship, larger social environment, and so forth.

Perseverance and Resignation: Role Enactment

We turn now to the second encompassing stage of caregiving careers, role enactment. This stage is examined in considerable detail in chapters 4 through 9, and as such needs only brief treatment here to highlight its place in the context of the caregiving career.

Role enactment, as we envision it, includes two distinct phases: in-home care and hands-on care provided following placement of a relative in a formal care facility. As we define it, therefore, this stage actually subsumes the transition from home to institution. Although our decision to view care provided at home and in an institutional setting as two phases of a single stage of the caregiving career may be questioned, it comes after some debate. On the one hand, home and institutions are different contexts of care joined by a deliberate transition. On the other hand, to treat home care and institutional care as separate stages would be to ignore the continuity of care between the two sites that we have observed. The scope of assistance might undergo considerable contraction, as we describe in chapter 9, but we find that most caregivers continue to provide some level of care to their institutionalized relatives. For some caregivers, role enactment occurs entirely within the home; for others, it is relocated to the institutional setting.

Figure 2.1 depicts the fact that caregivers do not necessarily occupy each of the substages. Some caregivers continue to provide in-home care until the dementia patient dies, moving directly from in-home care to bereavement. We refer to this pattern as *sustained caregiving* because in-home care continues for the entire duration of the illness. Other caregivers admit their impaired relatives to nursing homes and thereafter, the caregivers' activities diverge into several distinct patterns of caregiving. One pathway, which we label *comprehensive caregiving*, entails the continued provision of substantial amounts of hands-on care. As mentioned above, we treat this supplemental care as a facet of role enactment rather than role disengagement, because this assistance often is quite extensive and time-consuming, reflecting a continuing commitment to and responsibility for the well-being of the care recipients.

> If she gets too sick and goes into a nursing home, I wouldn't want to see her again—too painful.

Another pathway is formed by those who essentially cease caregiving when they admit their impaired relatives to nursing homes, a pattern we label *withdrawal from caregiving*. As we shall see in chapter 9, more caregivers remain invested in the care of their parent or spouse than withdraw from care.

Some caregivers who institutionalize their relatives, however, do not have the opportunity to continue with comprehensive caregiving or to withdraw. Instead, their relatives die shortly after admission. Whatever their intentions may be regarding involvement with the institutionalized patient, these intentions do not have sufficient time to materialize. We designate this pathway as *foreshortened caregiving*, referring to its abrupt end.

In chapter 10 we will explain how not all deaths immediately following admission may be attributed to poor patient health prior to admission. Consequently, many of these early deaths are unanticipated and abruptly alter caregivers' expectations about the future.

Grief and Readjustment: Role Disengagement

Role disengagement is the third and final stage of caregiver careers. Initiation into this stage is, for the most part, marked by the death of the impaired relative. In a few instances, however, disengagement comes about through the caregiver's own death or disability, or passing the baton to another family member. Although people with dementia can, and often do, live to be among the oldest old, they are typically already at an advanced age by the time they manifest the symptoms of the disease. Consequently, caregivers are likely to witness the demise of their relatives, to deal with the emotional aftermath of death, and to confront the challenges of picking up the worn threads of their pre-caregiving lives.

In some respects, this situation is not unlike that of disengagement from occupational life. Just as the impact of occupational retirement cannot be understood without knowing what occurred before retirement, the patterns of bereavement cannot be fully understood without knowledge of the conditions that preceded death. Similarly, just as caregiving is not merely something one does for a period of time, the experiences one has in the work force are likely to permanently alter one's life course trajectory. Thus, the postcare period may be seen on its own as a distinct stage of the caregiving career. The meaning and consequences of death have their origins in earlier stages of caregiving, as well as in the family history that precedes the onset of dementia. Although the postcare period is distinct in its own right, it is, nevertheless, very much a part of the caregiving career.

One might reasonably speculate that after years of caregiving and observing the inexorable deterioration of a loved one, the death of the beloved would be met with relief. Indeed, this seems to be the case for many caregivers. Grief and relief appear to be emotions that are frequently experienced independently: feeling one does not preclude feeling the other. No matter the amount of time since the onset of dementia, the length of time caregiving has gone on, or the age of the deceased relative, some period of grief is a normative response to the death.

> I was relieved when she finally died. I was thankful.

As we shall see in chapter 11, the duration of grief is quite variable. Some caregivers rapidly recover, whereas others relinquish grief only after a substantial passage of time. Also, most caregivers see themselves as recovered eventually, but some face enduring sorrow. The course of grief and social readjustment depends, at least in part, upon the conditions encountered during the role enactment stage of caregiving (Mullan, 1992).

Our treatment of role disengagement reflects our view that caregiving careers extend beyond caregiving activities. There is a distinction between exposure to the trials and tribulations of caregiving, on the one hand, and exposure to the consequences of caregiving that persist or surface after the cessation of caregiving, on the other hand. We conceive of the latter as being as much a part of the career as the former, a perspective that rests on the assumption that the effects of care-related experience are not coterminous with the duration of exposure to those experiences. The effects, moreover, are discernible for a lengthy period of time following the death of the relative, a point we are able to establish as a result of our multiyear follow-up interviews.

This long-term view of the final stage of the caregiving career enables us to distinguish grief from social readjustment. Grief, which may vary in its intensity and duration, is seen as an emotional response to the death of the family member. Readjustment or adaptation, by contrast, refers to the long-term ways in which people restructure their lives following the deaths of their relatives. We assume that grief and readjustment are related, either by grief interfering with adaptation or by adaptive failure interfering with the resolution of grief.

It is our guess that long after caregiving has ceased and people have dealt with their grief and made adaptations to loss, the long arm of the caregiving career continues to exert its influence on the remainder of the caregivers' life courses. For example, daughters who have left the workforce to care for their parents will not reenter it at the status they would have attained had they worked continuously, and are unlikely to reclaim lost advancement opportunities. Indeed, we see no end to this chain of influence. Our supposition that the caregiving career survives the death of the impaired relation is similar to Lopata's (1987) observation that keeping alive the memory of deceased family members constitutes an important filial duty. It is useful to look beyond the period immediately following death to consider how people reorder their lives after what had been a major role is eliminated from the larger configuration of their roles.

> I was isolated from society. I had forgotten my social mannerisms.

Thus, the notion of a caregiving career is useful in that it calls attention to the fact that the consequences of being thrust into a caregiver role may continue to reverberate long after the stage of active caregiving (i.e., during "retirement"). Being responsible for the institutional placement and care of an impaired relative and having to deal materially, socially, and psychologically with the death of that relative are, we believe, interconnected and interdependent. With each transition, a caregiver's life is, to some extent, restructured; the extent and direction of restructuring depends not only on the impinging conditions of the currently occupied stage but, perhaps, on the conditions faced at an earlier stage as well. Similarly, the postcare life-course trajectory differs from that which might have been anticipated if the need for care had not arisen. Thus, passage through the stages of caregiving tends to alter permanently the life-course trajectory, detouring caregivers towards alternate routes and destinations. One does not merely become a caregiver to an impaired relative: When one becomes a caregiver, one frequently finds that the entirety of one's life has been restructured, both its social exterior and its psychological interior.

Alternative Career Paths for Caregiving

By invoking the concept of a caregiving career, we do not mean to imply that all caregivers travel a single route, rather we seek to call attention to the diverse pathways traversed by caregivers. We have already described how the three major stages of the caregiving career, role acquisition, enactment, and disengagement, are encountered by virtually all role incumbents. These broad stages, however, encompass diverse personal experience.

Our specification of career seeks to differentiate major commonalities in the caregiving experience from the unique aspects of any one person's experience. Within this broad framework, clusters of caregivers share certain experiences that differ from the experiences of other caregivers. Each experiential cluster is analogous to a *career path*: a specific way of acting within career stages and a particular way of passing from one stage to another (Shafritz, 1980). The multiplicity of career paths in caregiving is similar to the subgroups formed by specialization within professions (e.g., internist vs. surgeon).

Career differentiation, however, is limited: The number of distinct career lines is far fewer than the number of caregivers. The numerous individuals who follow a single career line share similar experiences, which differ in some essential features from the collective experiences of those following alternate career lines.

The concept of distinctive career paths highlights a duality in the nature of caregiving: Some experiences are shared in common by most, if not all, caregivers; whereas other experiences uniquely specify distinct subgroups of caregivers. The evolving experiences of the subgroups coalesce as distinct trajectories over time, forming identifiable career lines.

If you recall, the four career lines were introduced earlier in the section on role enactment and illustrated in Figure 2.1. One line encompasses all three of the major career stages and the later two transitional events (comprehensive caregiving). The stage of role acquisition is followed by two phases of the role enactment stage, in-home care and institutional care, which are separated by the transitional event of admission of the care recipient to a nursing home. The phase of institutional care, when caregivers provide supplemental assistance to their spouses and parents who reside in nursing homes, is followed ultimately by the transitional event of the death of the dementia patient and, therefore, the stage of role disengagement, including bereavement and social readjustment.

Figure 2.1 depicts the remaining career lines with the interval of institutionalized care omitted. As may be seen, a second line resembles the first in all regards except one: The institutional care phase is so abbreviated that caregivers essentially move directly from nursing home admission to bereavement (foreshortened caregiving). The care recipient dies shortly after admission and, consequently, there is insufficient opportunity for caregivers to habituate themselves to the provision of institutional care, should they so desire.

The third career line also excludes the institutional care phase of role enactment, but for a different reason. In this scenario, when care recipients pass through the transitional event of taking up residence in nursing homes, caregivers exit from active role enactment and enter the social readjustment phase of role disengagement (withdrawal from caregiving). Withdrawal may be motivated by a host of conditions, such as exhaustion, inability to shoulder any further demands of caregiving, desire to recapture foregone opportunities, logistical obstacles to the provision of supplemental care, or sheer disinterest. As we shall see in chapter 11, the withdrawal pathway is followed by a substantial subgroup of caregivers, though it is by no means the most common mode of exiting from role enactment.

The fourth major career line not only omits institutional care, but it omits the transitional event of admission to a nursing home as well. In this instance, care recipients continue to reside at home until their deaths (sustained caregiving). Caregivers move from the in-home phase of role enactment to the bereavement phase of role disengagement following the transitional event of the death of their spouse or parent. This pathway, therefore, differs qualitatively from the previous three pathways insofar as this mode of role enactment consists solely of in-home care.

When caregivers embark upon a certain route, their ensuing journey is more likely to turn at some crossroads than others, but the course is not rigidly prede-termined. For example, change in the resources available to meet the demands of care, such as a precipitous decline in the health of the caregiver, may initiate a change in heading, catapulting the caregiver onto an alternate career line. The possibility of abrupt changes in career paths places caregiving careers clearly within the conceptual domain of "disorderly" or "chaotic" work histories (Wilen-sky, 1961).

The construct of a caregiving career is useful for a number of reasons. First of all, it calls attention to the extended and encompassing character of the role and its consequences. The concept of career also conveys a sense of movement and change that is more or less structured, not ruled by happenstance or random circumstances. This does not mean that there is a universal career course fol-lowed by all caregivers. On the contrary, there is a good deal of diversity among caregivers in the timing and direction of their careers. Moreover, because move-ment across career trajectories is more directly explained by the social, cultural, and economic contexts of caregiving than by idiosyncratic personality factors, the framework of career and its stages direct attention to patterns of diversity among groups of caregivers without becoming lost in a forest of individual differences.

Although the notion of career helps us to outline the structure of people's caregiving activities, chart changes across the trajectories of their careers, and discern commonalities among the situations in their lives, it does not inform us in detail about the structure of their day-to-day experiences, especially experiences that may have adverse effects on their well-being. In order to orient our research toward these kinds of issues, we rely heavily on the theoretical perspectives of the stress process. It is to the specification of this process that we now turn.

Caregiving and the Stress Process

There are many reasons why researchers are drawn to the study of caregivers: the high incidence of AD and other dementias within an aging population mark family caregivers as an increasingly important group; caregivers provide a rich case study of the development and functioning of informal care systems; care-givers are a source of information about the economic costs of chronic disease; and the population of caregivers is a meaningful focus of broad humanistic concerns. Our own research is most assuredly motivated by all of these consider-ations. In addition, however, we view caregiving as an opportunity to observe processes of enduring demand and hardship, the impact of these processes on caregivers' health and well-being, and the kinds of resources that may ameliorate their effects.

Caregiving, therefore, may be viewed as a situation capable of spawning an array of conditions and experiences having the potential to undermine the well-being of caregivers. It is a situation, too, in which there is considerable variation in the impact it exerts on people: Although the well-being of some is affected

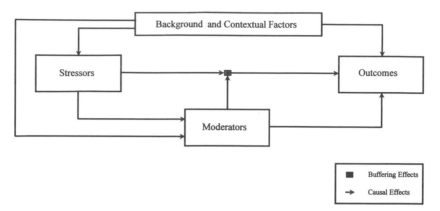

Figure 2.2   Stress process model.

adversely by caregiving, others seem to avoid or minimize damage to themselves. These observations to a large extent establish the two central analytic agendas of this book. One is to identify and describe the various conditions and experiences that generally affect the health and well-being of caregivers over time; the other is to explain variations in the effects of these conditions and experiences on subgroups of caregivers.

Our general model of the stress process, portrayed in Figure 2.2, is employed to serve both tasks. This model was originally developed from research into representative community samples (Pearlin, Lieberman, Menaghan, & Mullan, 1981) and has undergone considerable refinement since the initiation of our study of caregivers to persons with dementia (Pearlin, 1989; Pearlin, Mullan, Semple, & Skaff, 1990).

Figure 2.2, a simplified diagrammatic representation of the stress process, shows our conception of the process as having three components. *Stressors* are the problematic conditions and difficult circumstances experienced by caregivers (i.e., the demands and obstacles that exceed or push to the limit one's capacity to adapt). *Outcomes* refer to the consequences of stressors. We conceive of these outcomes rather broadly, including effects upon the individual's health and emotional well-being, especially internal affective states such as depression or anger; timing and sequencing of various transitional events like premature admission of the patient to a nursing home; behavioral changes, including the provision of supplemental care within an institutional setting; and the unfolding of the post-caregiving life course, such as the duration of grief.

The third component, *moderators*, is comprised of the social, personal, and material resources that help modify or regulate the causal relationship between stressors and outcomes. We consider these resources to be major factors in explaining subgroup variations in the effects of stressors on outcomes. The moderators that are primarily considered in this book are social support and mastery or self-efficacy. Moderators are shown in Figure 2.2 as altering the magnitude of associations between stressors and outcomes. In the literature on social stress, this conditional relationship usually is referred to as *stress buffering*. The key point is that the moderator transforms the basic stressor–outcome relationship, intensifying the impact of stress when resources are scarce and diminishing it when resources are plentiful. Resources are also thought to act as intervening links in the causal chain that connects stressors and outcomes. In this instance, resources serve as the conduit through which stressors affect various outcomes.

As illustrated in Figure 2.2, the stress process unfolds within the context of social, economic, cultural, and political factors. Individuals confront stressors not in isolation from other facets of their lives, but as the bearers of certain characteristics, the possessors of different statuses, and the occupants of positions within stratified social systems. These background and contextual factors influence the extent to which subgroups of the population are exposed to stressors, the kinds and levels of resources at their disposal, and the outcomes that emerge.

Because it is assumed that changes in one of the components of the stress process will result in changes in others, the utility of the model is best put to test in longitudinal investigations. Thus, the conceptual framework of the stress process is particularly useful in capturing the dynamic features of problematic life experience, caregiving being an excellent case in point.

To a greater or lesser extent, each of the stages of caregiving careers is examined in this volume from the perspective of the stress process model. Consequently, in the course of this examination we shall identify the multiple dimensions subsumed by each of the major components of the model and describe how they were measured. Of course, the substantive chapters address the complex interrelationships among these dimensions, as well as their stability and change over time. There is, however, one feature of the stress process that should be discussed in some detail at present: The generation of secondary sources of stress, which we refer to as stress proliferation.

The Proliferation of Stressors

Our notion of stress proliferation is based on the observation that a serious life problem usually does not exist apart from other life problems. This clustering arises not because an individual who falls victim to one stressor is somehow fated to be a target for other stressors. The reason, which we shall substantiate empirically, is that stressors tend to beget other stressors. As a result, individuals may be surrounded by constellations of stressors, some of them in areas of life other than those in which the stressors originally appeared.

In the case of caregivers, the stressors directly involved in providing care to impaired relatives may eventually give rise to stressors outside the boundaries of caregiving. It is this expansion of stressors to which the construct of stress proliferation calls attention. The original set of hardships are called *primary stressors* and those that arise as a result of them are labeled *secondary stressors*. The term *primary* emphasizes that these stressors originate within the enterprise

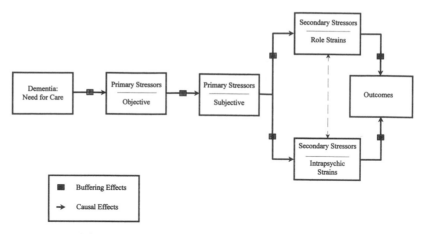

Figure 2.3   Stress proliferation and its containment.

of caregiving itself; whereas *secondary* calls attention to difficulties that flow from caregiving, but do not directly entail the provision of care. These terms, primary and secondary, do not reflect the relative capacity to produce deleterious consequences; once established, secondary stressors may be even more potent than primary stressors.

As indicated in Figure 2.3, primary stressors consist of those stressors that involve both the objective conditions of caregiving (e.g., managing the patient's behavioral problems) and certain subjective states prompted by these objective conditions (e.g., the sense of role overload). Similarly, secondary stressors include strains found in roles outside of caregiving (e.g., occupation) and a number of intrapsychic strains as well (e.g., doubts about one's competence). The various components and measures that constitute primary and secondary stressors are specified in greater detail in chapter 4.

One of the utilities of conceptualizing proliferation as an important feature of the larger stress process model is that it reveals more fully the points at which the moderating effects of resources may be observed. Thus, the moderating functions of social support and self-efficacy may not be limited to the relationships between all aggregated stressors and their outcomes. As indicated in Figure 2.3, they may also be detected in the relationship between objectively and subjectively assessed stressors, and similarly, between primary and secondary stressors. These kinds of functions are elaborated in chapter 7.

Our application of the stress process model to caregiving, then, emphasizes the role of moderators in containing the proliferation of care-related stressors. Moderators regulate not only the focal stressor–outcome relationship discussed above, we submit, but intermediary relationships as well, especially the processes whereby stressors beget more stressors. Thus, psychosocial resources may naturally intervene in the care-related stress process by interfering with the conversion of one source of stress into another. For example, self-efficacy may limit the progression of primary stressors by restricting the extent to which dementia creates objective tasks, or the extent to which these tasks are experienced subjectively as burdensome. Another example is that social support may limit the extent to which care-related stress overflows the borders of the care setting and interferes with other social roles and activities or damages the caregiver's sense of self. These resources may limit the translation of secondary stressors into various outcomes, such as elevated emotional distress, premature admission of the dementia patient to a nursing home, or protracted grief.

Although we may assert that there is a tendency for stressors to beget stressors, this premise leaves unidentified the particular conditions or mechanisms that underlie the proliferation of stress among caregivers. The most crucial basis for proliferation, we believe, is the fact that caregivers are not only caregivers, but are incumbents of other social roles as well. They may also be breadwinners and financial managers, actors in a web of family and kinship relations, employees and employers, and participants in voluntary associations and interest groups, and so forth. Each of these roles entails interactions with distinct sets of people, involves different activities, commitments, and obligations, and yields its own rewards and challenges. Each may also generate its own self-concept and identity. It is understandable that the secondary stressors that arise from the experiences of caregivers are often located within the panoply of these multiple roles. Under the most ordinary of circumstances, it may be difficult to integrate these roles in a way that enables the actor to avoid conflict both with others within a role set and between the competing demands of disparate roles. Where such conflict does arise, moreover, changes may occur in the ways people conceive of themselves; thus, they may begin to feel less competent, less worthy, less able to control their lives, and less optimistic about the future.

If, as we stated above, it may be difficult for people to integrate the diverse elements of their multiple roles under ordinary circumstances, it may be doubly difficult to do so under the extraordinary conditions of caregiving. It needs to be recognized, first of all, that the caregiver role is likely to have emerged after other roles have been in place long enough to have been accommodated into the flow of daily life. Caregiving is the new kid on the block. Once it emerges, furthermore, it does not simply take on a stable presence to which adjustments may be made through the fine-tuning of logistical arrangements. More typically, the caregiver role keeps expanding in its demands so that even with adjustments in other areas, it keeps a steady pressure on the boundaries of other roles in the constellation. Whereas other new roles (e.g., entering the labor force) might at first make inroads on adjoining roles before being accommodated within the organization of daily life, the initial demands of caregiving are modest, but continue to grow, making accommodation increasingly difficult. Among one's multiple roles, that of caregiver to a loved one with a progressive cognitive disorder typically stands out as the most relentlessly imperialistic.

Within the context of one's multiple roles, therefore, the new and expanding caregiver role has the capacity to create dislocations, frictions, and burdens in other areas of life. In other words, in the terminology of our theoretical perspectives, primary stressors of caregiving may result in clusters of secondary stressors. We believe that stress proliferation is a general phenomenon that may be discerned in other severely stressful situations, especially where the stressors are chronic. However, it is hard to imagine a situation where an integration of multiple roles is more difficult to establish and maintain than in caregiving. The intensity and changing character of the demands of caregiving make it troublesome to find and keep some equilibrium in relation to the demands of other roles. As a result, the stressors encountered by caregivers often extend far beyond the confines of their caregiving activities.

It is of considerable importance to assess stress proliferation and to distinguish primary and secondary stressors. Stress research commonly finds that people who appear to be exposed to similar stressors of similar intensity nevertheless experience different outcomes, such as divergent levels of depression. When findings like these are significant, it is commonly assumed that the differences in outcomes reflect variances in access to moderating resources, particularly coping resources or repertoires. For example, two caregivers who experience equivalent caregiving demands, but who differ with regard to the support provided by their networks, might exhibit depression at levels reflecting the differences in social support. As discussed earlier, these kinds of moderating effects may be of critical importance in helping to account for variations in outcomes.

However, they usually are unable to bear the entire analytic burden of explaining such variations. Part of the explanation, instead, lies with differences in the presence of secondary stressors, differences that may be overlooked entirely or only partly taken into account. That is, people may be identical with regard to the primary stressors to which they are exposed, yet be unalike in the secondary stressors they confront. Variances in the configuration and severity of secondary stressors, in turn, might help to explain differences in outcomes, such as depression. The systematic measurement and inclusion of potential secondary stressors, therefore, may appreciably add to the explanatory power of our studies of the dynamics of social stress.

Another reason to examine the secondary stressors that impinge on caregivers concerns intervention programs. It is probably a fair statement that most programs—for example, day care or respite care—are aimed at relieving primary stressors, those anchored directly in caregiving activities. Without belaboring the point, programs that are geared toward easing secondary stressors, such as economic hardships, the constriction of social and leisure life, or family conflicts, might be equally successful in relieving the caregiver of some of the deleterious outcomes associated with caregiving. At any rate, in attempting to understand the costs of caregiving and what might be done to reduce them, it is important to cast a wide net to capture the circumstances that significantly tax the lives of caregivers.

In closing, a final observation about the theoretical perspectives of the stress process is in order. Earlier we stated that the stressors to which caregivers are exposed, the moderating resources caregivers possess, and the outcomes caregivers experience, may vary with the social and economic characteristics of the caregivers and with features of the caregiving situation in which they are situated. These circumstances include attributes such as the caregiver's gender, age, and relationship to the impaired relative, composition of the household, distance from the care facility in which the relative is placed, and so on. We wish to highlight the importance of personal and situational characteristics here because their critical part in the stress process may be obscured by various analytic strategies. Concretely, the effects of these characteristics may be difficult to discern when change is being analyzed. The reason is that the presence of such characteristics is absorbed into initial states and then passed along through the stability of various conditions over time. In instances like these, however, the characteristics still exert indirect influence on the various outcomes being observed. The point that deserves emphasis, then, is that the socioeconomic and demographic contexts of caregiving are very much a part of the stress process that may have a deleterious effect on health and well-being, and the importance of the contexts cannot always be judged solely by their direct causal effects on specific outcomes.

The Synergistic Convergence of Caregiving Careers and the Stress Process

The concepts of the caregiving career and the stress process guide virtually all of the material that will be presented in the next chapters. The very organization of this book rests on the notion of career, with the chapters sequentially following the route of a modal trajectory. It is within each of the substantive chapters that a merging of our two theoretical perspectives may be found. In effect, we do not apply the stress process perspective to caregiving as a whole. Instead, it is applied in a manner appropriate to the examination of each of the various transitions and stages of people's careers. By employing the same basic theoretical orientation in the analyses of the different phases of caregiving, it is possible to derive a view of the changing aspects of people's lives as they traverse the span of their careers as caregivers. At the same time, the notion of career helps to frame our analyses in an integrated fashion. It is the basis for collecting, organizing, and attempting to make sense of an unusually large body of data bearing on complex issues. Separately and together, the two perspectives help to capture some of the critical experiences of caregivers and to bring to the outside observer an awareness of the meaning and consequences of these experiences.

Chapter 3

An Empirical Inquiry into Caregiving

Origins of the Theoretical Framework and Methods

The Formative Phase

The results presented in the ensuing chapters are the fruits of a multistage research program begun in the mid-1980s. At that time, gerontologists had recognized some of the burdens associated with providing family care to the frail elderly and had begun to tally the "hidden costs" of being a caregiver. The present research endeavor has its origins in the realization that caregiving represents a situation productive of multiple stressors and therefore, may be viewed from the vantage point of universalistic theory pertaining to the origins and impact of chronic social stress. The detailed investigation of this specific set of circumstances, we reasoned, could also shed light on chronic stress processes among the general population.

The first phase of the development of the inquiry was exploratory in nature. Although some burdens of care had been identified by other researchers, we believed the full scope of care-related stressors had not yet been fully mapped. Consequently, we conducted qualitative interviews with persons who were actively engaged in the provision of care to a spouse or parent suffering from dementia. The interviews asked about the demands directly tied to the provision of care, as well as about the impact of these demands on the caregiver's life in its entirety.

One theme that emerged with some regularity concerned the transformation of caregiving from a set of discrete tasks into a pervasive presence intruding into every nook and cranny of one's life. For some caregivers, this encroachment was felt most at the junctures between caregiving and other social roles: in collisions with the demands of paid employment, in competition with responsibilities towards one's own nuclear family, and in the constriction of one's social network. These observations supported our understanding of *stress proliferation*, an important perspective of this inquiry.

The developmental phase of the research focused on the articulation of central constructs in the theory of stress proliferation, especially those of primary and secondary stressors, and the translation of these constructs into sets of measures. First, the qualitative interviews were content analyzed to identify key elements of care-related stress processes. The constructs that emerged from the analyses were then operationalized into batteries of standardized questions suitable for interviews with large numbers of caregivers. The questions went through a series of pilot tests and revisions before being included in the full-scale implementation of the survey. Answers to the standardized questions subsequently were factor analyzed to form measures of our constructs. The development of the measurement strategy helped to crystallize our understanding of the multiple sources of stress encountered by caregivers. This work, which transpired over a period of several years, formed the foundation for moving our research into a large-scale quantitative investigation.

Implementation of the Fieldwork

The data for the investigation were collected by means of a multiwave panel survey. Four in-person interviews were conducted at 1-year intervals beginning in 1988,[1] thus the total time span encompassed by the interviews was 3 years. Personal interviews were conducted at the caregiver's home or in a setting of their choice.

The sample is comprised of family caregivers for persons suffering from Alzheimer's disease (AD) or a related dementia. Potential subjects were identified by conducting telephone screenings of all persons who contacted local Alzheimer's Disease and Related Disorders Associations (ADRDA) in one of two sites, the San Francisco Bay Area or greater Los Angeles. The screening determined whether an individual met eligibility criteria and was willing to participate in the study. Eligibility was defined as those individuals who were primary caregivers to noninstitutionalized spouses, parents, or parents-in-law suffering from dementia. Primary caregivers were defined as the one member of each family who spends the most time taking care of the cognitively impaired person. At the start of the study, all dementia patients resided in the community and, with the exception of a few, lived with their caregivers. Over time, some families placed their relatives in institutional care, and some impaired relatives died.

Caregivers were reinterviewed irrespective of whether they continued to provide in-home care at follow-up. Three separate, but overlapping, interview schedules wcrc used at the reinterviews. Each schedule was tailored to the specific circumstances of continuing in-home care or institutional care, or bereavement and adaptation

The remainder of this chapter provides detailed descriptions of the sample and its characteristics, caregiver transitions over time to institutional care and bereavement, contents of interviews and measurement techniques, and analytic strategies.

Caregivers and Their Impaired Relatives

Sample Selection

A total of 555 caregivers participated in the baseline interview, 300 in northern California and 255 in southern California. Over a thousand of the 1,740 persons contacted by phone did not meet our inclusion criteria. The large number of ineligible persons resulted from the fact that family caregivers are not the only persons who contact agencies like ADRDA. A total of 164 persons refused to be interviewed, often before the screening interview took place, thus rendering their eligibility status unknown. Eligibility also is unknown for those persons who were never successfully contacted (e.g., no answer after repeated attempts, disconnected telephone lines, and so forth). Therefore, it is not possible to calculate a meaningful response rate due to uncertainty about the total number of eligible persons.

At first it was hard because he didn't recognize me, but it's OK now.

It is worth noting the types of caregivers who may be underrepresented. Those not having affiliations with ADRDA are unlikely to be found in the sample simply because we used this organization to identify subjects. This potential bias is less severe than it might appear at first, however. Persons contacting ADRDA need not be members of the agency, nor do they need to participate in any of its functions. In addition, we traced primary caregivers from ADRDA contacts who were not themselves primary caregivers, which gave us access to persons who had no direct contact with this particular organization. For example, sons and daughters often called ADRDA on behalf of parents who were primary caregivers, presumably negotiating the bureaucratic maze of services for them. Using this contact, we were able to recruit primary caregivers who often lacked direct ties to dementia-related organizations. It should be noted as well that refusals might be more common among some types of caregivers, such as those for whom caregiving is so overwhelming that it inhibits participation or those for whom interest in the study is minimal because care responsibilities are not problematic. Moreover, the inclusion of only spouses and adult children obviously excludes several types of caregivers. Care is also undertaken by other relatives, such as siblings and grandchildren, and friends. Additionally, paid attendants may perform all of the tasks that would otherwise fall to informal caregivers. Thus, the sample should not be construed as fully representative of all dementia caregivers.

Our decision to limit the sample represents a compromise between scope and depth. Heterogeneity is desirable because results may be generalized to an entire class of caregivers, yielding a more complete picture of the caregiving situation. Diversity is not without cost, however, because the subgroups all represent unique sets of circumstances. For example, the dynamics of past family life are relevant to all caregivers with family ties to dementia patients, but the context of this past differs for siblings and spouses. Also, increasing the number of subgroups would decrease the number of subjects within each group, making it difficult to discern meaningful trends within or between groups. Given fiscal and practical realities, it would not have been possible to increase our overall sample size to maintain adequate numbers in these groups. Thus, being able to describe the experiences of more kinds of caregivers would have come at the price of being less precise in the description of each group.

We selected the two largest subgroups, spouses and offspring, in order to obtain sufficient numbers of subjects while retaining the critical contrast between generations. The latter feature permits the identification of circumstances that are unique to one group of caregivers and those that may be shared by different types of caregivers. Similarities and differences observed between spouses and adult children, therefore, give direction to the future expansion of this line of research to other caregiving contexts.

We turn now to a consideration of the characteristics of the caregivers, which, as we shall see, enhances confidence in the quality of our sample.

Socioeconomic and Demographic Characteristics

Despite its limitations, our recruitment strategy successfully generated a heterogeneous sample of caregivers and care recipients. Most caregivers were providing care to someone who had been diagnosed as having either AD or senile dementia of the AD-type (73.9%). Multi-infarct dementia (MID) (9.0%) and presenile, senile, or unspecified dementia (9.2%) were the next most common diagnoses. Other diagnoses present among the care recipients include organic brain syndrome, Pick's disease, and "old age memory loss." For simplicity, these various impairments are hereinafter referred to as *dementia* or *AD*.

Constance

Constance describes poignantly the transformation of her mother brought about by the destructive course of dementia:

I feel that the person I knew has gradually been disappearing, little bits and pieces gone as she loses her ability to do things, loses memory. What is still left are memories of my childhood. She remembers that. She loses track of the grandchildren. If I show her pictures from my childhood and mention names, I'll get a smile out of her. My mother's been dying for several years. Bits and pieces gone. By the end it's not the mother I knew or that knows me.

As may be seen in the first column of Table 3.1, a slight majority of the sample (58.7%) are spouses of the dementia patient, the remainder being adult children.[2] About two-thirds of the caregivers are female. The age distribution is bimodal because caregivers, in effect, represent two generations: Spousal caregivers tend to be elderly themselves, whereas sons or daughters typically are midlife.

The generational and gender attributes have implications for other caregiver characteristics. For example, two-thirds of the sample are not working outside of the home, reflecting the strong likelihood that spousal caregivers are retired or were never permanent participants in the labor force. Also, the vast majority of the caregivers are married (82.3%). Among the spousal caregivers, their partner is obviously the dementia patient and virtually all of these couples live together (99.1%). Sons and daughters also tend to be married, although some have never been married or were previously married. The majority of parental dementia patients live with their sons or daughters.

The socioeconomic status (SES) of the caregivers is quite varied. In some instances, the caregiver has very little formal education, a pattern more characteristic of spousal than adult–child caregivers. Other caregivers have college educations or postgraduate educations, levels of educational attainment more typical of the younger generation. Annual household incomes range from poverty level to affluent, with a median income of $27,500.

The sole sample characteristic that deviates substantially from population norms is ethnicity. The sample is predominantly non-Hispanic white: African Americans, Hispanics, Asian Americans, and other groups comprise less than a fifth of the total sample. The general population of California is extremely diverse. The relatively low number of caregivers from ethnic minority groups may reflect demographic disparities in the population structure by age due to group differences in life expectancy and immigration patterns. It is more probable, however, that non-Hispanic whites were simply most likely to be identified by our recruitment techniques.

Demographic characteristics are remarkably similar across the two study sites.

Table 3.1 Percent Distribution of Caregiver Characteristics at Time 1 and by Interview Status at Time 4

Caregiver characteristics	Time 1 (%) (N = 555)	Status at Time 4 (%)			
		In-home (n = 138)	Institutional (n = 131)	Bereavement (n = 188)	LTF[a] (n = 98)
Relationship to AD patient					
Wife	34.2	34.1	26.0	34.0	45.9*
Husband	24.5	26.8	22.1	22.9	27.6
Daughter	31.2	29.7	36.6	35.6	17.4
Daughter-in-law	3.2	2.2	6.1	2.7	2.0
Son	6.7	7.2	8.4	4.8	7.1
Son-in-law	0.2	—	0.8	—	—
Age: Spousal caregivers[b]					
Less than 65	22.8	32.1	22.2	15.0	23.9
65–74	45.5	44.1	50.8	46.7	40.9
75 and older	31.7	23.8	27.0	38.2	35.2
Age: Adult child[c]					
Less than 45	27.2	22.2	30.9	30.9	16.0
45–54	39.0	48.2	39.7	32.1	40.0
55 and older	33.8	29.6	29.4	37.0	44.0
Race					
Non-Hispanic white	83.8	81.2	82.4	89.4	78.6
African American	10.6	13.0	10.7	7.4	13.3
Hispanic	3.1	3.6	4.6	1.6	3.1
Asian American and other	2.5	2.2	2.3	1.6	5.1
Education					
Less than high school	13.4	10.1	9.2	13.3	23.7**
High school	19.9	19.6	20.6	18.1	22.7
Some college	33.7	39.1	33.6	34.0	25.8
College or more	33.0	31.2	36.6	34.6	27.8
Employment status					
Employed	33.3	37.0	36.6	33.5	23.5*
Not employed	66.7	63.0	63.4	66.5	76.5
Marital status: Adult child					
Married	57.2	48.2	67.6	55.6	53.9
Divorced or separated	19.2	25.9	10.3	23.5	15.4
Widowed	8.3	3.7	10.3	8.6	11.5
Never married	15.3	22.2	11.8	12.3	19.2
Lives with AD patient: Adult child[d]					
Yes	60.7	68.5	52.9	65.4	50.0
No	39.3	31.5	47.1	34.6	50.0

[a]LTF, loss-to-follow-up.
[b]n = 325, 1 subject missing.
[c]n = 228, 1 subject missing.
[d]n = 229.
*p ≤ .05. **p ≤.01: χ^2 test of loss-to-follow-up versus composite category of reinterviewed at Time 4.

One exception should be noted: Compared to San Francisco, the Los Angeles subsample is somewhat less well educated. Due to the overall pattern of similarity, a detailed comparison of the characteristics across the two sites is not presented here; however, it is available elsewhere (see Pearlin et al., 1990).

As may be seen in the last four columns of Table 3.1, the sample retains its diversity over time. The first three of these columns comprise those persons who participated in the study throughout all four interviews. At Time 4, 24.9% of the original sample continued to provide in-home care, 23.6% were caring for parents or spouses who resided in nursing homes, and 33.9% had lost their relatives to death.[3] Although there is some variation in caregiver characteristics across the three groups, the most notable feature of this comparison is the general similarity of the characteristics. Only one characteristic, spousal age, is related significantly ($p \leq .05$) to the status of reinterviewed subjects: By Time 4, the youngest husbands and wives are most likely to be providing in-home care, whereas the oldest are most likely to be bereaved. This pattern suggests that the ability to provide in-home care declines with age, reflecting the close correspondence between the ages of husbands and wives with regard to patient mortality. Subsequent chapters describe the impact of caregiver characteristics on the two career transitions that define these groups: institutional placement (chapter 8) and patient death (chapter 10).

Although overall sample attrition was limited, as illustrated in the final column of Table 3.1, we were concerned about a selective trend in those lost-at-follow-up. Consequently, the tests of statistical significance pertain to the comparison between the composite group of retained subjects versus those who attrited from the study so that we might identify possible differences between them. That is, we sought to determine if the rate of attrition varied across caregiver characteristics. The overall rate of sample attrition across the four interviews is quite low—17.7%. The attrited group is comprised of those who could not be located at any of the follow-ups, persons who refused to be reinterviewed, and caregivers who themselves were incapacitated or deceased. The latter is not an uncommon outcome given the advanced age of the spousal caregivers.

Table 3.1 also shows that loss-to-follow-up is associated significantly with three caregiver characteristics: kin relationship to the dementia patient, education, and employment status. The lost-at-follow-up group overrepresents wives and underrepresents daughters. Specifically, the rate of attrition is substantially lower for daughters (9.9%) than for wives (23.7%), husbands (19.9%), or sons (18.4%). Moreover, the attrited group comprises approximately the same number of persons from each of the four educational groups, but the total sample contains a relatively large number of highly educated persons. The rate of attrition is especially high for those with less than a high school education (31.1%), average for those with a high school education (20.0%), and low for those with some college (13.4%) or a college degree or more (14.8%). The rate of attrition also is substantially higher among those who are not working (20.3%) as opposed to those who are working (12.4%).

The educational and employment status differences in loss-to-follow-up may be attributed at least partially to the association of these statuses with kin relationship of the caregiver to the patient. Compared to adult children, spousal caregivers are understandably less likely to be employed and tend to have lower educational attainments. Consequently, we examined these associations within the subgroups of spousal and adult-child caregivers. The association between educational status and loss-to-follow-up is significant only among the spousal caregivers. This finding is due primarily to an exceptionally high rate of loss among the least-educated group (36.7%). The employment status and loss-to-follow-up association is not statistically significant within either subgroup, meaning the overall effect is spurious, attributable to the association between kin relationship and employment status.

In sum, SES and demographic characteristics are generally not associated with subject attrition over the multiple waves of the study. The two exceptions to this generalization are the exceptionally low rate of attrition among daughters and the exceptionally high rate of attrition among poorly educated spouses.

It is informative to consider not only the characteristics of caregivers, but also those of the impaired spouses and parents who are the care recipients. In general, the SES and demographic characteristics of the dementia patients converge with the characteristics of their caregivers, especially for husbands, wives, and adult children who live with their parents. Two distinctive patient characteristics are shown in Table 3.2. One is the age distribution of patients, which resembles that of the spousal caregivers. The majority of the patients are over age 70 years, with

Table 3.2   Percent Distribution of Patient Characteristics at Time 1 and by Interview Status at Time 4

Patient characteristics	Time 1 (%) (N = 555)	Status at Time 4 (%)			
		In-home (n = 138)	Institutional (n = 131)	Bereavement (n = 188)	LTF[a] (n = 98)
Relationship to caregiver					
Wife	24.5	26.8	22.1	22.9	27.6*
Husband	34.2	34.1	26.0	34.0	45.9
Mother	31.7	31.9	39.7	31.9	20.4
Father	6.1	5.1	5.3	8.5	4.1
Mother-in-law	2.9	2.2	6.1	1.6	2.0
Father-in-law	0.5	—	0.8	1.1	—
Age					
Less than 69	23.2	29.7	28.2	16.5	20.4
70–79	40.7	39.9	40.5	36.7	50.0
80 and older	36.0	30.4	31.3	46.8	29.6

[a]LTF, loss-to-follow-up.
*$p \leq .05$.

a mean age of 75.4 years ($SD = 8.7$). This age distribution, of course, reflects the fact that dementia is primarily a condition afflicting the elderly.

> She's young. She might live another 20 years.

Patient age is not related to loss-to-follow-up. However, when only those patients whose caregivers were interviewed at Time 4 are considered, there are notable differences in outcome, differences that are similar to those reported previously for caregiver age. Thus, among the youngest patients, continuing in-home and institutional care are the most common circumstances at Time 4, whereas the patient is most likely to be deceased at follow-up in the oldest age category ($p \leq .01$). The basis for this association is intuitively obvious: The risk of mortality increases with age.

The second distinctive patient characteristic that is apparent in Table 3.2 is kin relationship. For married couples, gender of the caregiver identifies the gender of the patient, and patients are more likely to be husbands than wives. This distribution of caregiver–patient pairs reflects major demographic trends: Husbands are typically older than their wives and women have a longer life expectancy than men. That is, wives, who are likely to be younger than their husbands, tend to be alive to care for ill husbands, but are likely to be widows if and when they themselves become ill.

The gender of the adult-child caregiver, however, is not informative about whether he or she is caring for a mother or a father. As illustrated in Table 3.2, most of the parents are mothers, reflecting the fact that their husbands had died. Indeed, mothers predominate irrespective of whether care is provided by a son (81.1%) or a daughter (84.4%). The most common pattern of intergenerational caregiving therefore, is that of daughters caring for their widowed mothers. This group represents 70.7% of the intergenerational dyads and 29.2% of all the caregiver–patient dyads ($n = 162$).[4] The other combinations are relatively infrequent: daughters caring for fathers ($n = 29$), sons caring for mothers ($n = 30$), and sons caring for fathers ($n = 8$).[5] These statistics, too, represent the impact of gender differences in mortality: Fathers are likely to be cared for by their wives, whereas mothers tend to be widowed and cared for by their daughters or sons.

The association between kin relationship and loss-to-follow-up, displayed in the column to the far right of Table 3.2, parallels the pattern previously reported for caregivers. This association, by and large, is due to the especially low rate of attrited daughters who are taking care of their mothers. Hence, the similarity between Tables 3.1 and 3.2 in this respect.

The joint distribution of gender and kin relationship poses some analytic difficulties. First, for spouses, gender of the caregiver is redundant information with gender of the patient. Second, the preponderance of daughter–mother pairs means, in essence, that the separate influence of adult-child gender and patient gender cannot be reliably estimated. Consequently, we use the following designation of caregiver-patient types for most analyses: wives caring for husbands (n

= 190), husbands caring for wives ($n = 136$), daughters caring for mothers ($n = $ 162), and others ($n = 67$). This approach is awkward at best because the "other" group has a hodgepodge quality. The main advantage of this technique is that the gender of the patient and the caregiver in the daughter–mother group is constant—female. This group may be compared to the other group composed of only female patients—wives cared for by husbands. It may also be compared to the other group composed of only female caregivers—wives caring for husbands. The clarity of gender in these contrasts at least partially offsets the loss of information associated with combining diverse pairs into the "other" category.

Transitions over Time

Although some caregivers continued to provide in-home care over the entire course of the study, this career pathway is not the most common one traversed by caregivers. Over the 3-year span of the study, many dementia patients were placed in nursing homes and many died either at home or in nursing homes. Figure 3.1 depicts the flow of care recipients from the start of the study, when all patients were receiving in-home care, until their death. Those who were alive at their last assessment are traced until that point, which is usually Time 4, but occurs earlier for those participants who were lost-at-follow-up. Patients could continue to receive in-home care (boxes), relocate to institutional care (hexagons), or die (ovals). As may be seen, some patients were admitted to nursing

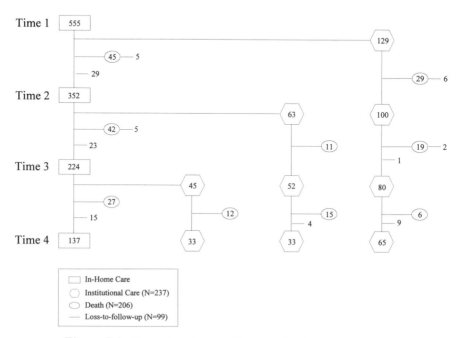

Figure 3.1   Dementia patient transitions over four interviews (3 years).

homes and died soon thereafter. At times, both of these transitions occurred in the interval separating adjacent interviews; in other cases, patients continued to reside in nursing homes at the next follow-up, but died some time thereafter.

The pathway to the far left of Figure 3.1 tracks the patients who continued to receive in-home care at each follow-up, a steadily declining number of persons. By Time 4, only 137 (24.7%) patients still resided at home. Thus, three-quarters traversed one of three alternative routes: 114 (20.5%) died while living at home, 237 (42.7%) were placed in nursing homes, and 67 (12.1%) were lost-at-follow-up prior to institutionalization or death. Those admitted to nursing home are distributed as follows: 131 continued to live in an institution through Time 4, 92 died, and 14 were lost-at-follow-up prior to death.[6] An additional 18 cases were lost-at-follow-up after patient death.[7] Thus, of those patients who survived until Time 4, about half were found at home and half resided in institutions.

Frank

The protracted course of in-home caregiving can exact an enormous toll from even the most dedicated of caregivers. Here, Frank, a devoted and loving husband describes the event that precipitated the institutionalization of his wife:

I'd like to tell you why I took her to a nursing home. A couple of years after round-the-clock care, I lost my temper and slapped her. I had had a bottomless end of patience. The next day I arranged for a nursing home. I was going downhill. Having a hell of a time. I lost my cool that once. It made me be very logical. I might do something much worse than that.

The flow of caregivers over the course of the study parallels that of the patients, but there are some important distinctions. First, when institutionalization and death both occurred between adjacent interviews, the caregiver completed only one interview, a bereavement interview and not a placement interview. However, the bereavement interview contained some retrospective questions pertaining to the institutional care stage, thus yielding some continuous coverage of the interval for cases of this kind.

Second, although Figure 3.1 shows patient careers ending in death, caregiving careers are conceptualized in Figure 3.2 as extending through the period of grief and social readjustment. Consequently, caregivers were interviewed after patient death. Indeed, there were three bereavement follow-up interviews for caregivers whose relatives died between Time 1 and Time 2, two for those whose relatives died between Time 2 and Time 3, and one for those whose relatives died between Time 3 and Time 4.

Caregivers providing in-home care at one interview move to one of five states at the following interview. First, they may have continued to provide in-home care, the straight horizontal pathway of boxes at the top of Figure 3.2. The ranks of those who continued to follow this track was reduced to 63.4%, 40.6%, and

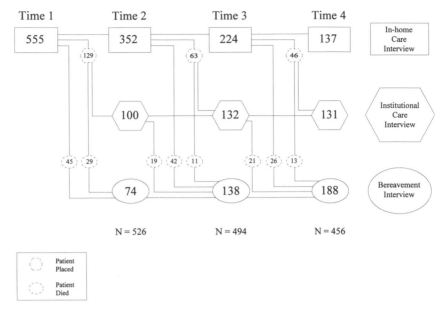

Figure 3.2   Interview status from Time 1 to Time 4.

24.7% of the original sample at Times 2, 3, and 4, respectively. Two additional tracks are established by way of admission of the patient to a nursing home (dashed hexagons): continued institutional care through the next interview (solid hexagons) and institutional care ended by death (dashed ovals) prior to the next interview in which the bereavement interview was used (solid ovals). The death of the dementia patient (dashed ovals) at home defines the fourth track. The fifth outcome associated with in-home care is loss-to-follow-up at the next interview, which is not shown in Figure 3.2 for simplicity of presentation. This composite category consists of those caregivers who we were unable to interview at follow-up because they had themselves died or become incapable of participating in the interview, or refused to be reinterviewed.

It's been a year and a half now that I can't leave him.

As depicted in Figure 3.2, caregivers whose spouses and parents resided in long-term care institutions at one interview encountered one of three potential circumstances at the next interview. The straight horizontal line of hexagons in the middle of the figure represents continued residence within an institution. This situation resulted in an additional institutional care interview, which provides longitudinal information about the postplacement period of the caregiver career. The primary alternate pathway is death of the dementia patient (dashed ovals), an event followed by a bereavement interview. Once again, loss-to-follow-up serves as a study endpoint, but is not shown in this figure. The follow-up of bereaved caregivers takes only two courses. Most were reinterviewed with the bereavement questionnaire, providing longitudinal information about life after caregiving. Other bereaved caregivers were lost-at-follow-up, which is not represented in Figure 3.2.

Patients may have been admitted to nursing homes at any time between Time 1 and Time 4. They may have died at any time during this interval as well. Consequently, the structure of the longitudinal data is quite complex. Sample attrition somewhat further adds to this complexity. The loss of subjects over time is depicted in Figure 3.3. Sample attrition is cumulative over time as we were unable to recover lost subjects at subsequent interviews. Thus, the total number of subjects interviewed, irrespective of type of questionnaires used in the interviews, declines over time to 456 at Time 4, which translates into a total attrition rate of 17.8% of the original sample.[8] This number represents an average of slightly less than 6% for each of the three interviews following the baseline interview. Earlier in this chapter, we saw that sample attrition is not related systematically to sample characteristics with the exception of potential age–gender mortality differences. Here, we note principally that this rate of attrition is low given the lengthy duration of the data collection, the large number of interviews, and the advanced age of the spousal caregivers, which contributes to the likelihood that they themselves will become sick or possibly die.

Caregivers who participated in all four interviews fit one of several distinct response patterns. The patterns are defined by questionnaire type and sequence. Indeed, all possible combinations of questionnaire sequences are present in the data, as illustrated in Table 3.3. Although at first glance it might appear that some combinations are omitted, some of these patterns are not logically consistent with

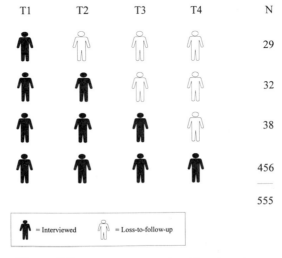

Figure 3.3   Loss-to-follow-up from Time 1 to Time 4.

Table 3.3   Number and Type of Interviews across Four Times[a,b]

Interview type at:					Number of interviews		
T1	T2	T3	T4	N	In-home care	Institutional care	Bereavement
H	H	H	H	137	4	0	0
H	H	H	I	33	3	1	0
H	H	H	B	39	3	0	1
H	H	I	I	33	2	2	0
H	H	I	B	15	2	1	1
H	H	B	B	48	2	0	2
H	I	I	I	65	1	3	0
H	I	I	B	6	1	2	1
H	I	B	B	17	1	1	2
H	B	B	B	63	1	0	3

[a]$N = 456$.
[b]T, Time; H, in-home care; I, institutional care; B, bereavement.

the sequence of career stages. For example, bereavement interviews were never followed by in-home or institutional care interviews and institutional care interviews were never followed by in-home care interviews.[9]

As may be seen in Table 3.3, the number of in-home care interviews numbers from one to four. Caregivers who provided in-home care at all four assessments obviously did not participate in any institutional care or bereavement interviews. In contrast, caregivers who participated in less than four in-home care interviews completed at least one institutional care or one bereavement interview. Thus, it is readily apparent that a sizable number of subjects participated in multiple types of interviews as well as multiple interviews of each type. A total of 104 caregivers participated in at least two institutional care interviews, providing longitudinal data on this career stage. Similarly, 128 caregivers participated in two or more bereavement interviews, providing long-term information about the course of grief and social readjustment. A small subgroup ($n = 38$) participated in all three types of interviews—in-home care, institutional care, and bereavement.

Two features of the data structure merit mention. First, for each type of interview, the number of subjects declines with each additional reinterview, such that the maximum sample size is made up of the number of caregivers who had the first interview of a given type. For example, the largest institutional care sample is for the first postadmission interview. This sample is formed by pooling caregivers who admitted their relatives to nursing homes between Times 1 and 2, Times 2 and 3, and Times 3 and 4 (see chapter 9). The greatest statistical power for longitudinal analysis, therefore, is found for the shortest follow-up interval: Time 2 for continuing in-home care, the first interview after placement, and the first interview after patient death.

Second, the smallest sample size consists of those caregivers who had the longest period of a specific type of follow-up: in-home care, institutional care, or bereavement. The longest follow-up, of course, always coincides with Time 4. That is, Time 4 captures 3 years of follow-up for those who continued to provide in-home care throughout the study, encompasses up to 3 years of follow-up for those who admitted their relatives to nursing homes between Time 1 and Time 2, and covers up to 3 years for those whose relatives died prior to Time 2. Statistical power clearly diminishes substantially for long-term analyses. On the other hand, these data are extremely valuable because they capture the longest period of time.

In essence, sample size and length of follow-up present a dilemma. We can be precise in our parameter estimates, but limited in the time span of our observations, or we can tolerate a greater margin of uncertainty, but encompass a lengthy interval of time. Throughout this volume we compromise, using both strategies in order to extract as complete a representation of the caregiver career as possible.

Why are the data so complex? One answer is that the sample is heterogeneous with regard to illness and duration of caregiving at the start of the study. Our first interview was not timed to coincide with some particular event, such as illness recognition, diagnosis, or admission to treatment. Instead, our interviews occurred randomly within each individual caregiver's career. This diversity is desirable because it generates variability in the duration of career stages and in the intensity of the care-related stress processes that are at the core of our investigation. On the other hand, it necessitates the use of several approaches to the data, which at times complicates our presentation of results.

Measurement Strategy

Developmental Stage

Our approach to the measurement of key constructs is contiguous with concepts that already have a presence in caregiving research, such as caregiver burden, yet the development of measures in this study emphasizes components distinctive to our conceptualization of stress processes. Consequently, we provide somewhat more information in this volume about our measures than would be the case if we relied solely on existing measures. Specific measures are introduced not in this section, but in conjunction with relevant substantive analyses. It should be noted that some of the information contained in the various interview schedules—in-home care, institutional care, and bereavement—is omitted entirely because it exceeds the scope of the central issues addressed in this single volume. In this section, we describe the procedures used in the development of specific study measures.

The measures created for this research were developed from firsthand accounts of care-related experiences. As explained at the beginning of this chapter, early on in our endeavor we conducted unstructured, qualitative interviews. Our concerns were more descriptive than analytic at that stage of the investigation: What types of problems are encountered during the ordinary course of providing care, and what strategies are used by caregivers in attempting to resolve these problems? Our intent was to capture the meaning of *adaptation* to caregiving as seen through the eyes of those who are doing the washing, feeding, bill paying, and worrying, in essence, the caring.

Several major conceptual themes were evident in the qualitative interviews, such as the pervasive encroachment of caregiving into all corners of life, the gradual atrophy of social involvements beyond caregiving and the family, the synergistic layering of problem upon problem, and the metamorphosis of self-concept. The qualitative interviews also helped to reveal the diverse experiences entailed in caregiving. Although certain themes were echoed repeatedly, no single theme emerged as a uniform element of caregiving. For example, many caregivers experienced a constriction of social ties as their care-related respon-sibilities escalated, forcing out nonessential elements of daily life. Nonetheless, some caregivers deviated from this pattern, retaining, or perhaps even expanding, the scope of their social involvements. By way of example is the husband who seeks emotional and instrumental assistance within a self-help group, or the daughter who becomes politically active, lobbying on behalf of dementia patients and their families. Thus, the realization that individuals respond differently to seemingly similar difficult circumstances arose quite early in this research. With regard to measurement, the chief consequences of this realization were the inclu-sion of constructs likely to mediate the psychosocial impact of care-related stress, constructs like mastery or self-efficacy and social support.

Overview of Key Measures

As described above, four interview schedules were used in our data collec-tions: the baseline interview, when all caregivers were providing in-home care, and three follow-up interviews tailored to the unique circumstances of continuing in-home care, institutional care, and bereavement and social readjustment. Table 3.4 summarizes the measures used to operationalize key constructs. Specific measures are described in greater detail as they become relevant to the analyses reported in the following chapters. The list of measures, therefore, refers the reader to the chapter that introduces each construct and describes its psycho-metric properties. In addition, Table 3.4 indicates whether the measure was included in each of the four types of interviews.

As may be seen, some measures were shared in common across all interviews, whereas others were specific to a given type of interview. Demographic charac-teristics were assessed at the baseline interview; only changes in marital and employment status were assessed at follow-up. In general, characteristics of the patient were assessed across interview types, except for the bereavement inter-views, when these questions were no longer relevant. Likewise, elements of care-related stress that pertain to interactions between the caregiver and the care recipient were asked at all interviews exclusive of the bereavement interview. However, secondary stressors, in the forms of role strains and intrapsychic strains, were assessed in all types of interviews as they are not necessarily

Table 3.4 Description of Measures: Chapter Location and Interview Type

Measures	Chapter	Type of interview			
		Baseline	In-home care	Institutional care	Bereavement
Demographic characteristics	3	♦	—	—	—
Dementia characteristics					
Illness duration	4	♦	—	—	—
Length of care	4	♦	—	—	—
Diagnosis	3	♦	♦	♦	—
Patient health status	8	♦	♦	♦	—
Primary stressors: Objective					
Cognitive impairment	4	♦	♦	♦	—
Problematic behavior	4	♦	♦	♦	—
ADL dependencies	4	♦	♦	♦	—
Patient resistance	4	♦	♦	♦	—
Primary stressors: Subjective					
Role overload	4	♦	♦	♦	♦
Role captivity	4	♦	♦	♦	—
Loss of intimate exchange	4	♦	♦	♦	♦
Secondary stressors: Role strains					
Family conflict	4	♦	♦	♦	♦
Work strain	4	♦	♦	♦	♦
Work reduction	4	♦	♦	♦	♦
Not employed	4	♦	♦	♦	♦
Financial strain	4	♦	♦	♦	♦
Secondary stressors: Intrapsychic strain					
Loss of self	4	♦	♦	♦	♦
Lack of caregiver competence	4	♦	♦	♦	♦
Absence of caregiving gains	4	♦	♦	♦	♦
Guilt	9	♦	♦	♦	♦
Extraneous stressors	4	♦	♦	♦	♦
Psychological distress					
Depression	6	♦	♦	♦	♦
Anxiety	8	♦	♦	♦	♦
Severe anger	8	♦	♦	♦	♦
Social support					
Instrumental support	7	♦	♦	—	—
Socioemotional support	7	♦	♦	♦	♦
Health and social services	7	♦	♦	♦	♦
Mastery or self-efficacy	7	♦	♦	♦	♦
Placement					
Anticipatory worry	8	—	♦	—	—
Date of placement	8	—	—	♦	♦

Table 3.4   (continued)

Measures	Chapter	Baseline	In-home care	Institutional care	Bereavement
				Type of interview	
Reasons for placement	8	—	—	♦	♦
Help in decision making	8	—	—	♦	♦
Problems during placement	8	—	—	♦	—
Worries during placement	8	—	—	♦	—
Visitation	9	—	—	♦	—
Satisfaction with facility	9	—	—	♦	♦
Problems with facility	9	—	—	♦	—
Bereavement					
Date of death	10	—	—	—	♦
Grief	11	—	—	—	♦
Help with funeral	11	—	—	—	♦
Longing	11	—	—	—	♦
Preoccupation	11	—	—	—	♦
Painful affect	11	—	—	—	♦
Dissociation	11	—	—	—	♦

confined to the life span of the dementia patient, but may continue indefinitely. The same is true for extraneous stressors.

Attributes of the caregiver generally were assessed at baseline and all follow-up interviews. These characteristics include indicators of key outcomes, especially psychological distress. Potential stress mediators or moderators, including social support, mastery, and the use of health and social services, were also assessed at each interview. Questions pertaining to institutional care and bereavement generally were confined to these two types of interviews, respectively. The in-home care follow-up interviews, however, contained items concerning the anticipation of institutionalization; specifically, worries about the future welfare of the patient and practical obstacles surrounding admission to a nursing home. When patients were admitted to nursing homes and died shortly thereafter, their caregivers participated in the bereavement interview only. In these instances, some retrospective questions about the institutional care period were asked in order to provide continuous coverage of all caregiving career stages.

As noted previously, not all of the information contained in these interviews will be presented within this volume. The omitted domains, which do not appear on the list in Table 3.4, include the structure and functioning of the family as a group, coping cognitions and behaviors, role-specific indicators of distress, the structure of informal social networks, and the quality of the caregiver's relationship with the care recipient prior to the onset of the dementia. These constructs were not included in this volume primarily because our analyses are already multivariate and at the upper bound of complexity. Also, in some instances, most notably coping and the structure of social networks, we were not yet satisfied with our attempts at creating composite measures that are both reliable and theoretically coherent. Our selection of some domains over others reflects our overriding concern with processes of stress proliferation and the social psychological factors that lead to stress containment.

Data Analysis Strategies

The techniques used to analyze the data are, by and large, standard statistical procedures, including descriptive statistics such as measures of central tendency and dispersion. More typically, given our theoretical approach, we employ multivariate explanatory procedures like ordinary linear regression and logistic regression. We attempt to make these results easier to grasp by presenting findings graphically whenever possible. Where technical details that might be of interest to those conducting similar research are glossed over, more detailed information is presented in chapter notes.

There are two analytic techniques we employ that have not had extensive previous applications in gerontological, caregiving, or stress research: *hazard models* and *canonical correlations*. Consequently, these methods are described briefly in this section. The purpose of the descriptions is not to present the methods in statistical detail, but to provide sufficient explanation for interpreting the findings presented in the ensuing chapters.

Hazard Models

In some instances, time is viewed best not as study time (i.e., Time 1 through Time 4) but as the duration of a stage in the caregiving career. Each stage is defined by the occurrence of the transitional events marking its start and finish. For example, in-home care is bound by the initiation of assistance at one end and by the institutionalization or death of the dementia patient at the other. Similarly, illness duration is defined as the interval separating symptom recognition from death.

The shift in perspective from study time to event time required reorganization of the data around the occurrence of relevant events. That is, time is measured with reference to the transitional events that mark the beginning and ending of the career stage, with time starting to accrue when the initial event occurred and continuing to accrue until the concluding event occurred. For example, the duration of institutional care—time from admission to a nursing home until death—is counted as the number of months from the date of admission until the date of death. Time zero, the date of admission, may have taken place at any time in the interval separating the Time 1 interview from that of Time 4; similarly, death may have occurred at any subsequent point in this interval. In essence, the reorganization entails "stacking" data for identical transitions that were recorded at different interviews. The details of specific applications of data reorganization are discussed in conjunction with the analyses to which they pertain. Here, we provide only an overview of this technique.

In order to count some time intervals, we had to rely upon retrospective data provided at the baseline interview to identify the start of a career stage. Specifically, we used baseline reports of the time since symptom recognition and the time since the start of care to establish initial values for illness duration and in-home care duration. The initial values were then incremented until specific events occurred following the Time 1 interview. In contrast, the start of institutional care was demarcated by the date of admission to a nursing home, an event that necessarily transpired after the baseline interview.

The end of a career stage also is marked by a transitional event. The two events emphasized in our analyses signaling pivotal transitions in caregiver careers are admission of the patient to a nursing home and death of the patient. For example, one application, discussed in detail in chapter 8, concerns factors influencing the length of in-home care prior to institutional placement. This interval was calculated as the summation of the duration of care reported at baseline and the elapsed time between the baseline interview and nursing home admission. A second instance of this approach is found in chapter 10, which examines illness duration (i.e., the time from symptom recognition until death).

The chief complication in the analyses that prompts our use of hazard models is the passage of time; specifically, the length of time an individual has been at risk for the occurrence of an *exit* event. We could examine whether or not the exit event occurred prior to Time 4, the end of our observations, but this approach is flawed because some of those who had not exited from a stage by Time 4 eventually will do so. For example, some of those caregivers who were providing in-home care at Time 4 subsequently will admit their relatives to nursing homes. These caregivers are observed as being negative, rather than positive, on this exit event merely as a result of not being observed for a sufficient period of time; these cases may be thought of as being misclassified on the true outcome.

Error in classifying an exit event is especially problematic because the caregivers in this study have been "at risk" for transitional events for varying periods of time. The interval of risk for an exit event is the length of time that has passed since entry into the career phase. For example, for admission to a nursing home, the interval of risk is the length of time the caregiver has been providing in-home care. Compared to caregivers who have just started to assist their spouses or parents, those who have put their shoulders to this task for years have had many more opportunities to institutionalize their relatives (i.e., to exit from the in-home care phase).

When caregivers have not been observed long enough for an event to have occurred, the data are right-censored. The length of time the caregivers will occupy a career stage is not yet known. Ignoring these censoring problems introduces serious bias in parameter estimates (Singer & Willett, 1991). To illustrate this point, consider again the example of the duration of in-home care bound by the start of care and institutionalization. Limiting analysis to caregivers who did indeed place their relatives prior to Time 4 would tend to bias downwardly the estimates of the duration of care because the groups that are excluded disproportionately contain those who have been providing in-home care for the longest time: caregivers who provide in-home care until the patient dies and those who are still providing in-home care at Time 4.

Consequently, we employed analytic techniques that take into account censored cases. These procedures used information about the duration of a career stage up until the time when the case became censored, capitalizing upon the fact that we knew the case had "survived" at least that long. Chapter 8 uses these techniques to examine the duration of in-home care and the risk of institutionalization. These techniques are used again in chapter 10 to examine illness duration and the risk of death.

A brief comment is warranted concerning the interpretation of the regression coefficients for hazard models. In this type of analysis, positive regression coefficients indicate an increase in the hazard function, which is equivalent to a negative effect upon survival time. The exponential of the regression coefficient may be interpreted as a partial odds ratio (i.e., the multiplicative effect of a unit change in the covariate on the odds of event occurrence). We present these transformed values because they are substantively easier to interpret than the linear coefficients calibrated to the log odds.

We should also point out that the hazard models for institutional placement and patient death use two types of covariates: fixed and time-varying. Fixed covariates have values that remain constant over the entire period of observation, such as gender. Other covariates may change in value over the course of observations, variables like declining cognitive functioning, hence, they are time-varying covariates. For example, cognitive impairment is initialized to its baseline value, which is used to predict whether exit events occur between Time 1 and Time 2. If the event does not occur in this interval, the Time 2 level of cognitive impairment is then used to predict whether exit events occur in the interval between Time 2 and Time 3.[10] This procedure is repeated for the next interval and so on. Thus, the covariate is updated during analysis to the value most proximal to the transitional event.

These analytic techniques, more commonly used in demography and population studies, have had recent application to the risk of institutionalization among the elderly. For example, Liang and Tu (1986) estimated a lifetime probability of entering a nursing home as .297 or 29.7%. Greene and Ondrich (1990) took a more explanatory approach, using a discrete-time hazard model to assess risk factors for admission to a nursing home.

Finally, we note that in some of our analyses the passage of time is treated as an independent variable. The two events of primary interest are institutionalization and death of the patient. For example, in chapter 9 the duration of institutional care is examined as a factor affecting adjustment. A second application probes the impact of time upon grief and social reintegration, as reported in chapter 11.

Canonical Correlations

In some analyses, we are concerned not with a single outcome, but with multiple outcomes. The technique of canonical correlations is well suited to these circumstances: It describes simultaneous associations between multiple independent and multiple dependent variables. As described in Afifi and Clark (1984, chap. 15), canonical variables are computed for the independent and dependent variable sets; the resulting canonical variables are linear combinations of the variables comprising each set. The new variables are then correlated with one another. This technique is used in chapter 4 to examine linkages among various conceptual domains, such as primary and secondary stressors.

The first linear combination maximizes the correlation between the canonical variable for the independent variables and the canonical variable for the dependent variables. More than one canonical variable may be extracted when there is more than one variable in each set. In instances like these, the maximization criterion is conditional: The canonical variables for the independent variables are not correlated with one another, nor are the canonical variables for the dependent variables correlated with one another. Although variable sets are referred to as independent or dependent, it is not necessary to impute a causal order among these sets, which is similar to the use of simple correlations.

Canonical correlation coefficients are analogous to multiple correlation coefficients, but pertain to multiple dependent variables considered as a set. The standardized weights indicate the relative contribution of each variable in the set (independent or dependent) to the canonical variable. We apply this technique to describe associations among various sets of variables, such as the linkages among primary and secondary stressors introduced in the next chapter.

Summary

• The data reported in the following chapters were collected by way of four personal interviews conducted annually with 555 primary caregivers to a spouse or parent afflicted with AD or a related dementia.
• The sample is heterogeneous in its socioeconomic and demographic characteristics: A slight majority are spouses of the dementia patient, two-thirds are female, one-third work outside of the home, and the median income is $27,500. However, ethnic groups other than non-Hispanic whites are somewhat underrepresented.
• Over the course of 3 years, 237 (42.7%) dementia patients were placed in a nursing homes and 206 (37.1%) died either at home ($n = 114$) or in institutions ($n = 92$).
• At the end of 3 years, 137 (24.7%) of the dementia patients continued to reside at home and 131 (23.6%) continued to live in institutions.
• Total loss-to-follow-up from all sources—caregiver death, inability to locate the caregiver, and refusal—was low (17.7%) and generally unrelated to the characteristics of the caregiver or care recipient.
• To accommodate the progression of the caregiving career, three separate, but overlapping, interview schedules were used at follow-up. Each schedule was tailored to the unique circumstances of continuing in-home care, institutional care, or bereavement and readjustment.

- The interviews assessed (1) characteristics of the caregiver and the dementia patient, (2) primary and secondary sources of care-related stress, (3) potential mediators or moderators of care-related stress, and (4) mental health consequences of the care-related stress process.
- The institutional care interview also assessed problems associated with the admission of the care recipient to a nursing home, satisfaction with institutional care, and level of involvement with the patient and with his or her care following institutionalization.
- The bereavement interview also asked about the circumstances surrounding the death of the dementia patient, experience of grief and mourning, and subsequent changes in the caregiver's life.
- For the most part, the data were analyzed using familiar statistical procedures. However, we employed two techniques that have had only limited application in previous caregiving research: hazard models and canonical correlations.

The application of the methods described in this chapter has resulted in a set of data that is necessarily complex because it captures the intricacies of the caregiving career as it evolves over time. We turn to the results of our investigation in the following chapters. The presentation is organized around the stages and transitions of the caregiving career and focuses on the care-related stress process.

Notes

[1]Two additional waves of data have been collected, but are not processed completely for analysis at this time. Consequently, we limit our analyses to the first four interviews.

[2]There are too few caregivers who are in-laws of patients to permit separate statistical analysis. Consequently, in-laws are combined with daughters or sons for analysis. Thus, unless otherwise specified, we use daughter to mean daughter and daughter-in-law, and son to mean son and son-in-law.

[3]The bereaved group includes caregivers who institutionalized their relatives prior to their relatives' death, as well as those who continued to provide in-home care at the time of death.

[4]This figure includes 16 daughter-in-laws caring for their husbands' mothers.

[5]This figure includes one son-in-law caring for his wife's father.

[6]One patient who returned to in-home care following two periods of institutional care is counted as loss-to-follow-up because this trajectory is unique in the sample.

[7]Although more patients died at home than in nursing homes, the death rate is substantially higher among nursing home residents because all patients are at risk of in-home death while they live at home, but only those admitted to nursing homes are at risk of dying there. See chapter 10 for further information.

[8]This figure includes one patient who returned home following institutionalization.

[9]The sole individual who returned home from a nursing home is treated as loss-to-follow-up.

[10]Censored cases are removed from subsequent analysis and, therefore, are updated in this manner only until the time of censoring.

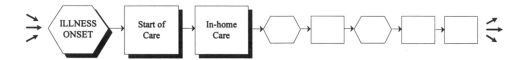

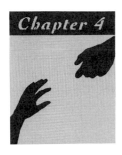

Chapter 4

The Organization of Stressors in the Lives of Caregivers

We turn now from theory and method to the actual experiences of individuals as they go about the business of taking care of their cognitively impaired husbands, wives, mothers, and fathers. This chapter concerns the earliest phases of the caregiving career: the start of care and the active provision of care within the home. The baseline data are used to describe the types of impairment present among dementia patients at the beginning of the study, the demands these impairments as primary stressors impose upon caregivers, and the consequences of the primary stressors on other aspects of life (i.e., the creation of secondary stressors). The measures used to operationalize primary and secondary stressors are presented in this chapter along with their psychometric properties. We examine patterns of association among primary and secondary stressors as well. Our goals are, first, to translate abstract constructs into concrete observations, and second, to demonstrate that care-related stressors do not necessarily exist independently of one another. We reason that if one stressor or cluster of stressors exists, then others are likely to coexist.

The Onset of Caregiving

The story of caregiving begins when a parent or spouse is stricken with Alzheimer's disease (AD) or a related dementia, the crossroad at which established patterns of family life begin to be irreversibly altered. Like many chronic conditions, the onset of dementia is often insidious and virtually imperceptible. Consequently, the recognition and acknowledgment that something is wrong typically occurs some time after the true onset of the underlying disease. *Symptom recognition,* the realization that one's parent or spouse is acting in ways that deviate markedly from their usual demeanor, marks the social beginning of the condition, the onset of the illness as distinct from the onset of the disease. Yet the caregiver's own story often begins somewhat later, when he or she becomes actively engaged in providing care.

Valerie

The interior of Valerie's large home is somewhat in disarray, cluttered, dusty, with lots of interesting mementoes—framed theatrical prints, merry-go-round horse, doll house, stained-glass hangings, costumes, and an eclectic mix of chairs and furnishings. Its old, worn, dusty—homey. Valerie dresses in a Bohemian style in natural fabrics, grey slacks, blue blouse, woven vest, stone beads, turquoise silver ring, round glasses, soft short curly grey hair, and flat buckled shoes. She is articulate, outgoing, and open. She cares for her severely impaired husband Donald at home:

Someone's gotta do it. I'm the logical one, the obligated one. He'd do it for me. He's very nurturing. He'd do it better for me than I do for him.

It's never been love. I've never been in love with him. He says he loves me. You know how in a marriage one person loves more than the other. I love him less. I never loved him. I've been in love . . . this is not it. He's my very best friend.

The bitterness is almost always there. Our lives could have been different. And my life after this disease — I'm not going down with the ship. There'll be a life, dammit! Not let the disease get both of us!

I worry, what if I get sick? Who would take care of me?

Throughout these analyses, therefore, we used two yardsticks to measure time. The first, *illness duration*, was gauged with the question: "How long ago did you realize that something was wrong with your (relative)?" When caregivers were asked what made them realize something was wrong, the most common reasons were forgetting recent events (31.7%), personality change (14.8%), and getting lost (8.1%). The second measure of time is *duration of care*, which we discerned by asking: "How long ago did you *first* have to start helping (him/her) do things that (he/she) was no longer able to do for (himself/herself)?" The times were initially assessed at the baseline interview and incremented at each reinterview.

> Our oldest boy called me up at work and asked, "What's wrong with Mom? When I call her on the phone she acts like she's drunk."

The distributions of time since symptom recognition and time since the start of care at the baseline interview are displayed in Figure 4.1. The shapes of these two distributions are quite similar: comparatively few caregivers are found at the very short or very long durations. However, the time since first recognizing symptoms is greater than that since the initiation of care, reflecting the fact that symptom recognition typically precedes the initiation of care. The semiquartile range, encompassing the middle 50% of the sample, is 3–7 years for symptom recognition; for start of care, this range is 2–4.5 years. At baseline, the average caregiver in our sample had known something was wrong for slightly more than 5 years and had been providing care for about 3 years.

Thus, although some caregivers were novices at the start of the study, the typical caregiver was a veteran of several years service. The broad span of time

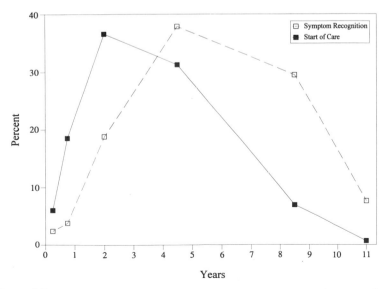

Figure 4.1   Percent distribution of time from symptom recognition and from start of care.

since the start of in-home care reflects the wide range of illness duration, which, in turn, reflects variation in the timing of the onset of dementia. As we shall see, these different histories produce a prismatic spectrum of care-related stressors, running the gamut from minor inconvenience to total disruption of day-to-day life.

Another question we asked caregivers was how long it had been since their relatives had first been seen by a doctor for memory problems, an event that had transpired on average 3.5 years before their first interviews. As mentioned in the previous chapter, the most common diagnosis was AD (73.9%), followed by multi-infarct dementia (MID) (9.0%) and unspecified dementia (9.2%). Some caregivers (4.7%), however, had not received any specific diagnosis at the time of the baseline interview.

The times at which caregivers experienced symptom recognition, diagnosis, and start of care are associated with one another, but there is considerable variability in the sequencing of the events (Aneshensel, Pearlin, & Schuler, 1993). We refer to the most common order as a protracted *moratorium* to call attention to the lengthy interval in which acquisition of the caregiving role was help in abeyance. In this pattern, symptom recognition and diagnosis coincided in time, but caregivers started to provide help much later than when they first noticed something was wrong and consulted a physician ($n = 160$). The second pattern began with a single occurrence, symptom recognition, followed by the joint occurrence of consulting a physician and starting to provide help ($n = 112$). We refer to this career line as *indeterminate* to emphasize the interval of uncertainty between symptom recognition and diagnosis. Third, approximately one in five caregivers noticed something was wrong, started to provide help, and had their relative consult a doctor at about the same point in time ($n = 100$). We label this pattern *compressed* role acquisition to highlight the temporal convergence of these three milestones.

Collectively, the three sequences—moratorium, indeterminate, and compressed—account for approximately two out of three caregivers. We also identified nine other sequences that account for the remaining third of the sample ($n = 183$). Three of these sequences are represented by 5–10% of the sample: symptom recognition, diagnosis, and care separated by lengthy intervening intervals ($n = 49$); symptom recognition and help coinciding and preceding diagnosis ($n = 42$); and symptom recognition followed by care and then by diagnosis ($n = 41$). No other single configuration of the events represented more than 2% of the sample.

In summary, a key feature differentiating caregiving career lines is the manner in which one enters the role. There are two important points to emphasize about the transition into the role acquisition stage. First, there are variations among caregivers in the order of transitional events, and second, there are common patterns of sequences of transitional events that caregivers follow. Three sequences of events predominate, accounting for the experiences of a majority of caregivers. It should be noted that each of these typologies subsumes additional variation in the time between events, meaning that the duration of the intervals varies within type. All configurations entail the lengthy passage of time between at least two events with the exception of the compressed pattern. The transition into role acquisition, then, typically is protracted. Variability in how caregivers take up the role reflects the importance of other contextual factors, such as characteristics of the patient, of the caregiver, of their past and present relationship, of the larger social environment, and so forth.

The Primary Stressors of Caregiving

Were we interested merely in demonstrating that caregiving can, and often does, generate conditions experienced as excruciatingly stressful, we might have ended our inquiry in the exploratory phase of this study. Yet the graphic narratives provided by the caregivers made us realize that caregiver stress flows from multiple founts. The physical tasks of providing care push some individuals beyond the limits of their physical or emotional stamina. Many find the junctures between caregiving and other adult social roles troublesome, especially when conflict arises between caregiving and employment. This multiplicity of pressure points is a reflection of the multidimensional character of the stressors confronting caregivers. The assessment of these stressors, therefore, needs to capture a broad spectrum of care-related hardships and difficulties that come to intrude into other social, economic, and personal pursuits. As described in chapter 2, our efforts to identify the ways in which caregiving becomes problematic ultimately led us to differentiate between those stressors directly caused by caregiving activities, primary stressors, and those indirectly caused by caregiving activities, secondary stressors.

By stressors we mean the conditions, experiences, and activities that are problematic for people, threatening them, thwarting their efforts, fatiguing them, and defeating their dreams. As we shall see, stress resides not solely in the external conditions of an individual's life, but in the interaction of these conditions with an individual's internal state; that is, with an individual's needs and desires; ability to mobilize energy; assessment of what is important in life; sense of self, including how he or she views him or herself in relation to others; and plans, aspirations, and hopes for finding his or her lot in life.

This orientation is not novel, but reflects the general approach to stress that predominates within the field. Thus, we approach stress as a state of arousal resulting from the presence of conditions that tax or exceed an individual's usual ability to adapt, or the absence of the means for an individual to attain sought-after goals (Lazarus, 1966; Menaghan, 1983; Pearlin, 1983). This definition captures two essential elements: the external stimulus and the internal catalyst. Stressors have the potential to arouse stress, which typically manifests itself as tension, uneasiness, anxiety, alarm, worry, fear, dread, upset, and physical illness.

It must be emphasized that stress is not an inherent consequence of external conditions, but emanates from discrepancies between those conditions and characteristics of an individual (Aneshensel, 1992). That is, stress does not stem exclusively from either environmental demands or from an individual; instead, it arises from the intersection of an individual and his or her environment. This distinction is critical to understanding why caregivers respond differently to situations that appear to be identical: The way caregiving is experienced depends upon the personal factors of a caregiver's life, such as the quality of the predementia patient–caregiver relationship, the social meanings attached to this history, expectations about the future of the relationship, and so forth. Thus, the emergence of stress is inseparable from the meaning caregivers give to the circumstances of their lives.

Caregiving stress, therefore, arises when the demands imposed by the patient's condition collide with the caregiver's subjective ability to respond to these demands, or when these demands obstruct the pursuit of other objectives. Stress escalates as demands increase, as resources decrease, or as both of these changes occur. We may be certain, too, that change will occur as it is part and parcel of the inescapable degenerative course of dementia. Thus, caregiving should be viewed not as a system that achieves and maintains a state of equilibrium, but as a continually shifting terrain that plunges caregivers into turmoil, not allowing them to maintain firm footing.

The degenerative course of dementia is the nucleus of the care-related stress process. The onset of the illness, the realization that current behavior deviates from normal functioning and the identification of this deviation as a disease, represents an initial jolt to existing family relationships. This thrust sets in motion a series of dislocations and readjustments that evolve over a rather lengthy period of time. Recall, at the baseline interview, the typical patient had been ill for more than 5 years and the average caregiver had been helping the patient for about 3 years. As the status of the patient deteriorates over time, the need for help and supervision escalates, coalescing into a set of conditions we refer to as primary stressors.

The stressors are "primary" in the sense that they are inseparable from the root of the problem, the impaired condition of the patient. They evolve from difficulties that flow directly from the needs of the patient and the scope of care necessitated by these needs. In essence, the stressors are primary because they are integral components of the underlying illness that has created the demand for caregiving. Our conceptualization of care-related stressors differentiates between the actual tasks of caregiving and the meaning these obligations have for the individual caregiver.

Objective Conditions of Caregiving

We refer to the actual demands of caregiving as primary stressors. These conditions are designated as "objective" insofar as they pertain to concrete manifestations of the patient's impairment. The core element in this cluster of stressors is the patient's state of cognitive impairment, which creates dependencies and the need for assistance. The second component pertains to tangible actions taken by the caregiver to tend to the patient and to safeguard his or her well-being.

Cognitive Impairment

A key sign of dementia is the state of cognitive impairment. The range and difficulty of caregiving activities and the ability of a caregiver to manage his or her relationship with the impaired relative are strongly influenced by the patient's memory loss, communication deficits, and recognition failures. Although reported by the caregivers, our evaluation of the patients' cognitive status is based on standard tests typically used in the clinic (Folstein, Folstein, & McHugh, 1975). Specifically, we asked,

> Now, I'd like to ask you some questions about your (relative's) memory and the difficulty (he/she) may have doing some things. How difficult is it for your (relative) to: remember recent events, know what day of the week it is, remember (his/her) home address, remember words, understand simple instructions, find (his/her) way around the house, [and] speak sentences?[1]

The response categories for these signs and symptoms ranged from *not at all difficult* (0) to *can't do at all* (5).

The validity of these assessments was assessed for a subsample of 75 participants whose impaired relatives were clients of the Northern California Alzheimer's Disease Center. Independent clinical evaluations using the Mini-Mental Test, probably the most widely accepted measure of cognitive impairment, are strongly correlated with the ratings made by caregivers ($r = .65$). Thus, caregivers appear to evaluate the cognitive abilities of their relatives with a high degree of accuracy. These determinations have considerable internal reliability as well ($\alpha = .86$). Scale scores are the summation of the weighted item responses divided by the total number of possible impairments, 7, which yields the average rating of the patient across all impairments.

How cognitively impaired are the dementia patients who are being cared for by our respondents? The distribution of the *number* of cognitive impairments present (any rating except *not at all difficult*) is highly skewed, with an average approaching six of the seven possible impairments (5.81), and a mode of seven (42.5%), which is the upper limit of the count. Each of the impairments, then, is present for the majority of the patients.

The *severity* of the impairments (a count of the number of symptoms rated as *can't do at all*), however, reveals somewhat greater diversity, suggesting two impairment profiles. More than half of the care recipients (59.5%) have *only* mild to moderate symptoms (i.e., do not have any symptoms rated in the most severe category). The remainder have at least one severe impairment, with about 10% of the sample being rated as severely impaired on a majority of the cognitive tasks. The cognitive impairment scale exhibits the full range of disability from 0 through 4, with a mean of 2.20, which is close to the midpoint of the scale. Thus, there is considerable variability in the cognitive functioning of the care recipients, averaging impairment in the moderate range.

The most common type of deficit is difficulty remembering recent events, rated as present for all but four patients. Almost all care recipients also have trouble recognizing the day of the week (96.4%) and understanding simple instructions (91.5%). At the other extreme, the two impairments least likely to be present are difficulty finding his or her way around the house (59.3%) and trouble speaking sentences (69.3%). It should be noted, however, that even though these are the least common impairments, they are present in the majority of the cases. In general, about 10% of the sample is rated as severely impaired in each of the discrete tasks, although only one in five patients is rated as severely impaired in remembering recent events, and about one-third cannot recall any addresses or the day of the week.

If we were to describe the typical care recipient, then, we would paint two pictures. One type of patient is limited in his or her cognitive abilities, and this deficit is manifest across a broad array of tasks: The individual remains functional, albeit in a restricted manner. The other kind of patient exhibits more pervasively severe impairments. Rather than having moderate difficulty in many activities, this person tends to be completely unable to do most things. Looking ahead, we can anticipate that the second type of patient will remain severely impaired over time, while the first sort, those with less severe impairment, still face the debilitating decline characteristic of degenerative diseases.

Problematic Behavior

A second and somewhat related objective primary stressor of caregiving entails troublesome and disruptive behavior on the part of the patient, and the surveillance, control, and exertion such behaviors require of the caregiver. The vigilance that must be maintained and the "damage control" that must be exercised to ensure that patients harm neither themselves nor others constitute a formidable stressor (Pruchno & Resch, 1989). Moreover, these behaviors serve as a constant and painful reminder of the changed persona of the patient.

In order to measure problematic behavior, we asked,

> In the past week, on how many days did you *personally* have to deal with the following behavior of your (relative)? On how many days did (she/he): keep you up at night; repeat questions/stories; try to dress the wrong way; have a bowel or bladder "accident"; hide belongings and forget about them; cry easily; act depressed or downhearted; cling to you or follow you around; become restless or agitated; become irritable or angry; swear or use foul language; become suspicious, or believe someone is going to harm (him/her); threaten people; [and] show sexual behavior or interests at wrong time/place?

The response categories were *no days* (1), *1 or 2 days* (2), *3 or 4 days* (3), and *5 or more days* (4). This 14-item scale demonstrates strong reliability ($\alpha = .78$).

It must be emphasized that the problematic behavior scale refers to the *caregiver*; specifically, how often he or she had to deal with each of the behaviors, as distinct from how often the dementia patient exhibited these behaviors. This perspective differs from the cognitive impairment measure, which refers only to the capabilities of the patient. Being the one who manages troublesome behavior reflects not only the presence of the behavior, but the extent to which this behavior engages the time, energy, and emotions of the caregiver.

She shadows me.

Our caregivers are generally caught up in the surveillance and control of care recipients' behavior, which may be described as potentially injurious to the care recipient or others; provocative in the sense of evoking irritation, embarrassment, or anger; or just simply troublesome. At the start of the study, almost all of the patients exhibited at least some negative behaviors in interactions with their caregivers. Only 12 caregivers did not have to deal with any of these acts during the week prior to the baseline interview. Given that our list of 14 behaviors is a brief inventory of the ways in which a patient's behavior may deviate from normative adult standards, we may assert confidently that virtually all caregivers have to struggle with the control of behavior that is defined as socially inappropriate.

Rosemary

Rosemary—who possesses a delightful, lighthearted sense of humor—often giggled as she recounted one of the more embarrassing incidents regarding her husband's bizarre behavior:

Two years before he died we were invited to a Christmas party and we went. When we got there, I could see that he'd be totally lost and irresponsible in the cocktail crowd preceding dinner. He began drinking wine and he had no memory of having had a glass of wine so he kept on drinking glass after glass. It was purely a matter of having no realization beyond the present moment. So I persuaded him to sit down at the table and wait.

Laughingly, she continues:

I left him at the table and he proceeded to eat everything in sight, all the salads, drank a lot of wine, and wrecked the whole surrounding area of the table. He filled his wine glass with cranberry sauce and then put wine in his coffee cup, which he later added cream and sugar to and drank. When I came back to the table and saw what he'd done there was nothing I could do. I got the waitress to fix a lot of the damage and I asked everyone around to keep the wine away from him. I was impressed that people were so understanding and cooperative. They were wonderful.

The average number of behaviors reported for the week before the baseline interview is 6.1, or almost half of those about which we specifically inquired. Approximately half of the caregivers experienced two or fewer behaviors on a daily basis, whereas the remainder reported dealing with at least three behaviors more or less all the time.

The most common problems encountered by caregivers are patients who are restless, angry, depressed, clinging, verbally repetitive, or apt to misplace objects. About two out of three caregivers had to deal with these situations during the week prior to the interview. In contrast, only one in ten caregivers confronted inappropriate sexual behavior, and one in five had patients who threatened other people. Overall control of patient behavior, therefore, is a pervasive aspect of the caregiving experience; however, the specific problems confronted are quite varied.

Although the typical caregiver may be caught up with a considerable burden of surveillance and control, these responsibilities are more varied than might have been anticipated on the basis of the patient's level of cognitive impairment. As you may recall, two profiles of impairment were observed: mild to moderate impairment and pervasively severe impairment. The profiles for problematic behavior are less clearly delineated. These problems do not increase as a simple response to the progression of the disease. Instead, the nature and quality of these problems ebbs and flows over time (Haley & Pardo, 1989).

Activities of Daily Living Dependencies and Patient Resistance

Measurement of the third and fourth primary stressors, activities of daily living (ADL) dependencies and patient resistance, share their orientation with the measurement of problematic behavior in the sense that they, too, inquire about the burden encountered by the caregiver, rather than the needs of the patient. The distinction between assistance that is given and that which is required is critical because one adaptation caregivers make to an escalating need for assistance is to involve others in the provision of that assistance—other family members, paid attendants, respite care, and ultimately, nursing home care. Dementia patients require greater assistance as time goes on, but the load carried by the caregiver may not increase: It may decrease or remain stable over time depending on how much of this burden is shared with others. In any event, it cannot be assumed that needed care is the equivalent of provided care, at least that provided by a single family caregiver.

The basic question we asked was, "I'd like to ask you about your (relative's) ability to perform some daily activities. I'm going to read from a list and ask you how much your (relative) depends upon you *personally* for help." The list contained the following 15 items: (1) eating, (2) bathing or showering, (3) going to the bathroom, (4) dressing or undressing, (5) brushing teeth or hair, (6) cooking or preparing food, (7) handling money, (8) getting in or out of bed, (9) walking around the house, (10) driving or taking the bus to where (he/she) needs to go, (11) going for a walk in the neighborhood, (12) taking medications, (13) using the telephone, (14) doing housework like sweeping floors or dusting, and (15) getting going in an activity. Each item was rated from *not at all* (1) to *completely* (4) according to the degree of dependency upon the caregiver. Our composite ADL scale evidences strong reliability ($\alpha = .89$).

At Time 1, the average patient relied upon the caregiver for assistance in 9 to 10 of these 15 ADLs. Almost all patients depended completely on the caregiver for at least one activity (93.7%); on average, this dependence is complete for five to six activities. The tasks for which virtually all caregivers—9 out of 10—provided at least some assistance were meal preparation, financial management, and transportation. Indeed, about three-quarters of the patients relied completely on the caregiver for help with these three activities. About half of the patients were completely dependent upon the caregiver for walks, use of the telephone, housework, and initiating activities; two-thirds were completely dependent with regard to medications. The least-common dependencies were assistance with walking around the house and getting in and out of bed.

These types of limitations, of course, have a prominent place in previous gerontological research, including studies of caregivers. Some of the research suggests that the condition of the patient lacks a strong or consistent relationship to caregiver stress (e.g., George & Gwyther, 1986). The magnitude of the work load by itself may be less important as a source of stress than the degree of resistance encountered from the patient. That is, having to satisfy dependencies may be in itself less difficult than having to satisfy them with a recalcitrant relative. Consequently, we include in our assessment of daily dependencies a single question regarding the patient's overall resistance to help: "When you try to help your (relative) with ([an activity]/these activities), does (he/she) generally make it *very* difficult for you by resisting your help?" If the caregiver responded affirmatively (43.6%), a follow-up question probed for the specific activities that elicited resistance. Patients were most likely to resist with showering or bathing and with dressing or undressing.

In summary, objective stressors refer to tangible conditions and actions. On the one hand, are patient behaviors like the routine communications and transactions of normal adult life that he or she can no longer enact, and inappropriate, troublesome, and sometimes dangerous actions. On the other hand, there is the caregiver's response to the patient's inability to take care of him or herself, including assistance with ADLs and monitoring overt behavior that poses a threat to the patient or others. These stressors are "objective" in the sense that they involve phenomena that may be observed independently of the caregiver's assessment of them.[2]

The relationship of the objective stressors to one another is portrayed in Figure 4.2. This graphic presentation is based upon bivariate correlations among the variables. The shaded portions reflect the extent to which the constructs overlap; operationally, this overlap is R^2, the amount of shared variance expressed as a proportion. As may be seen, the most extensive correspondence occurs for cognitive impairment and ADLs ($r = .62$, $p \leq .001$). Although problematic behavior does not vary systematically with cognitive impairment ($r = .05$, $p > .05$), it tends to co-occur with ADLs to a modest extent ($r = .23$, $p \leq .001$). This pattern is consistent with the natural history of AD in that troublesome behavior does not necessarily increase with illness severity (Haley & Pardo, 1989; Zarit, Todd, & Zarit, 1986).

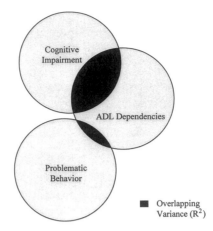

Figure 4.2   Association between objective primary stressors.

The course of the objective stressors over time is displayed in Figure 4.3. The vertical axis represents the average level of impairment or demand; the horizontal axis represents illness duration (i.e., time since symptoms were first recognized).[3]

The most striking feature of these profiles is the similarity in the course of cognitive impairment and ADL dependencies coupled with the distinctly different course of problematic behavior. Confronting troublesome behavior essentially is independent of illness duration: the bivariate correlation of this stressor with onset does not differ from zero. The specific behaviors that emerge may well

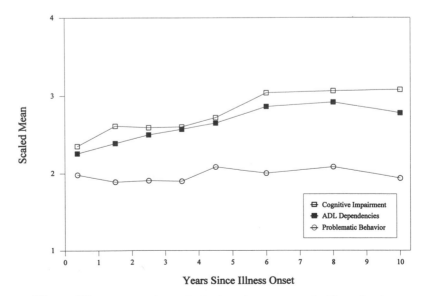

Figure 4.3   Mean magnitude of objective primary stressors by illness duration.

vary over time, but the typical day-to-day burden on the caregiver remains relatively constant over the course of caregiving.

Most of the specific behaviors we examined did *not* vary systematically with illness duration, although some clearly ebbed while others flowed. Troublesome behaviors that appear to increase with time include having bowel or bladder accidents and threatening other people. In contrast, repeating questions and hiding things become less common as the illness progresses. For most behaviors, however, there is a marked lack of time dependency.

The degenerative course of dementia may be seen quite clearly in the cognitive impairment trajectory, a course that generates a similar pattern of ADL dependencies upon the caregiver. The average level of cognitive impairment increases over time, but the rate of cognitive deterioration varies with time. Our measure of cognitive impairment detects the most rapid deterioration during the period of onset and after about 5 years. The apparent plateau after 6 years probably represents a ceiling effect in our instrument (i.e., our instrument may not be able to detect disability progression in the most severe stages of the disease). The course of ADL dependencies parallels that of cognitive impairment, although the trajectory of ADL dependencies suggests a more constant rate of change over time.[4] Thus, increasing cognitive impairment appears to translate rather directly into increasing dependency upon the caregiver.[5]

> Now we're better because he's worse.

Deteriorating cognitive function is an objective indicator of the health status of the patient and the progression of the disease. These conditions generate dependencies and troublesome behaviors that impinge upon the caregiver as he or she goes about the business of supervising, protecting, and nurturing the dementia patient. The primary stressors form the nucleus around which other elements of caregiving stress arise and adhere to one another. The scope and difficulty of caregiving activities also come to symbolize the changes that have begun to predominate the lives of both the dementia patient and the caregiver.

Subjective Reactions to Caregiving

The stressors we have examined thus far are anchored in the patient's cognitive impairment; functional limitations, such as the inability to feed oneself; and actions undertaken by caregivers to assist and monitor the patient. These objective primary stressors describe concrete sets of behavior—patient behavior on the one hand and responsive actions by the caregiver on the other. As imposing as these difficulties may be, they convey only the surface manifestations of caregiving stress. The demands imposed by dementia not only require behavioral responses, but elicit internal cognitive, attitudinal, and emotional responses as well. We classify these responses as primary stressors also as they are located within, and are inseparable from, the domain of caregiving. They are designated as

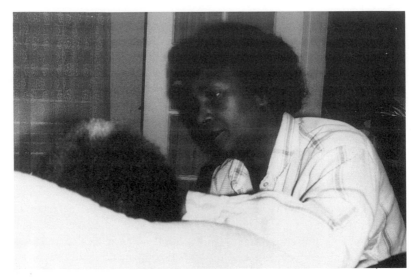

Photograph 1

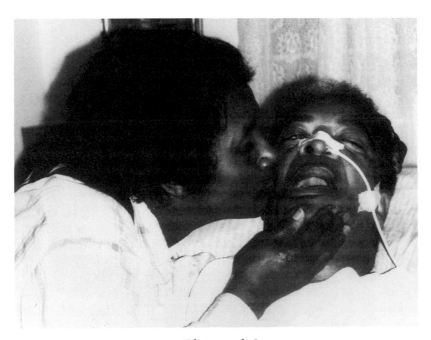

Photograph 2

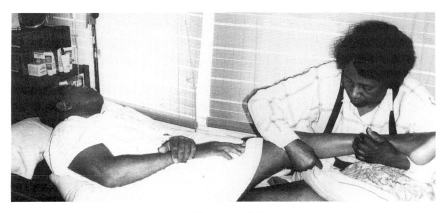

Photograph 3

"subjective" stressors because they refer to the caregiver's internal responses and to the personal meanings evoked by external stimuli. The subjective impact of caregiving is evident in the expressions of this woman as she shaves and turns her husband, actions that require the use of a special harness (see photographs 1–4).

Our indicators of these subjective primary stressors bypass the condition of the patient and inquire directly about the internal responses to hardships experienced by caregivers. It is not possible to enumerate exhaustively all of the potential thoughts and feelings of caregivers as they go about monitoring, feeding, clothing, and cleansing their spouses or parents. Instead, we emphasize a

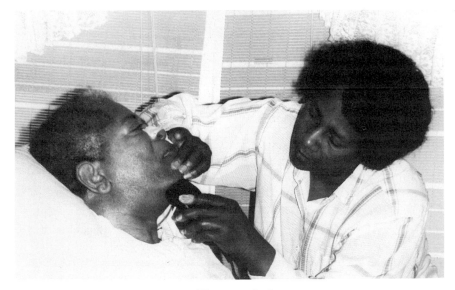

Photograph 4

select set of manifestations that emerged during our preliminary analyses as especially important to understanding the several stages of caregiving and the transitions between these stages: role overload, role captivity, and loss of intimate exchange.

Role Overload

The construct of role overload refers to the internal experience of being overwhelmed by care-related tasks and responsibilities. It differs from the objective stressors discussed previously by addressing not the extent of activities performed by the caregiver, but the feeling that these activities are too much to endure. The items constituting the measure bespeak the level of fatigue felt by caregivers as well as the relentless and uncompromising nature of its source:

> Here are some statements about your energy level and the time it takes to do the things you have to do. How much does each statement describe you?: you are exhausted when you go to bed at night, you have more things to do than you can handle, [and] you don't have time just for yourself?

The response categories ranged from *not at all* (1) to *completely* (4). This three-item scale is a highly reliable ($\alpha = .78$) indicator of the subjective experience of being worn down, worn-out, and overloaded.

Role Captivity

The second internal primary stressor is role captivity: The sense of being an involuntary incumbent of the caregiver role. This feeling of being trapped exists when a person feels compelled to be and to do one thing, while preferring something else. Role captivity refers less to the demanding responsibilities associated with care, which are captured by role overload, and more to the fact that these responsibilities are experienced as obligatory. The distinguishing characteristic of role captivity, therefore, is not that the role is difficult or stressful, but that the role is unwanted (Aneshensel et al., 1993; Pearlin, 1983; Pearlin & Turner, 1987).

Role captivity refers to the tension between what one must be and do and what one wants to be and do. We assessed this construct with a three-item scale ($\alpha = .83$), which asked caregivers how well the following statements describe their feelings and thoughts about being a caregiver: "wish you were free to lead a life of your own, feel trapped by your (relative's) illness, [and] wish you could just run away." Ratings were made on a 4-point scale that ranged from *not at all* (1) to *very much* (4).

Loss of Intimate Exchange

AD and other dementias are not merely debilitating, they erode the very essence of the afflicted individual. They destroy memories of the lifetime that make each person unique and alter personality until an individual cannot be recognized as the person they once were. The transformation of these fundamental elements of personhood unavoidably shatters the very foundation of the caregiver–patient relationship because one of the role partners has become someone else. In essence, as the impairment progresses, caregivers often come to feel increasingly separated from those parts of their affective lives that had been shared with the care recipients.

> But Father doesn't become a stranger. He becomes a nobody.

The items that measure the third subjective primary stressor emphasize the sense of having already lost closeness and intimacy because of the patient's cognitive decline:

> Caregivers sometimes feel that they lose important things in life because of their relative's illness. To what extent do you feel that you personally have lost the following? How much have you lost: being able to confide in your (relative), the person that you used to know, [and] having someone who really knew you well?

Responses were rated on a 4-point scale with *completely* (1) on one end and *not at all* (4) on the other. The scale is quite reliable ($\alpha = .76$).

The measures of the subjective stressors are modestly associated with one another, with an average correlation of .25 (minimum .22, maximum .30). Thus, they tap largely separate aspects of the domain of subjective primary stressors.

In sum, the three subjective primary stressors differ qualitatively from one another. Role overload quite clearly taps the *presence* of an undesirable state, an excess of demands, whereas loss of intimate exchange refers to the *absence* of a desirable state, the positive aspects of the predementia relationship with the patient. Role captivity bridges these cross-pressures, reflecting both the presence of unwanted activities and the absence of sought-after conditions.

The Link between Objective and Subjective Primary Stressors

The subjective experience of care-related stress emanates from the objective demands of caregiving, but is distinct from these demands. The connection between these two domains is manifest as two canonical correlations between the objective and subjective stressors that are significantly different from zero ($F = 7.90$, $df = 6$, $p \le .001$). The second correlation is independent of the first, meaning that there are two separate and unique links among these dimensions of care-related stress, as illustrated in Figure 4.4.

A word of explanation about canonical correlations is in order. As described briefly in chapter 3, canonical variables are linear combinations of the measures within each of two domains; in our study, objective versus subjective primary stressors. The relative contribution of each measure to its canonical variable is expressed as a standardized weight. These weights maximize the correlation between the two domains (i.e., the canonical correlation). Each canonical correlation reflects an independent link between the two conceptual domains.

In Figure 4.4, each circle represents a distinct conceptual domain that is

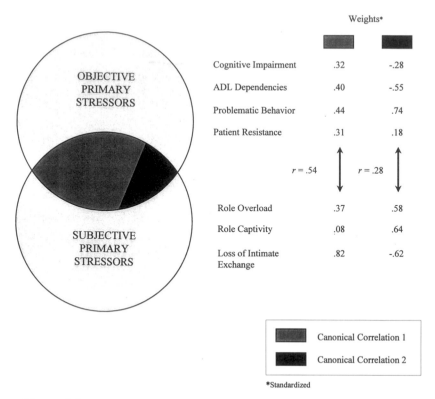

Weights*

Cognitive Impairment	.32	-.28
ADL Dependencies	.40	-.55
Problematic Behavior	.44	.74
Patient Resistance	.31	.18

$r = .54$ $r = .28$

Role Overload	.37	.58
Role Captivity	.08	.64
Loss of Intimate Exchange	.82	-.62

	Canonical Correlation 1
	Canonical Correlation 2

*Standardized

Figure 4.4   Canonical correlation among objective and subjective primary stressors.

operationalized by the measures listed to the right. The extent to which these conceptual domains coincide with one another is depicted as an area of shaded overlap between the circles. This shared variance is partitioned into components representing separate canonical correlations; in this case, two distinct correlations. The correlations are differentiated from one another by the gradation of shading within the area of overlap. The value of each canonical correlation is given to the right.

The first canonical correlation indicates that increasing impairment and assistance are manifest most in feelings of having lost one's intimate relationship with one's parent or spouse. The correlation between the first two canonical variables is quite strong ($r = .54$), reflecting substantial overlap between the objective and subjective stressors. As illustrated in Figure 4.4, all of the objective stressors contribute at least moderately to the first canonical variable. For the subjective stressors, however, loss of intimate exchange is a substantially more important component than the other two stressors.

The second canonical correlation suggests that feelings of being overwhelmed by and trapped within the caregiver role are likely to accompany troublesome behaviors, especially among patients who are comparatively unimpaired and who require relatively little assistance from the caregiver. The second canonical correlation reflects a much weaker link than the first ($r = .28$). Although three of four variables contribute at least moderately to the second objective canonical variable, these loadings are of differing signs. Patients who are high on all objective stressors, therefore, would score low on this canonical variable, whereas those who exhibit behavioral problems in the absence of impairment would attain high scores. Role overload and role captivity make moderate positive contributions to the second canonical variable; loss of intimacy has a negative loading.

In sum, all four dimensions of objective stress—cognitive impairment, ADL dependencies, problematic behavior, and patient resistance—contribute to loss of intimate exchange, but problematic patient behavior appears to be especially important to feelings of role overload and role captivity.

In conclusion, primary stressors are conceptualized as emanating from the demands associated with providing care to a spouse or parent suffering from dementia. The nucleus of this constellation of stressors is the condition of the patient, which imposes demands on the caregiver to assist the patient and to monitor his or her behavior. These tasks, in turn, generate experiences of being overwhelmed, of being prevented from pursuing preferred life goals, and of having lost intimacy with the person for whom care is being provided. The conditions of care have the greatest impact on this last element, the sense that one's husband, wife, mother, or father has become a stranger. Thus, it is not simply the case that providing care is burdensome. Instead, the specific configuration of hardships encountered by caregivers corresponds to distinct subjective strains.

The Creation of Secondary Stressors

Thus far, the stressors we have considered are located within the enterprise of caregiving itself: the need for care arising from the cognitive deterioration of the dementia patient, the behavioral responses of the caregiver to assisting and monitoring the patient, and the subjective meaning of these circumstances to the caregiver's life. These stressors are common experiences for caregivers, and these shared circumstances define the caregiving career. The demands associated with providing care and the constraints imposed upon other activities separate the day-to-day life of caregivers from the routines of those not caught up in caregiving. At the same time, however, many caregivers continue to be engaged in aspects of adult life that are not specific to caregiving, and it is to these involvements that we now turn in considering secondary sources of care-related stress.

The participation of caregivers in activities unrelated to care represents aspects of social, economic, and personal life that caregivers share in common with other adults, that is, with adults who are *not* caregivers. Of course, caregivers differ from one another in their engagement in noncare activities. This involvement depends, in part, upon the extent to which care-related responsibilities make other activities too difficult to pursue. Some caregivers, for example, are so overwhelmed that their lives come to revolve almost exclusively around the provision of care. Participation differs according to social and economic circumstances as well. For instance, access to various resources alleviates some caregiver burdens, thereby facilitating engagement in extracare activities. Moreover, involvement in noncare activities is differentiated by characteristics like generation and gender. For example, adult children are more likely than spousal caregivers to be employed.

Although caregivers share various forms of social and economic participation with persons who are not caregivers, their experiences within these other social roles is shaped at least partially by their roles as caregivers. Employed caregivers, for example, frequently find their work interrupted by care-related crises, which, in turn, generate a type of on-the-job stress not encountered by those who are free of the caretaking responsibilities. The extent to which caregiving intrudes into noncare elements of life, therefore, is a form of stress unique to caregiving. We label these stressors as *secondary* to emphasize that they are not caused directly by caregiving, but arise as consequences thereof.

> When she started to get ill, I didn't even know how to run the washing machine.

Expanding our view of the domains of caregiver stressors to include secondary as well as primary stressors is critical to understanding why caregiving is more damaging to some caregivers than others. Previous research indicates that caregiving and some of its burdens elevate the risk of emotional distress (Baumgarten, 1989; Schulz et al., 1990; Wright et al., 1993). Yet many caregivers, including many whose care-related burdens are heavy, do not manifest exceptionally high levels of distress. Conversely, some caregivers who have comparatively light caregiving burdens are exceedingly distressed.

One potential explanation for this variation is that some caregivers have ready access to resources that alleviate the adverse consequences of caregiving, resources such as economic means, social support, and personal attributes. For example, a caregiver may be relatively unscathed because he or she is able to pay for an attendant; kin participate in the care and management of the patient; or the caregiver possesses inner resolve and fortitude, or an effective coping repertoire.

Explanations relying upon the dynamics of differential *vulnerability* to stress are misguided, however, if variation in the outcome is instead a result of differential *exposure* to secondary stressors. Caregivers who appear to be excessively affected by the demands of care may not be unresourceful copers, for example; instead, they may have been exposed to an exceptional array of secondary stressors. We run the risk of mistakenly attributing the effects of differential exposure to the effects of vulnerability if we fail to account for the full range of adverse circumstances impinging upon caregivers *because* they are caregivers.

It should be emphasized that secondary stressors are not "secondary" in terms of their potency. Once established, secondary stressors are every bit as powerful as those that are primary in the sense of emanating directly from the demands of care. Indeed, as we shall later show, secondary stressors often serve as the conduit through which primary stressors come to damage emotional well-being.

The Encroachment of Care-Related Stress into Other Social Roles

It is not possible to enumerate exhaustively all of the potential problems that might be encountered by caregivers, especially difficulties that are affected by caregiving, but do not directly entail the provision of care. The universe of such problems is infinite in its permutations. Consequently, it is necessary to sample from this universe, to select those elements that seem particularly important to understanding how caregiving permeates social and economic life. Our approach is to emphasize key aspects of everyday life: family relations, work, and finances.

Family Conflict

The degenerative course of dementia coupled with escalating care-related responsibilities inevitably alters not only the relationship between the provider and the recipient of care, but also the relationships that these two individuals have with other family members. These transformations occur within the context of relationships and modes of interaction that had been established long before the onset of dementia and the initiation of caregiving. Family members must adapt to the new persona and behaviors of the dementia patient under the backdrop of the family's history and the biographies of its members. The magnitude of the resultant reorganization might be equated with that of a significant earthquake: The upheaval may leave the structure, organization, and functioning of the family in disarray and disequilibrium.

Three dimensions of family conflict were identified in our qualitative interviews and developed into a composite measure for use in the analyses of the large-scale survey. One type of conflict between caregivers and other family members arises out of disagreements about the extent of patient impairment: beliefs about the disability of the patient, its seriousness, and the appropriate strategies for dealing with it. A second conflict, also between the caregiver and other relatives of the disabled person, concerns whether other family members pay adequate attention to the patient. The third dimension of dissension concerns the attention and acknowledgment accorded the caregiver for the assistance he or she gives to the impaired relative.

He has the ability to cover up his disease so the family doesn't know how bad it is.

The core question asked about friction over the severity of the patient's condition was as follows:

Family members don't always see eye-to-eye when it comes to their relative who is ill. How much disagreement have you had with anyone in your family concerning any of the following issues? The specific items are as follows: the seriousness of your (relative's) memory problem, the need to watch out for your (relative's) safety, what things your (relative) is able to do for (him/herself) [and] whether your (relative) should be placed in a nursing home.

The second dimension of conflict, the involvement of other family members with the dementia patient, was ascertained by posing this question:

Family members may differ among themselves in the way they deal with a relative who is ill. Thinking of all your relatives, how much disagreement have you had with anyone in your family because of the following issues? How much disagreement have you had with anyone in your family because they: don't spend enough time with your (relative), don't do their share in caring for your (relative), don't show enough respect for your (relative), [and] lack patience with your (relative)?

Friction over others' treatment of the caregiver, the third kind of family conflict, was elicited by asking,

I've just asked you how your relatives act toward your (relative). Now I'd like to ask how they act toward you, the caregiver. Again, thinking of all your relatives, how much disagreement have you had with anyone in your family because of the following issues? How much disagreement have you had with anyone in your family because they: don't visit or telephone you enough, don't give you enough help, don't show enough appreciation for your work as a caregiver, [and] give you unwanted advice?

Response categories for all of the family conflict items ranged from *no disagreement* (1) to *quite a bit* (4). Although these are three distinct dimensions of family conflict, they are strongly correlated with one another (average $r = .59$), meaning that the common thread uniting these discrete elements is substantial relative to the unique aspects of each element. Our focus is on the global aspects of care-related stress, rather than the particularistic dynamics of family relations. Consequently, we employ the composite measure instead of its subscales ($\alpha = .90$).

Conflict among caregivers and other family members is less common than we had anticipated given the ubiquitously difficult circumstances confronted by these persons. The modal response category for each of these items was the low endpoint, *no disagreement*, which was selected by two-thirds to three-quarters of the caregivers for each item. This pattern was consistent across the three dimensions of conflict: the seriousness of the illness, the treatment of the patient, and the treatment of the caregiver. Indeed, one-third of the caregivers reported no conflict on *any* of the specific areas of disagreement.

On the other hand, some families are beset by pervasive and serious conflict. Approximately one-quarter of the caregivers reported *quite a bit* of disagreement, the high endpoint, for at least one item. Serious discord was found along all three dimensions: approximately 15% of the caregivers selected the most extreme response category for one or more indicators of dissension. When the entire set of items is considered in total, one in four caregivers reported at least one area of intense strife.

Work Conflict

The indirect effects of caregiving are not confined to family life, they intrude upon roles external to the family as well. Although caregiving is a full-time occupation for many, other caregivers, especially adult children, also work outside of the home. Time spent at work is time away from caregiving, which may either be beneficial or detrimental to the caregiver (Scharlach & Boyd, 1989; Stoller, 1989). Moen, Robison, and Fields (1994) found that working does not detract from women's caregiving responsibilities: Women add on new roles, rather than replace or alter old ones.

The positive potential of employment for caregivers resembles the benefits women may accrue from working outside of the home in contrast to being exclusively homemakers. Work provides an escape from the immediate care situation, which often entails unpleasant, repetitive, and boring tasks that are not highly esteemed. Paid employment differs from caregiving precisely because it is paid, an indicator of its social evaluation. In addition, the income derived from working may alleviate some of the financial burdens associated with caregiving. Employment also provides the opportunity for normal social exchanges with friends and peers, interaction that is often in short supply in the lives of caregivers.

On the other hand, employment entails labor: more tasks to be performed, more hours to be active, and more demands heaped upon an already full plate. In addition to sheer overload, work and caregiving may come into direct conflict. While at work, caregivers worry about the well-being of their relatives; conversely, work-related pressures sometimes interfere with the provision of care at home. Again, this situation is akin to the competing demands of being a homemaker, especially a mother, and having paid employment outside of the home.

The balance between the costs and benefits of employment varies across work and caregiving contexts. Employment is not inherently positive or negative for caregivers; instead, its impact depends upon the conditions encountered at work and how these conditions intersect with caregiving. Thus, it is important to consider not only whether or not the caregiver is employed, but if he or she is employed, the extent to which work and caregiving complement or collide with one another.

Approximately a third of the caregivers in this study were working at the start of the study. Of the 370 caregivers who were *not* working, 53.5% describe themselves as retired and another 39.2% say they are homemakers. These two categories account for 61.8% of all caregivers. Only 27 persons described themselves as unemployed or otherwise occupied.

About a quarter of the sample reported having changed their work situation *because* of their relative's memory problem ($n = 134$). Some of these individuals, however, did not experience a net change; they exchanged one situation for a roughly comparable one (14.2%). Other caregivers decreased their work involvement in one way or another: Some reduced the hours they worked from full- to part-time (12.7%); others stopped working full-time (46.3%) or part-time jobs (16.4%). Increasing work involvement was relatively uncommon (10.4%). In all, almost one in five caregivers reduced or eliminated their previous level of employment specifically to accommodate caregiving ($n = 101$).

Among employed caregivers, we measured *work strain*, or job–caregiving conflict, with a five-item scale ($\alpha = .75$):

> From your own personal experience, how much do you agree or disagree with the following statements about your present work situation? In the last 2 months or so: you have had less energy for your work; you have missed too many days, you've been dissatisfied with the quality of your work; you worry about your (relative) while you're at work, [and] phone calls about or from your (relative) interrupt you at work.

The response categories ranged from *strongly disagree* (1) to *strongly agree* (4). The emphasis of this measure, therefore, is upon the negative impact of caregiving on work performance, especially cross-pressures from these two domains.

The level of hardship reported for work appears greater than that reported for family relations. Two items were endorsed by about half of the employed caregivers: insufficient energy and worry about the patient. The remaining three items were reported by about one in four or five workers. Four in five working caregivers (79.3%) reported the presence of at least one difficulty at work, compared to the presence of family conflict for two out of three caregivers. However, only one-third of the employed caregivers rated any serious difficulty at work. The mean value of the work strain scale, which has a range of 1 to 4, is only 2.15; the semiquartile range is 1.6 through 2.6. Thus the distribution of caregivers on this measure is skewed towards the low end. Although some caregivers experience very high levels of work-related strain, most experience less intense problems. These difficulties, nonetheless, appear to be somewhat more common than those incurred within the family.

In sum, a substantial minority of caregivers are working outside the home. About a third of those who are working experience intense work-related problems. In addition, many have changed their work life to accommodate caregiving, usually reducing their work involvement.

Financial Strain

Caregiving may also impose formidable strain on family finances because of the expenditures of providing care and decreased earnings. These losses are assessed by three indicators. First are reductions in total household income over time, an objective measure of tightening finances.[6] Second are increases in expenditures related to the care and treatment of the patient:

> These questions ask about your household expenses and your standard of living. Think back over your financial situation as it was *just before* you began to take care of your (relative). Compared to that time, how would you describe your monthly expenses? Are they: *much less now* (5), *somewhat less now* (4), *about the same* (3), *somewhat more now* (2), or *much more now* (1)?[7]

Third, we asked whether there is enough money to make ends meet month-to-month: "In general how do your family finances work out at the end of the month? Do you usually have: *some money left over* (1), *just enough to make ends*

Table 4.1   Mean Income by Financial Strain

Financial strain	N	%	Income (thousands)
Relative expenses			
Less or much less	63	11.5	$27.18**
About the same	189	34.5	38.10
Somewhat or much more	296	54.0	35.59
Monthly budget			
Some money left over	299	54.9	41.67***
Just enough	188	34.5	26.62
Not enough	58	10.6	22.40

*p < .05.   **p ≤ .01.   ***p ≤ .001.

meet (2), or *not enough to make ends meet* (3)?" The distribution of responses to these questions and the average level of income for each level of financial strain is shown in Table 4.1.

In general, the caregivers in this study are experiencing some financial burden, but extreme financial duress is found only in a selectively small subgroup. As may be seen in Table 4.1, the majority of caregivers reported that their monthly expenses have increased since they began providing care. Only about 1 in 10 decreased in expenses; these individuals have by far the lowest annual family income. It may be that low income[8] necessitates a reduction in other expenses to accommodate care-related expenditures, or that expenses that would have been incurred by the patient are foregone in the face of strong economic constraints. Most caregivers also reported that they have some money left over at the end of the month. Only about 1 in 10 reported not having enough money to make ends meet on a month-to-month basis. Also, family income is substantially lower among those with a monthly shortfall than those who are breaking even or enjoying a surplus.

I'm frugal.

In sum, roughly a quarter to a third of the sample experiences at least one source of financial stress. One in four has run out of money, had sharply increased expenses, or experienced both of these conditions. When low income is added to the picture, this group expands to one in three caregivers. In general, then, the majority of the sample has sufficient financial resources or better, but a substantial minority are in precarious financial straits.

The Independence of Secondary Role Strains

The three domains of secondary stress—family, work, and finances—appear to exist rather independently of one another. The indicators of strain for them have only modest levels of bivariate association with one another. The multivariate links among the three were assessed by way of canonical correlation analysis for pairs of domains (e.g., financial- and work-related strains). The results demonstrate that stressors tend to covary across family, work, and economic life, but not in an especially powerful manner.

The single canonical correlation between family conflict and work-related stress is of modest magnitude ($r = .23$, $p \leq .001$), with a substantial positive loading for work strain and a substantial negative loading for not working. That is, family conflict is elevated in conjunction with problems at work and is somewhat lower among those who are not working. The canonical correlation between family conflict and financial strain also is of modest magnitude ($r = .17$, $p \leq .001$). Family conflict coincides somewhat with having trouble meeting monthly expenses, but is relatively distinct from increases in these expenses.

Work and financial strains are linked by two canonical correlations ($F = 5.29$, $df = 2$, $p \leq .01$). The first canonical correlation ($r = .21$) links insufficient financial resources to strain among those who are working and to a reduction in employment due to caregiving. The second canonical correlation ($r = .14$) links *decreased* expenses with reduced hours at work or decreased work strain.

Thus, family, work, and finances emerge as distinctive sources of stress for caregivers. When things go poorly in one area of life, things tend to go poorly in other areas as well. Such overlap is to be expected, of course, because caregivers' lives are not compartmentalized into the crisp conceptual categories used in theory and research. Nonetheless, the magnitude of these connections among domains is rather modest. Consequently, work, finances, and family life stand on their own as quasi-independent sources of caregiver stress.

The Link between Primary Stressors and Secondary Role Strains

The preceding findings suggest that the demands of caregiving are manifest as discrete sets of consequences. That is, the secondary role strains stand as independent entities, representing alternative responses to the demands of care. Two patterns of response may be anticipated. First, the *same* primary stressors may produce financial strain for some caregivers, family conflict for other caregivers, and work-related strain for still others. Second, the *various* primary stressors may have quite unique effects, generating specific types of secondary stressors. For example, problematic patient behavior may tend to cause conflict in some families rather than financial strain.

In the following chapter, we trace the linkages between primary and secondary stressors over time. Here we assess the correlations between secondary role strains and primary stressors with baseline measures. The seven primary stressors considered are cognitive impairment, problematic behavior, ADL dependencies, patient resistance, role overload, role captivity, and loss of intimate exchange. The six secondary stressors are family conflict, work strain, unemployment,[9] reduction in work commitment, increased expenses, and lack of enough money to

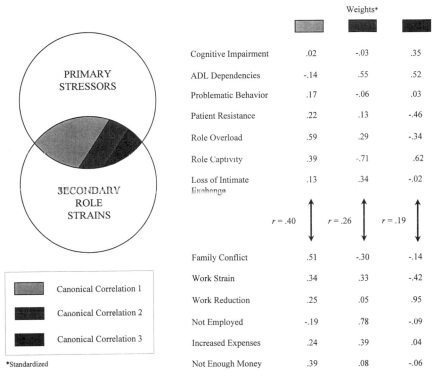

Figure 4.5   Canonical correlation among primary stressors and secondary role strains.

meet monthly expenses. The method of analysis, once again, is canonical correlations because we wish to capture the multiple dimensions inherent in each of these conceptual domains.

Three of the six possible canonical correlations attain statistical significance ($F = 1.58$, df 20, $p \leq .05$). As shown in Figure 4.5, the correlation among the first canonical variables is .40; this value is .26 for the second canonical variables and .19 for the third. Thus, the first linear combination of primary stressors accounts for 16.3% of the variance in the first linear combination of secondary role strains. The amount of shared variance drops off substantially for the second and third sets of linear combinations, being 6.7 and 3.5% respectively. As such, the primary stressors are linked to the secondary role strains along three dimensions; collectively, these links are modest in magnitude, with the first set of associations being substantially stronger than the others.

The first dimension captures, by and large, a diffuse and pervasive association among the two types of stressors. Role overload and family conflict make the strongest contributions to the first canonical variables, representing primary stressors and secondary role strains, respectively. Among the primary stressors, role captivity also makes a moderate contribution to the first canonical variable;

modest contributions are made by problematic behavior and resistance as well. Among the secondary role strains, experiencing care-related strain at work and having insufficient economic resources contribute moderately to the first variable; reducing one's work commitment and increasing expenses additionally make modest contributions.

In contrast, the second and third canonical correlations represent rather specific points of intersection between primary stressors and secondary role strains. Being out of the workforce and not feeling trapped by caregiving make the strongest contributions to the second canonical variables. ADL dependencies also contribute to this variable, essentially linking the actual work of caregiving to not working outside of the home. Thus, not working outside of the home is associated with providing extensive help to the patient, especially when the patient's impairment and need for care is *not* accompanied by a sense of role captivity.

The third canonical variable relates ADL dependencies and role captivity on the one hand to work reduction on the other hand. The third correlation, then, is somewhat similar in substantive meaning to the second correlation. Severe patient impairment and a heavy burden of care are associated with a reduction in work outside of the home, and this reduction is likely to be accompanied by feelings of being trapped by one's care responsibilities.

The pivotal distinction among the three canonical correlations revolves around role captivity. On one side of the coin, caregivers who experience conflict between work and care demands are likely to feel they are captives of caregiving. On the other side of the coin, caregivers who are not working tend to provide substantial care to their severely impaired patients, but do not feel particularly involuntarily constrained by their responsibilities unless they have left the labor force as a direct consequence of caregiving. In essence, then, care-related obligations appear to hinder caregivers least when they do not conflict with work roles or when the caregiver is voluntarily not working outside of the home.

These associations reflect the interplay between the conditions of providing care and the contextual circumstances of caregivers' lives. High levels of primary stressors are not uniformly accompanied by high levels of secondary stressors, although this tendency certainly exists in some cases. Once this pervasive relationship is taken into account, the burdens of providing care are associated selectively with secondary role strains.

The Care-Related Erosion of Self-Concept

The underlying premise of our conceptual scheme is that stressors tend to beget other stressors. As with role strains, the stressors we will be discussing in this section, *intrapsychic strains*, are identified as "secondary" because they are by-products of the ongoing conditions encountered in providing care. Intrapsychic strains, for the most part, involve dimensions of self-concept. Although role strains focus upon external conditions, like the quality of the caregiver's involvement with various social actors and institutions, intrapsychic strains pertain to internal states.

Conditions of enduring hardships tend to damage self-concepts, and when this happens, people are likely to suffer emotional distress (Pearlin et al., 1981). Caregiving to chronically disabled relatives illustrates this scenario. The relentless and expanding demands of caregiving, coupled with ensuing role strains, are capable of diminishing positive elements of "self"; in turn, people are left increasingly vulnerable to stressful outcomes (i.e., intrapsychic strains).

Self-concepts are formed early in life and molded by ensuing experiences throughout the entire life course, including the experiences of caregiving. Chapter 7, which deals with stress mediators, considers the impact of caregiving on global elements of self-concept. Here we focus on elements of self that are anchored directly in the caregiving situation, the measurement of which reflects this context: loss of self, lack of caregiving competence, and absence of care-related gains.

Loss of Self

Self-concept is a social phenomena, shaped by the nature and quality of social exchange with those individuals who figure prominently in one's life. Mothers, fathers, husbands, and wives certainly fall within the inner circle of relationships contributing to self-definition. As we described earlier, the degenerative course of dementia erodes personality, altering the persona of one of the two individuals involved in the husband–wife or parent–child relationship. To the extent that the identity and life of the caregiver has been closely bound to that of the patient, the caregiver may experience a loss of his or her own identity as the patient's persona becomes fragmented and blurred. This loss of self is exacerbated when caregiving comes to exclude other activities and roles in which the caregiver previously found self-validation (Skaff & Pearlin, 1992).

Self-loss is measured by a simple two-item scale: "How much have you lost: a sense of who you are [and] an important part of yourself?" Each item was rated from *not at all* (1) to *completely* (4). The items are highly correlated ($r = .76$). This measure is isomorphic to the loss of intimate exchange measure that was described previously as a subjective primary stressor.

Lack of Caregiver Competence

We also asked caregivers to evaluate how they viewed themselves as caregivers. For most individuals, caregiving constitutes a new social role, one not previously occupied, at least not with regard to another adult. Identification with the role often coincides with role incumbency and with the development of self-evaluation of how well one performs the role.

We measured self-appraised competence by asking,

Here are some thoughts and feelings that people sometimes have about themselves as caregivers. How much does each statement describe your thoughts about your caregiving? How much do you: believe that you've learned how to deal with a very difficult situation [and] feel that all in all, you're a good caregiver?

The response categories for these items ranged from *not at all* (1) to *very much* (4). We then asked,

> Think now of all the things we've been talking about: the daily ups and downs that you face as a caregiver; the job you are doing; and the ways you deal with the difficulties. Putting all these things together: How ———— do you feel?: competent, self-confident? How much do you believe that you've learned how to deal with a difficult situation [and] feel that all in all, you're a good caregiver?

Each of these items was rated from *not at all* (1) to *very* (4). This four-item scale is quite reliable ($\alpha = .74$). Of course, a sense of competency is not considered stressful; instead, it is the *lack* of this positive self-regard that is troublesome.

Absence of Caregiving Gains

Many caregivers feel that caregiving, difficult though it is for them, has contributed positive elements to their lives, especially self-enrichment and personal growth. To assess whether the caregiver's self-concept has expanded in this manner, we asked,

> Sometimes people can also learn things about themselves from taking care of a close relative. What about you? How much have you: become more aware of your inner strengths, become more self-confident, grown as a person, [and] learned to do things you didn't do before?

The response categories ranged from *not at all* (1) to *very much* (4) ($\alpha = .76$). Again, as is the case with caregiving competence, it is the *lack* of this sentiment that is considered stressful.

The Convergence of Intrapsychic Strains

Most caregivers appear to retain a clear sense of personal identity over the course of caregiving: About one in three did not report *any* loss of self and less than 10% reported the *complete* loss of important components of identity. Actually, many caregivers reported positive changes in their self-concepts as a consequence of caregiving. Most notably, caregivers felt they had become more aware of inner strengths: greater than half (56.8%) gave this item the strongest endorsement, whereas less than 1 in 10 (8.1%) did not feel this way at all. Most caregivers also reported at least some increase in self-confidence, personal growth, and skill enhancement.

In general, then, caregivers are more likely to report positive than negative changes in self-concept as a result of caregiving. Nonetheless, a subgroup of caregivers experienced marked diminishment of personal identity. It must be emphasized that these two components of self—losses and gains—are distinct reactions to caregiving, not opposite ends of a single continuum. They are virtually independent of one another ($r = .005$, $p \geq .90$). Thus, a caregiver may experience both losses *and* gains at the same time.

I feel I've become much stronger as
a person in coping with problems.

The two components are associated with self-perceptions of competence in providing care, albeit in opposite directions. Gains in self-concept tend to accompany a sense of having done a good job in certain aspects of caregiving ($r = .32$, $p \le .001$). Those caregivers experiencing a loss of identity, in contrast, also are likely to feel unable to deal with difficult situations, that they are not good caregivers, and that they are neither competent nor self-confident as caregivers ($r = -.13$, $p \le .005$).

Self-perceptions of how well one does the job of caregiver, therefore, are somewhat more strongly associated with increments in self-concept than with the erosion of identity. Also, because the caregivers are, for the most part, veterans of several years service, they tend to be self-confident in their ability to do what must be done. In sum, then, although the typical caregiver appears to withstand threats to self-concept, others, nonetheless, feel diminished by their caregiving experience.

The Link between Primary Stressors and Secondary Intrapsychic Strains

The self-perceptions of caregivers regarding the personal impact of caregiving are strongly associated with their actual experiences in providing care. Two of the three canonical correlations between the seven primary stressors and three intrapsychic strains are statistically significant ($F = 6.02$, $df = 12$, $p \le .001$). These two intersections are illustrated in Figure 4.6.

The first set of canonical variables yields a rather strong correlation ($r = .55$), with approximately 30% overlap between the components of primary stressors and intrapsychic strains. Among the primary stressors, the first canonical combination is defined less by the objective demands of caregiving than by the subjective responses to these demands. Loss of intimate exchange with the dementia patient is the strongest contributor. Among the intrapsychic strains, only one variable figures in this first link: loss of self (i.e., the erosion of personal identity). Thus, caregivers who feel overwhelmed and constrained by the tasks they perform are likely to feel that they have lost touch with themselves, especially if they also feel bereft of the intimacy they previously shared with their spouses or parents.

The second set of canonical variables yields a somewhat smaller, but nonetheless moderate association ($r = .33$) between the demands of caregiving and self-perceptions as a caregiver. Here, the influence of objective conditions is more evident. Both cognitive impairment and ADL dependencies contribute importantly to the second canonical variable. Role captivity also adds to this variable, but its sign is negative. Caregiver competence and, to a lesser extent, self-gains contribute to the intrapsychic side of this picture. Thus, those who are providing substantial assistance to severely impaired relatives are likely to feel positively

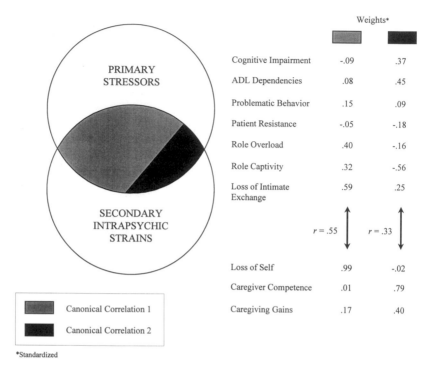

	Weights*	
Cognitive Impairment	-.09	.37
ADL Dependencies	.08	.45
Problematic Behavior	.15	.09
Patient Resistance	-.05	-.18
Role Overload	.40	-.16
Role Captivity	.32	-.56
Loss of Intimate Exchange	.59	.25
	$r = .55$ $r = .33$	
Loss of Self	.99	-.02
Caregiver Competence	.01	.79
Caregiving Gains	.17	.40

PRIMARY STRESSORS

SECONDARY INTRAPSYCHIC STRAINS

Canonical Correlation 1

Canonical Correlation 2

*Standardized

Figure 4.6   Canonical correlation among primary stressors and intrapsychic strains.

about the jobs they have done as caregivers and to enjoy a sense of personal growth, especially if they do not feel trapped by caregiving. Alternately stated, those who feel involuntarily constrained by few demands from comparatively unimpaired relatives generally do not feel good about themselves as caregivers and do not accrue a sense of personal growth from performing this role.

In sum, both the objective demands of care and the subjective responses of caregivers to these demands contribute to caregivers' perceptions of themselves. Those with the most exacting situations are also likely to feel most competent in their role performance. Those with negative subjective reactions to the demands, however, are likely to feel a diminishment of self. Intrapsychic strains do not arise as a blanket response to caregiving; rather, they are specific reactions to the precise array of care-related stressors that impinge upon the caregiver.

The Link between Secondary Role Strains and Intrapsychic Strains

The way in which caregivers see themselves as caregivers is linked not only to the primary stressors associated with caregiving, but to secondary role strains as well. Figure 4.7 illustrates that two of the three canonical correlations between

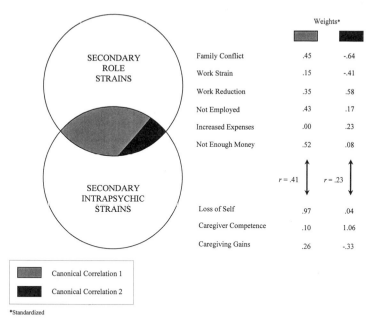

		Weights*
		▢ ■
Family Conflict	.45	-.64
Work Strain	.15	-.41
Work Reduction	.35	.58
Not Employed	.43	.17
Increased Expenses	.00	.23
Not Enough Money	.52	.08
	$r = .41$	$r = .23$
Loss of Self	.97	.04
Caregiver Competence	.10	1.06
Caregiving Gains	.26	-.33

▢ Canonical Correlation 1

■ Canonical Correlation 2

*Standardized

Figure 4.7   Canonical correlation among secondary role strains and intrapsychic strains.

the two sets of secondary stressors are statistically significant ($F = 3.40$, $df = 10$, $p \leq .001$).

The first canonical variables link aspects of family conflict, employment status, work-related stress, and economic strain to loss of self. Among the secondary role strains, the strongest contributor to this first intersection is having insufficient funds to pay monthly expenses. Intense conflict with family members and being out of the labor force also add moderately to the first canonical variable; reducing work commitments makes a somewhat smaller contribution. These role strains are most closely associated with a loss of personal identity; the other two intrapsychic strains make virtually no contribution to this linkage with role strains. The first correlation is of moderate strength ($r = .41$).

The second canonical correlation is substantially smaller in magnitude ($r = .23$). Several of the role strains that added to the first canonical variable also play a part in the second, but the configurations in the second are distinctive. Reducing one's labor force participation loads positively on this variable, whereas family conflict and work-related strain have negative loadings. On the other side, caregiver competence is the prime contributor to the second link between the secondary stressors. Caregivers tend to feel good about themselves as caregivers when they are getting along with other family members and when they are either not working or experiencing little on-the-job stress. Alternately stated, caregivers who encounter conflict with others in the family and problems at work tend to view themselves as not doing a particularly good job at caregiving.

In sum, the two sets of secondary stressors exhibit two separate links to one another. The first link is forged by a pervasive set of role strains that is manifest as a diminishment of personal identity. The second link represents the context of feeling good about oneself as a caregiver, a sentiment that is accompanied by little conflict in other social roles, especially family and work roles.

> In retrospect, I don't know how I did it, but you find inner strength.

Our approach to intrapsychic strains emphasizes the diminishment of self-concept, especially the development of self-disparagement as a caregiver. Dementia jeopardizes the caregiver's identity because it destroys the personality of the patient, leaving the caregiver, in essence, without a role partner. Moreover, the patient is not just any role partner, but part of a primary relationship in the caregiver's life, one half of the unique social bond to a parent or spouse. Thus, the lost role partner is not easily replaced; the vacuum created in self-concept is not easily restored. Incumbency of the caregiver role may compensate, at least partially, for the erosion of the child or spousal identity. Those who do not experience this replacement of identity stand in double jeopardy.

Quite obviously, our focus on self-concept captures only a small portion of the internal strife that may be occasioned by dementia and caregiving. Yet, we believe it to be among the most important for two reasons. First, the transformations of the role relationship that accompany dementia and caregiving are, as we just described, a potent threat to self-concept, and it is possible to observe this damage if it occurs. Second, self-evaluations play a pivotal role in stress processes. Recall that stress does not reside just in the external environment, that is, not exclusively in the demands of caregiving, rather it dwells in how these demands stack up against the individual's perceived ability to master the challenges presented by the illness. Any erosion of self comprises not only a threat in and of itself, but increases the perceived potency of other threats.

Extrinsic Stressors

The domain of secondary stressors does not include each and every stressor indirectly encountered by the caregiver in his or her activities of providing care. Caregivers can, and certainly do, experience various stressors that have nothing to do with their roles as caregivers. For example, death of a close friend is a major life event that intrudes upon the lives of both those who are and those who are not caregivers. Any association with caregiver status is probably tangential:

Being a caregiver may reduce the total odds of experiencing the death of a friend because one's circle of friends is constricted, but it does not influence the probability that any given friend will die. We refer to these kinds of problematic life circumstances as *extrinsic stressors*.

These stressors might appear irrelevant to caregiving stress, but this is not the case. At minimum, they increase the total burden carried by the caregiver. Furthermore, these stressors contribute to the overall context within which caregiver stress unfolds. Thus extrinsic stressors may magnify the impact of care-related stressors, both primary and secondary, or intensify the proliferation of stress. A caregiver may be managing the demands of care and its intrusion into other aspects of life, for example, until some unexpected event tips the balance out of control. Although not a major feature of our investigation, we do examine how these supplementary stressors influence the magnitude and impact of care-related stress.

Constance

Constance's recent life has been marred by crises: her husband suffered a heart attack, her best friend died, her daughter suffered a miscarriage, and her mother, the person for whom she is caring, broke her pelvis. This last event precipitated the institutionalization of her mother.

Our assessment of such stressors necessarily is abbreviated because of our extensive assessment of care-related stressors. The composite measure used in the analyses of extrinsic stressors is a count of the major events occurring in the life of the caregiver or someone close to the caregiver, such as a friend or relative. The first item asked is, "In the past *two years* has anyone close to you, a friend or a relative, passed away?" More than half of the caregivers (52.8%) had lost someone—a rather high rate that probably reflects the advanced age of the spousal caregivers. The second event was illness to someone else: "In the *past year*, has a close friend or relative had a serious illness or injury?" Illness was far less frequently reported than death, but was by no means an uncommon occurrence (35.7%). Less common still was having a close friend or relative divorce or separate from their spouse in the past year (17.3%). The final item cast a very wide net: "Are there any other stressful things that have happened to you or your family or friends in the *past year*?" About a third of the caregivers (34.2%) responded in the affirmative to this catchall question.

The average number of extrinsic stressors encountered by the caregivers is quite high (1.4 events), considering that we asked about a rather small, select set of events. About a quarter of the caregivers (22.0%) did not report any events, including negative responses to our open-ended probe. On the other hand, almost half of the sample (44.3%) reported two or more events. Clearly, caregiving does not insulate people from exposure to other problems of daily life.

The occurrence of the extrinsic stressors does not depend substantially upon the occurrence of care-related stressors. The number of stressful events was regressed upon all of the primary and secondary stressors discussed in this chapter. This regression equation is statistically significant ($F = 3.56$, $df = 16$, 532, $p \leq .001$), but accounts for only 9.7% of the variance in stressful life events. Only two of the individual regression coefficients are significantly different from zero: Role overload is associated with a large number of events, and loss of intimate exchange is associated with a small number of events.

The most important aspect of this analysis is the lack of any significant association between the objective demands of care—cognitive difficulty, ADL dependencies, problematic behavior, and patient resistance—and the occurrence of these events. Not only are these factors unimportant in the multivariate analysis, they lack any bivariate association to event exposure as well.

The Social Context of Caregiving

The stresses and strains of caregiving do not occur in a vacuum, of course, but are shaped by the caregiver's life course trajectories and his or her contemporary life circumstances. Consequently, we expect that exposure to at least some sources of stress are tied to characteristics of the caregiver and the caregiving relationship.

Our general expectation is that advantaged social standing will be accompanied by moderation of the burden of care; specifically, caregivers with access to socioeconomic resources are able to shield themselves from the full brunt of providing care by converting their material assets into some form of relief. Because dementia is a "democratic" disease—striking without much regard to economic circumstances, ethnicity, or gender—severity of impairment should be unrelated to social standing. However, it would seem that varying caregiver characteristics (e.g., socioeconomic status [SES]) likely play a role in the conversion of dementia into additional difficulties.

This possibility was evaluated by regressing baseline exposure to stressors on caregiver characteristics. All independent variables were entered into equations simultaneously: kin relationship, age of the patient, ethnicity, income, education, employment status, duration of care, and site of care, (San Francisco or Los Angeles). The results pertaining to primary stressors are displayed in Table 4.2. For simplicity, only statistically significant coefficients are presented.

Cognitive impairment depends upon the duration of care and little else. The length of care, of course, is determined by disease progression; this association, therefore, primarily captures the course of the dementia. When duration is taken into consideration, education is inversely associated with impairment. This association is of modest magnitude and the bivariate association is not significant. We interpret this relationship as an education effect on the appraisal of impairment, rather than impairment per se. At the bivariate level, low levels of impairment are found among patients attended to by wives, younger persons, and those who reside in Los Angeles. Because these characteristics are not statistically signifi-

Table 4.2 Impact of Socioeconomic and Demographic Characteristics on Exposure to Primary Stressors

Standardized regression coefficients

Characteristics	Objective primary stressors				Subjective primary stressors		
	Cognitive impairment	Problematic behavior	ADL dependencies	Patient resistance	Role overload	Role captivity	Loss of intimate exchange
Relationship to dementia patient							
Husband	—	-.140**	.150***	-.153***	-.287***	-.393***	—
Wife	—	-.112*	—	-.095*	—	-.215***	.100*
Daughter to mother[a]	—	—	—	—	—	—	—
Patient age	—	—	.096*	—	-.083*	-.134**	—
Non-Hispanic white (/all others)	—	—	—	—	—	.128**	—
Family income (thousands of dollars)	—	-.157***	-.126**	-.106*	-.152***	—	—
Caregiver education (in years)	-.091*	—	—	—	—	—	—
Caregiver unemployed (/employed)	—	—	.088*	—	—	—	—
Duration of care (in years)	.280***	-.087*	.083*	—	—	—	—
Site of care: San Francisco (/Los Angeles)	—	—	.133**	—	—	—	—
R^2	.082***	.041***	.095***	.028**	.103***	.119***	.010*

[a]The excluded category is 'Other' (sons and daughters caring for fathers).
*$p \leq .05$. **$p \leq .01$. ***$p \leq .001$.

cant in multivariate analysis, their association with impairment appears to be an artifact of their covariation with how long the caregiver has been caring for his or her spouse or parent.

The remaining primary stressors depend upon at least one caregiver characteristic. Each characteristic, in turn, is associated with at least one primary stressor. The kin relationship of the caregiver to the patient and family income have the most pervasive sets of associations with primary stressors.

Husbands have comparatively low rates of exposure to the following four of six stressors: problematic behavior, patient resistance, role overload, and role captivity. With the exception of role overload, wives similarly have low rates. In contrast, husbands have elevated scores for ADL dependencies, whereas wives score especially high on loss of intimate exchange. Daughters caring for mothers do not emerge as significantly different from the reference category, "other" caregivers (sons and daughters caring for fathers) in multivariate analysis. These differences emerge even when patient age is taken into account statistically, meaning that it cannot be attributed to implicit differences in the caregiver's age.

In sum, there is a generational difference in exposure to primary stressors: spouses generally encounter somewhat less stress than adult children. There are two exceptions to this finding: husbands have an especially high burden of ADL dependencies and wives feel the loss of their impaired husbands most intensely.

It should be emphasized that although generation matters to the primary stressors in one way or another, it essentially is immaterial to the state of cognitive decline. Thus, spouses and adult children provide care to dementia patients with similar levels of impairment; however, the impairment is manifest as different types of care-related burdens.

Family income is inversely related to four of the primary stressors in the multivariate analysis: problematic behavior, ADL dependencies, patient resistance, and role overload. Income is not related to cognitive impairment, though. At similar levels of patient impairment, therefore, those with more financial resources typically encounter somewhat fewer care-related demands.

The remaining demographic characteristics have very specific effects on select stressors. Patient age is positively related to one objective stressor, ADL dependencies, and inversely associated with two subjective stressors, role overload and role captivity. Being non-Hispanic white is associated with elevated levels of role captivity, even when the rest of the characteristics are taken into consideration. With all other conditions equal, unemployment is associated with a heavy burden of ADL dependencies.

Although demographic characteristics contribute significantly to variation in the primary stressors of caregiving, the magnitude of the associations ranges only from weak to modest. At the low end, loss of intimate exchange depends upon only one characteristic, being the wife of a patient, and accounts for a mere 1% of the variance in this stressor. Problematic behavior and patient resistance also fall at the low end of this continuum. At the high end, role overload and role captivity depend upon demographic characteristics to a somewhat greater extent, 10 to 12% of the variance, which is a reliable but modest link between social standing and exposure to primary stressors. Most of this explained variance may be attributed to two factors: relationship to the patient and family income. Cognitive impairment and ADL dependencies fall in approximately the same range of explanatory efficacy, 8 to 9%; almost all of the effect of cognitive impairment is due to the impact of illness duration.

Table 4.3 presents the results of a similar analysis for secondary stressors and extraneous stressors. Here, too, we see the influence of social position upon exposure to stress. With the exception of work strain, which is not significantly related to any of the demographic characteristics even at the bivariate level, secondary role and intrapsychic strains are contingent upon the SES of the caregiver and his or her kin relationship to the dementia patient.

In those instances in which relationship matters to exposure, the pattern is similar to that for primary stressors: exposure varies by generation. Relative to adult children, husbands and wives have the lowest levels of conflict with other family members. Although husbands are least likely to experience a loss of personal identity, this loss is most common among wives. On the other hand, wives are most likely to feel they have gained something from the experience of caregiving. This sentiment is less common among husbands and adult children.

When kin relationship is taken into account, patient age is related to four secondary stressors. Three of these associations are inverse; specifically, as patient age increases, family conflict, reduction of work involvement, and loss of self are less likely to occur. In contrast, age is associated with increased expenses. It should be noted that the duration of care is controlled in these analyses, as is kin relationship of patient to caregiver, meaning that the age differences are not mere artifacts of illness duration or generation.

Income contributes to economic strain, such that low income translates into insufficient money to meet monthly expenses. High income also is inversely related to reducing the number of hours worked and leaving the labor force entirely. However, caregivers with high incomes are most likely to experience a loss of personal identity and feel they have *not* gained anything from their roles as caregivers. Those with more advanced education are most likely to reduce work involvement, lack sufficient funds, and lack a sense of competence as a caregiver. These educational differences are independent of income, even though education and income covary.

It should be emphasized that these characteristics are not significantly related to cognitive impairment. Thus, at similar levels of patient disability, there are generational and socioeconomic differences in exposure to secondary role and intrapsychic strains.

Duration of care and city are the other two characteristics with multiple ties to secondary stressors. The longer a caregiver has been at the task of caregiving, the higher the probability he or she will experience economic strain both in terms of increased expenses and having insufficient funds to meet monthly expenses, and have reduced involvement in the work force. In contrast, doubts about one's skill as a caregiver decline as time marches on. Caregivers in Los Angeles tend to have greater financial strain and doubts about their abilities as caregivers than

Table 4.3 Impact of Socioeconomic and Demographic Characteristics on Exposure to Secondary Stressors

Standardized regression coefficients

Characteristics	Secondary role strains						Secondary intrapsychic strains		
	Family conflict	Work strain[a]	Work reduction	Increased expenses	Not enough money	Loss of self	Lack of caregiver competence	Absence of caregiving gains	Extraneous stressors
Relationship to dementia patient									
Husband	-.421***	—	—	—	—	-.103*	—	—	—
Wife	-.376***	—	—	—	—	.135***	—	-.088*	—
Daughter to mother[b]	—	—	.109*	—	.115**	—	—	—	—
Patient age	-.240***	—	-.120**	.091*	—	-.199***	—	—	—
Non-Hispanic white (/all others)	—	—	—	—	-.104**	—	—	.141***	-.095*
Family income (thousands of dollars)	—	—	-.145**	—	-.382***	-.094	—	.112*	—
Caregiver education (in years)	—	—	.091*	—	.117**	—	.105*	—	—
Caregiver unemployed (/employed)	—	—	—[c]	—	—	—	.189***	—	—
Duration of care (in years)	—	—	.139***	.152***	.128**	—	-.155***	—	—
Site of care: San Francisco (/Los Angeles)	—	—	—	—	-.186***	—	-.092*	—	.109*
R^2	.155***	—	.057***	.035***	.204***	.089***	.044***	.048***	.020**

[a] $N = 181$.

[b] The excluded category is 'Other' (sons and daughters caring for fathers).

[c] Not included because work reduction is antecedent to being unemployed at baseline.

*$p \leq .05$. **$p \leq .01$. ***$p \leq .001$.

those residing in San Francisco. Note that duration of care and education, two characteristics in which the sites differ from one another, are controlled statistically in this analysis. Thus, location appears to make an independent contribution to financial strain and self-perception.

Ethnicity did not emerge as an especially salient characteristic in the analysis of primary stressors, but does contribute to our understanding of several secondary stressors. In particular, non-Hispanic whites encounter a lower level of monthly economic hardship than caregivers from other ethnic groups. However, whites are least likely to feel they have gained something from the experience of caregiving, other conditions being equal.

Characteristics of the caregiver make the strongest contribution to explaining shortages in economic resources relative to costs. Other secondary stressors are reliably related to these characteristics, but at a far more modest level. Much of this explanatory burden is carried by relationship to the patient, income, education, and ethnicity.

Finally, the occurrence of extraneous stressors is largely independent of caregiver characteristics. Only two factors attain statistical significance in either bivariate or multivariate analysis: ethnicity and site of care. Compared to non-Hispanic whites, caregivers from other ethnic groups encounter a greater number of stressors that are unconnected to caregiving per se. These stressors are also somewhat more common among caregivers in northern than southern California.

Summary

In this chapter, we have described the key elements of care-related stress and the linkages among primary and secondary stressors. The key findings from the cross-sectional analyses of the baseline data are as follows:

• At the start of this study, the average caregiver had known something was wrong with his or her relative for about 5 years and had been providing care for about 3 years.

• Two major profiles of cognitive impairment predominate among those receiving care: partial impairment across a broad spectrum of activities and pervasive, complete incapacitation.

• The average caregiver must respond to an array of troublesome patient behaviors that keep him or her in a state of vigilance.

• The typical dementia patient relies completely upon the caregiver's assistance with several ADLs.

• Cognitive impairment and ADL dependencies are moderately associated with one another and increase with illness duration. These two primary stressors, however, are rather distinct from a third primary stressor, problematic patient behavior, which does not vary consistently with illness duration.

• The objective demands of care are manifested subjectively as a loss of intimate exchange with the dementia patient (i.e., the feeling that one's spouse or parent has become a stranger).

• Two subjective stressors, role overload and role captivity, correspond with high levels of troublesome behavior among minimally impaired patients.

• Among the secondary role strains that we considered in this study, family conflict is not widespread, although some caregivers experience intense strife; work-related stress is quite widespread among employed caregivers, but generally not intense; one in five caregivers have reduced or eliminated employment to accommodate caregiving; and, although most of the caregivers have adequate financial resources, one in three or four caregivers are beset by financial difficulties.

• There are three links joining primary stressors to secondary role strains: a diffuse and pervasive overall association; a discrete link between not working and a heavy objective burden of care; and a heavy objective burden of care associated with reduced employment and feeling hemmed in by caregiving.

• Secondary intrapsychic strains also are limited: Although caregivers are more likely to report positive than negative changes in self-concept as a consequence of caregiving, some caregivers experience a marked diminishment of personal identity.

• An erosion of identity more closely corresponds to subjective than objective primary stressors: The experience of being overwhelmed and held captive by caregiving parallels loss of self, especially when accompanied by loss of intimacy with the care recipient.

• Negative sentiments about oneself as a caregiver are most pronounced among those who are providing extensive care to persons with limited impairment.

• Secondary role strains and intrapsychic strains are linked along two dimensions.

• Caregivers are exposed to extraneous stressors that occur independently of the objective demands of care, stressors that may alter the impact of care-related stress.

• The primary and secondary stressors of caregiving depend, at least in part, upon social position: kin relationship to the caregiver and income have the most consistent links to stress exposure.

• Although statistically significant, the contribution of SES and demographic characteristics is of relatively modest magnitude. The more pronounced effects are found for insufficient economic resources, family conflict, role captivity, and role overload.

• Caregivers providing care to similarly impaired relatives differ in their exposure to other care-related stressors as a function of their own characteristics.

Discussion

Although being a caregiver to a parent or spouse with dementia is indeed stressful, the nature, intensity, and configuration of problems encountered on a day-to-day basis are not uniform. Instead, they vary with disease progression and with the social circumstances surrounding the caregiver–patient dyad. This heterogeneity is apparent in the distributions of various stressors at the time of the baseline interviews, because our participants had been providing care for periods ranging from months to more than a decade. The baseline assessments reported in this chapter, therefore, give a snapshot of caregiving across time by portraying the experiences of those who have occupied the role for different periods of time. This cross section illustrates the complex and dynamic processes through which the objective conditions of caregiving generate problems in areas of life removed from the actual tasks of caregiving.

The differentiation of primary and secondary stressors plays a key role in illuminating how the patient's impairment becomes translated into caregiver stress. It does this by separating problematic circumstances that are part and parcel of caregiving from those that are inadvertent consequences of caregiving. The total burden of care endured by the caregiver encompasses both components. The underlying impairment generates stress by imposing objective demands and constraints on the caregiver, which, in turn, evoke subjective states of being overwhelmed and obstructed. These primary stressors correspond to secondary stressors encountered in the enactment of other social roles and in deficient evaluations of oneself as a caregiver.

Primary and secondary stressors are related to one another: Those who provide extensive care to severely impaired relatives, on average, tend to encounter the most difficulties in family, work, and economic life. The magnitude of this association, however, is at best moderate, indicating substantial differences across caregivers in the extent to which the demands of care generate additional life problems. The linkage between primary and secondary stressors, therefore, emerges as pivotal to the question of why caregiving exerts a more pernicious impact upon some caregivers than others. As we shall see in chapter 6, variation in the impact of caregiving may be attributed, at least in part, to variation in the proliferation of stress into other areas of life.

Notes

[1]One additional item, "recognize people that (he/she) knows," was included in the impairment battery, but was dropped from the summary scale because it did not make sense for AD patients living in institutions. Including this item in the baseline measure, therefore, was problematic for the analysis of the longitudinal data. The high reliability of the scale renders the deletion of this one item immaterial to the substantive analyses.

[2]Although we rely entirely upon the caregiver's reports, these stressors may be assessed by other means, such as direct observation.

[3]These three stressors have distinctive sets of response categories. For cognitive impairment, the highest score of 4 represents tasks the dementia patient cannot do at all; for ADLs a score of 4 represents complete dependency upon the caregiver; for problematic behavior, this value means that troublesome behaviors were confronted by the caregiver on at least 5 days during the past week. Thus, it is not meaningful to compare absolute mean values across these measures. In order to facilitate relative comparisons, these three measures were scaled to a common metric, the interval of 1 to 4.

[4]The decline in ADL dependencies at the longest illness duration, 10 or more years, is too slight to be substantively meaningful. As such, this trajectory should not be seen as a leveling off of the patient's need for help, but as a possible leveling off of the amount of help provided by the caregiver. This may result from the fact that the ADL questions refer not solely to the level of disability, as is the case for cognitive impairment, but to the extent to which the caregiver takes on various tasks.

[5]Each primary stressor was regressed upon illness duration and the square of illness duration to determine whether the relationship was nonlinear (i.e, quadratic). For both cognitive impairment and ADL dependencies, the coefficients are statistically significant; for problematic behavior, neither coefficient is significant. Thus, the course of cognitive decline and ADL dependencies shows deterioration over time, but not a constant rate of decline, whereas the course of problematic behaviors does not vary consistently with illness duration.

[6]Changes in family income are assessed with the follow-up data. This dimension of financial strain, therefore, is discussed in more detail in the following chapter, which examines changes over time.

[7]At follow-up, this question referred to a year ago (i.e., at the time of the preceding interview).

[8]Low income is defined as more than one standard deviation below the mean income for the sample.

[9]Work strain had valid values only for the employed; its use would limit the analysis to this subgroup. Consequently, we substituted the mean value for those who are not employed and used this imputed variable in conjunction with a dummy variable for unemployment, which removed the effects of mean substitution. Thus, the coefficient for work strain applies only to those who are working; the unemployed variable captures the impact of not working.

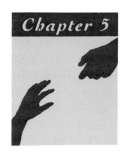

The Natural History of Care-Related Stress

One of our central objectives is to identify factors that intensify care-related stressors over time and those that constrain this process of stress proliferation. The expansion and contraction of primary and secondary stressors as caregiving continues over lengthy intervals, we submit, is consequential to the caregiver's well-being. In addition, we expect that these processes are important to an array of potential outcomes. For example, in chapter 8 we consider the impact of changes in care-related stressors on the risk of premature admission of the dementia patient to a nursing home.

Mom's illness has taken a chunk out of my life.

It is necessary to have some understanding of how these stressors are configured over time in order to appreciate their impact upon one another and upon other outcomes (e.g., depression). This chapter presents just such a descriptive picture, tracing the expansion and contraction of care-related stressors over the course of in-home caregiving, encompassing the entire 3-year interval separating Time 1 and Time 4. Although the following chapter examines how change in some of these stressors generates change in other stressors, and how these shifting configurations affect the caregiver's mental health, our present concern is more circumscribed: We attempt to delineate how each care-related stressor relates to itself as time progresses.

The Course of Primary Stressors over Time

Describing the natural history of care-related stressors over the course of this study is complicated both by the movement of patients into institutions and patient deaths.[1] At each reinterview, the number of caregivers who continued to provide in-home care declined, while there was an increase in the number who admitted their spouses or parents to nursing homes, became bereaved, or experienced both of these transitions. The pattern of stress exposure over time among those who continued in-home care, therefore, was influenced by the ebb and flow of various stressors, as well as by the selection of caregivers *out* of this phase of role enactment.

Consequently, we examine average levels of stress exposure from two vantage points. First, we look at all those providing in-home care at the time of each interview, and second, we consider only the subsample who provided in-home care across multiple points in time. This latter strategy delineates the impact of selection out of active, in-home caregiving and thereby enables us to extract a more accurate picture of the course of primary stressors among those who continued to provide such care.

It should be noted that the ensuing description of care-related stress applies to caregivers as a group rather than the experiences of individual caregivers, which are examined later in this chapter. Although the composite picture of the group is the sum total of the individual experiences, this is not informative about experience at the individual level. For example, caregivers together may appear to encounter little change over time, but some individual caregivers may incur severe worsening of their situations, whereas others have their burdens lifted.

This approach is depicted in Figure 5.1 for one objective primary stressor, cognitive impairment. The solid line plots the average level of cognitive impairment among all patients being cared for in the home at each interview. The dashed lines represent subsamples of those who provide in-home care longitudinally: at Times 1 *and* 2 ($n = 352$), at Times 1, 2, *and* 3 ($n = 224$), and at Times 1, 2, 3, *and* 4 ($n = 137$).

The difference between the solid line and the dashed lines indicates quite clearly that those who exited from in-home care were more cognitively impaired at the start of the study than those who continued to receive in-home care over the course of the study. The selection effect is most pronounced for those patients who remained at home throughout the entire course of our observations (i.e., until at least Time 4). This pattern suggests that initial levels of cognitive impairment affect the subsequent probability of being admitted to a nursing home or dying, either in an institution or at home. That is, what appears here as a selection effect, emerges in later chapters as a potential contributor to institutionalization (chapter 8) and death (chapter 10).

The most notable feature of the data presented in Figure 5.1, however, is the clear course of deterioration in cognitive functioning over time regardless of the caretaking course. Declining abilities are evident among those who subsequently exit this situation, but are most apparent among those who continue to be cared for at home, especially those who remain at home for the duration of our observa-

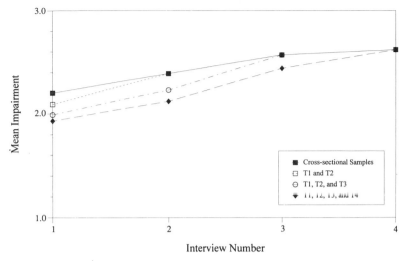

Figure 5.1   Mean level of cognitive impairment over time.

tions. This trajectory, of course, reflects the degenerative course of the underlying dementia. It should be noted that our assessment of change in cognitive impairment is constrained by ceiling effects in our measure (i.e., maximum impairment scores cannot be observed to deteriorate further even if a patient's condition worsens). At extreme levels of impairment, the measure is not sensitive to change. More generally, the lower the initial score, the more room there is for decline over time. In essence, patients may continue to worsen, though in ways not measured.

The longitudinal trajectories for the other primary stressors—both objective and subjective—were also examined. These primary stressors follow two distinct courses. The first is an increase in the mean level of the stressor over time, similar to that illustrated in Figure 5.1 for cognitive impairment. Only one other primary stressor parallels the course of cognitive impairment, the loss of intimate exchange with a patient, which is a subjective stressor.

The second course reflects minimal fluctuation in the mean level of stress encountered over time. This pattern is illustrated in Figure 5.2 for role overload. As may be seen, the mean level of role overload reported by those who continued to provide in-home care is rather stable over time. Selection out of in-home care into institutional care and bereavement is evident as well: Those caregivers who continued to provide in-home care over time tended to have slightly lower initial levels of role overload than those who subsequently exited this career stage, either by admitting their relatives to nursing homes or by becoming bereaved.

The other objective primary stressors besides role overload that follow the second longitudinal trajectory of flat mean distributions over time are problematic behavior, ADL dependencies, and patient resistance. On the subjective side, two stressors follow this plateau: role overload and stressors. As mentioned

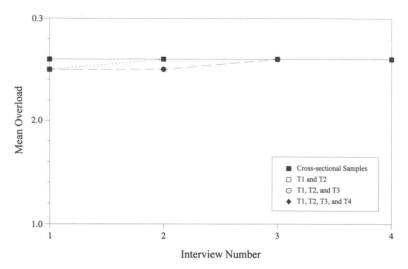

Figure 5.2   Mean level of role overload over time.

previously, the third subjective stressor, loss of intimate exchange, follows the first pattern (i.e., deterioration over time). It should be noted that some stressors seem to abate slightly as time passes, but this trend is quite small and may well reflect selection effects.

Thus, the degenerative course of dementia does not necessarily portend an intensification of primary stressors. Some caregivers undoubtedly do face deteriorating conditions as they provide in-home care. It appears, however, that the daily demands of caregiving remain steady for some caregivers, while they ease for others. The types of primary stressors encountered over time are illustrated by this caregiver who has been assisting his wife for more than a decade with virtually all aspects of daily life, including eating, personal hygiene, walking support (see photographs 5–8).

The Course of Secondary Stressors over Time

A central element of our conceptual model concerns the extent to which primary stressors generate or exacerbate secondary stressors. As stated in chapter 4, secondary stressors are of two broad types: role strains—pressures encountered in other social roles, (e.g., family, work, and finances); and intrapsychic strains—perceptions of oneself in the position as caregiver (e.g., loss of self, lack of caregiver competence, and lack of caregiving gains). Our description of stress exposure over time considers one additional element as well, extraneous stressors, life events independent of caregiving. Again, this description concerns caregivers as a group, which is composed of individual caregivers; individual trajectories, however, cannot be discerned in this composite picture, but are discussed later in this chapter.

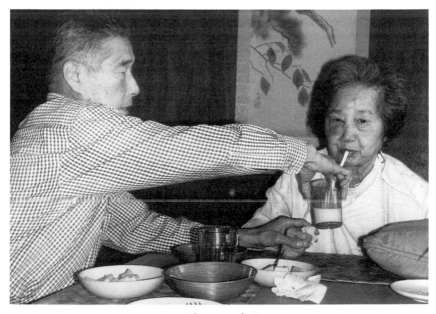

Photograph 5

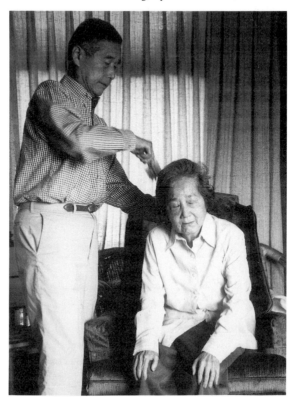

Photograph 6

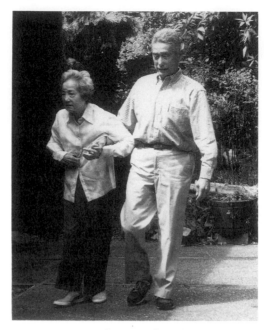

Photograph 7

Only one longitudinal trajectory emerges for all secondary stressors, the flat distribution just described for most of the primary stressors. Among those who continued to provide in-home care, there are no discernible differences in the average level of exposure at baseline compared to any of the follow-up interviews. Because none of these stressors follow the pattern of deterioration described previously for cognitive impairment and loss of intimate exchange, the degenerative course of dementia and its associated loss of persona are not necessarily associated with intensified problems in other social roles or self-perceptions.

Moreover, the flat pattern is the same for the complete sample of in-home caregivers and longitudinal subsamples of those who continued to provide care for 1 to 3 years after baseline. Secondary role strains and internal strife with regard to caregiving did not differ appreciably between those who continued to provide in-home care and those who ceased to be engaged in this type of care. Thus, there is no evidence of selection effects due to caregivers who exited active in-home care.

Parenthetically, extraneous stressors also follow a flat trajectory over time with no evidence of selection effects.

It is useful to consider the multiple domains of life encompassed by our measures of secondary stress. First, for role strains, in addition to considering problematic conditions experienced within the family, around work, and in finances, we examine transitions out of the workforce and in family income.[2] Second, the average levels of intrapsychic strains reflect minimal fluctuations

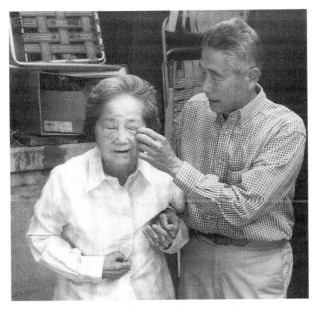

Photograph 8

across time. These measures comprise a rather broad spectrum of potential secondary consequences of caregiving. Yet it is quite evident that in-home caregivers, *as a group*, do not uniformly follow a downward spiral of deteriorating conditions in other social roles or in their self-concepts.

> He's been home for over 5 years—tired,
> boring conversations with him every day.

In sum, the degenerative course of dementia does not inevitably portend an intensification of secondary stressors; instead, for those caregivers who continued to provide in-home care, these pressures remained at more or less the same average intensity over time. This conclusion does not imply that all caregivers face a steady state in areas of their lives other than caregiving or in their sentiments about themselves. Contrarily, these secondary stressors are likely to ebb and flow over time in individual caregivers' lives. Although some caregivers are gaining the upper hand over these problems, others are being overwhelmed by seemingly similar conditions.

Individual Patterns of Stability and Change

Although exposure to most aspects of care-related stress appears rather stable when caregivers are viewed collectively, this composite picture masks offsetting patterns of expansion and contraction in these hardships. Average levels of exposure remain constant not because the experience of individual caregivers is invariant, but because deteriorating conditions among some caregivers are counterbalanced by improved circumstances among others. Furthermore, at the individual level, an expansion of care-related difficulties at one point in time may be followed by a contraction of these burdens at another point in time. Alternately, catastrophic disruption may arrive on the heels of an interval of relative tranquility. Care-related stressors, therefore, comprise a dynamic, rather than a static, system.

Valerie

The drain on the strength and energy of the those providing in-home, hands-on care is illustrated by Valerie's description of nights with her husband Donald:

He's up and down all night and I don't get much sleep. At least we have a big king-sized bed. I'm going to get two separate mattresses on top with two separate sets of bedding so that I don't have to change the whole thing all the time.

She finds some relief from the burdens of caregiving during brief intervals when Donald is lucid:

He still has a great sense of humor. That's the one thing we do share. I make jokes. When we share a laugh, that's a good thing. I'll do anything — dance, anything, to entertain him. For a while I found all the old letters I'd written my mother about him, and when the baby was born. I read them to him. He loved it. Those were stories he could relate to.

These moments contrast dramatically to the changes in Donald's behavior that have resulted from his dementia. In a matter of fact manner, she reports:

He's attacked me three or four times. The last time was a week ago. Donald came after me, tried to bite me. I was able to hold him away from me. I get icy calm when that happens. I don't get upset. The first time was a couple of months ago. I thought he was trying to kill me, but that's not it. He's expressing his anger. He's never picked up anything. I've hidden all the knives, pokers. Now I think I can handle it. At first I totally panicked . . . There's times I've wanted to hit him. I can feel myself getting abrupt, pushing him.

Change evaluated at the individual level is illustrated in Figure 5.3 for cognitive impairment, our most direct indicator of disease progression. Two sets of difference scores are plotted for those who continued in-home care: short-term change (Time 2 minus Time 1, $n = 352$) and long-term change (Time 4 minus Time 1, $n = 137$). The cognitive impairment scores range from 0 through 4. Difference scores of 0 indicate no change over time, positive values signify deterioration, and negative values connote improvement.

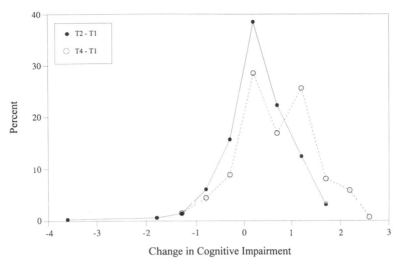

Figure 5.3   Change in cognitive impairment over time.

Recall that cognitive impairment is one of two primary stressors that deteriorate for in-home caregivers as a group. This decline also is evident in Figure 5.3 insofar as the two distributions are centered somewhat to the right of 0. The mean change over the 1-year interval is .30, and is .69 for the 3-year span. Positive values clearly predominate over negative ones. The few negative values observed probably reflect subjective variation in caregiver appraisals of the patient, rather than actual improvement in functioning. Finally, cognitive decline is more marked over 3 years than 1 year. The observed distributions in cognitive change scores, then, match the degenerative and irreversible course of the underlying dementia.

The deterioration in cognitive functioning observed over the course of the study is important, given the known progression of dementia. Figure 5.3 demonstrates that our data conform to expectations based on the nature of the disease. This correspondence substantiates our methods as accurately capturing the course of dementia and, hence, the course of caregiving. Such validation is especially critical because other elements of care-related stress processes do not follow the same pattern of inevitable decline as does cognitive impairment.

Consider family conflict, for example, which is illustrated in Figure 5.4. Compared to cognitive impairment, the family conflict change scores are centered more closely around 0, the value indicative of no change. With scores ranging from 1 to 4, the mean change over the 1-year interval is -.01, and -.07 for the 3-year span. Furthermore, these distributions are evenly divided between positive and negative scores. In particular, for some caregivers, relations with other family members improved over time and improved by a substantial amount. On the other hand, these relations deteriorated substantially for other caregivers. Similar patterns emerge for 1 and 3 years. That is, over both the short- and long-term, there is

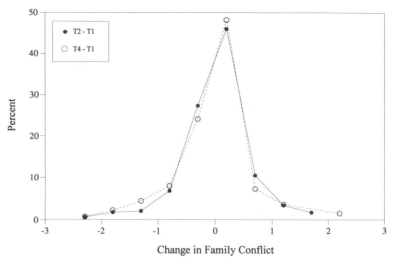

Figure 5.4   Change in family conflict over time.

considerable flux in the nature of relationships between caregivers and members of their extended families. Stationary circumstances are matched by shifts for the worse and for the better.

Two time trends dominate the course of average exposure to care-related stressors. The first is deterioration over time; that is, an escalation in the burden that falls on the caregiver as time passes. In addition to cognitive impairment, loss of intimate exchange with the patient deteriorates over time. The remaining primary, secondary, and extraneous stressors follow the second pattern, the pattern typified by family conflict (i.e., a relatively stable average level of stress exposure for those who continued to provide care over time, bound by marked improvement on the one end and marked deterioration on the other).

Never put off to tomorrow what you can do today. Don't feel that it's going to get better. It's not as bad now as it will be then.

The distributions of change scores seem to suggest that exposure to care-related stress is somewhat haphazard, but this is not the case. Instead, the amount of stress encountered at one point in time depends strongly upon previous conditions and strongly determines subsequent circumstances. Because this point is not immediately apparent from the data presented up to this juncture, we conclude our presentation of the natural history of care-related stressors with a summary of stability coefficients, which are shown in Table 5.1.

The correlation of each care-related stressor with itself tends to be somewhat higher for the 1- than the 3-year span. In most instances, however, this apparent erosion of stability is not as large as one might expect, given the threefold increase in the time interval.

Table 5.1   Auto-correlations of Care-Related Stressors

Care-related stressors	Time interval	
	1 year[a] (n = 352)	3 years[b] (n = 137)
Cognitive impairment (0–4)	.75***	.62***
Problematic behavior (1–4)	.61***	.50***
ADL dependencies (1–4)	.62***	.43***
Patient resistance (/no)	.31***	.06
Role overload (1–4)	.66***	.52***
Role captivity (1–4)	.66***	.67***
Loss of intimate exchange (1–4)	.63***	.38***
Family conflict (1–4)	.56***	.45***
Work strain (1–4)[c]	.47***	.54**
Work reduction (/no)	−.04	−.13
Not employed (/employed)	.81***	.71***
Increased expenses (1–5)	.16**	.05
Not enough money (1–3)	.61***	.46***
Income (thousands of dollars)	.87***	.81***
Loss of self (1–4)	.52***	.45***
Lack of caregiver competence (1–4)	.57***	.52***
Lack of caregiving gains (1–4)	.62***	.56***
Extraneous stressors (0–2)	.29***	.20*

[a]Time 1 and Time 2.
[b]Time 1 and Time 4.
[c]n for 1 year = 110; 3 years = 37.
*p ≤ .05.   **p ≤ .01.   ***p ≤ .001.

Most of these stressors display moderate to high levels of stability over both the short- and long-term. This pattern characterizes all of the primary stressors, both objective and subjective, except for patient resistance, which is only somewhat stable over the short-term and displays no long-term stability. The secondary stressors, role strains as well as intrapsychic strains, also tend to have strong levels of stability over both 1- and 3-year intervals. There are two exceptions to this generalization. First, reducing one's involvement in work is not at all stable over time: Once caregivers decrease their hours at work, the only further reduction possible is leaving the workforce, after which no further reductions are possible. Second, having had increased expenses as a result of the care-recipient's condition is only slightly related to subsequent augmentations in expenses and at this, they are only over the short-term.

Finally, exposure to extraneous stressors tends to have a slight impact on subsequent exposure to the same types of stressors both over 1 year and 3 years.

In summary, the primary and secondary stressors of caregiving are typically quite stable over time. This stability does not mean that individuals stay at a steady state. Instead, correlations indicate that individuals usually maintain their ranking relative to one another on each stressor. Thus, elements of care-related stress tend to be self-perpetuating (i.e., sustain themselves over time). Nonetheless, the auto-correlations presented in Table 5.1 are far from perfect ($r = 1.00$), indicating the presence of increases and decreases over time.

Summary

This chapter has traced the natural history of care-related stressors as they evolve over the course of providing in-home care.

• Caregivers as a group tend to maintain a relatively uniform level of stress exposure as time passes. The exceptions to this finding are those primary stressors directly tied to the degenerative course of dementia: cognitive impairment and loss of intimate exchange.

• There is considerable variability in exposure at the individual level; however, some caregivers face deteriorating care situations, whereas others find some relief over time.

Discussion

Why do some primary stressors worsen over time whereas others remain, on average, at about the same intensity? A clue to these divergent patterns may be found in the nature of the conditions that deteriorate (i.e., cognitive impairment and loss of intimate exchange with the patient). These two factors are tied directly to the degenerative and irreversible course of dementia. Waning cognitive abilities are inevitable as time marches on and as cognition fades, so too, does the persona of the individual.

In contrast, the other primary stressors are less closely tied to the degenerative course of dementia. For example, although some problem behaviors increase over time, others abate (Haley & Pardo, 1989). Moreover, some stressors are potentially reversible even if the disease is not. For example, as dementia progresses, the patient requires more assistance with activities of daily living (ADLs), which might well increase the ADL dependencies that fall on the shoulders of the primary caregiver. However, caregivers may seek assistance from other informal caregivers or obtain formal assistance in managing patients at home, thereby containing or even reducing the direct demands they themselves encounter. Such a scenario also is likely to prevent increases in role overload and role captivity.

Similarly, selection effects may be discerned for most primary stressors, but not for secondary role strains, secondary intrapsychic strains, or extraneous stressors. One explanation may be that the objective demands of care prompt exits from in-home care, but role strains, internal strife about oneself as a caregiver, and ambient problems do not. Alternately, difficulties directly associated with the status of the patient may be predictive of patient death, whereas other problems are not, precisely because these other problems are not directly tied to the degenerative course of the disease. These possibilities are examined directly in chapter 8 and chapter 10.

This chapter has examined the natural history of care-related stressors over time, demonstrating that there is considerable stability in the array of stressors impinging upon caregivers as they continue to provide in-home care over lengthy intervals of time. The data also reveal considerable fluctuation in exposure to primary and secondary stressors over time at the individual level of analysis. We turn in chapter 6 to a consideration of the forces that drive increases and decreases in exposure to stress over the course of in-home caregiving.

Notes

[1]Loss-to-follow-up presents similar selection effects.

[2]Work reduction, leaving work or decreasing hours, is substantially more pronounced at baseline than at any follow-up. This is because the baseline assessment covers the entire duration of the illness prior to this assessment, whereas the follow-up assessments cover only the past year.

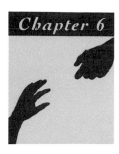

Stress Proliferation

In the previous chapter, we reported that most stressors are fairly stable over time, with average levels of exposure remaining at about the same intensity for caregivers as a group, but with some individual caregivers encountering marked improvement and others marked deterioration. The two exceptions to this generalization, cognitive impairment and loss of intimate exchange, steadily increase over time as dementia progresses. The clear distinction between the course of these stressors and other care-related stressors demonstrates that the system of stress proliferation is not driven solely by the underlying dementia. Also, although the system of care-related stressors tends to perpetuate itself, it clearly is not static.

Instead, stressors experienced in one domain of life, including those that remain at about the same level of intensity, often engender stressors in other domains, a phenomenon we refer to as stress proliferation. As the routines of daily caregiving relentlessly continue, areas of life extending beyond caregiving may be fundamentally restructured. This reordering of ordinary life, although driven by the necessity to provide care, frequently is most evident outside the confines of the care recipient–caregiver dyad. The effects of such change on the well-being of caregivers may be no less potent than conditions residing directly in care-related tasks and responsibilities.

In this chapter, we examine stress proliferation as it is found within the continuing in-home care segment of the caregiving career. The core issue we address concerns the impact of one domain of experience on another, especially the extent to which primary stressors, strains anchored in caregiving activities, generate secondary stressors, problems occurring outside the boundaries of caregiving. This issue was introduced in chapter 4 with regard to the cross-sectional data. The analyses demonstrated the presence of associations among objective and subjective primary stressors on the one hand, and secondary role and intrapsychic strains on the other. In this chapter, we extend the earlier analyses by examining the longitudinal data. First, however, we shall briefly elaborate a conceptual question we first raised in chapter 2: Why should stressors proliferate?

Structural and Interpersonal Foundations of Stress Proliferation

As we outlined in chapter 2, we believe stress proliferation is the result of a basic structural circumstance, the interrelatedness of multiple social roles. Caregivers are not only caregivers: They may also be parents, children, and siblings within a larger family system; workers and breadwinners; and parishioners, club members, friends, and neighbors. In the ordinary organization of daily life, these activities and relationships tend to be temporally and spatially segregated from one another, an arrangement that helps to avoid confusion and competition among the total array of expectations and responsibilities arising within the various domains. In the case of caregivers, for example, those who are employed typically engage in their work at one time and place, and in their caregiving at another time and place. To the extent that it exists, this kind of structural separation probably inhibits the diffusion of problems from one area of life to another, however, it does not necessarily prevent such diffusion. The reason, of course, is that although there are multiple roles separated in time and space, there is but a single actor playing them. When that actor experiences severe and sustained problems within the boundaries of one role, his or her actions and interactions in the other roles may be affected.

It is not an automatic certainty that the problems caregivers experience as caregivers will create problems in their other roles and domains of activity. Nonetheless, there are several distinctive features of caregiving that increase the likelihood of contagious effects. One, clearly, is the emergence and expansion of caregiving as a central commitment, which may alter the priorities that order an individual's multiple roles. For example, occupational activities previously commanding the central interests of the caregiver may now seem less compelling and less worthy of personal investment, or the idiosyncracies of family and friends that were once met with patience and humor are now irritants not to be tolerated in the face of more urgent affairs.

Another feature of caregiving that contributes to stress proliferation concerns the sheer limits on time and energy imposed by the role and its demands. This property is distinct from, but perhaps related to, the reordering of priorities. Indeed, shifting priorities sometimes serves as a means of rebudgeting or redirecting energies that are insufficient to satisfy mounting demands. This social readjustment, in turn, may have consequences for the self-concepts of caregivers, the ways they perceive themselves as people. Thus, when role activities are no longer driven by the same vigor and commitment, or when energy and time are spread so thin that it is necessary to withdraw altogether from some activities, the ways in which caregivers view themselves may also undergo alterations. For instance, they may experience a loss of identity or come to think of themselves as failures, no longer upholding the expectations others have for them or the expectations they have for themselves. Understandably, as experiences that previously might have confirmed and sustained knowledge of one's self come to be altered, so, too, will the self-knowledge that had been supported by those experiences.

It is evident from this discussion that an individual does not play a social role in isolation; instead, he or she invariably acts as part of a role set composed of other social actors. Thus, one cannot be a family member without relatives; one usually is not a worker without supervisors, subordinates, fellow workers, or clients; and one is not able to be a friend unless there is another person. We call attention to the interpersonal contexts of multiple roles because the contagion of problems from one role to another is likely to be accompanied by disruption of the relationships among the actors comprising that role set. In affected roles, whether these be family, occupational, or other social roles, the troubled caregiver whose actions no longer fulfill established expectations may evoke from others signs of disappointment, remonstration, or even hostility. These kinds of responses from significant others, independent of the conditions that prompted them, may create problems for the caregiver in their own right.

What should be underscored is that the multiple roles of caregivers constitute the structural underpinnings of stress proliferation. To the extent that the demands of caregiving impinge upon the enactment of other social roles, caregivers may rearrange their priorities and reallocate their energies. One does not restructure daily life without affecting the lives of other people with whom one interacts. Consequently, there is a risk that these kinds of alterations will set in motion a chain of negative actions and reactions between the caregiver and others. Eventually, the valued self-concepts of individuals may be casualties of these interconnected changes. The entire constellation of altered circumstances, finally, may come together to undermine the health and well-being of the caregiver. This description is admittedly a rather bleak and grim picture of stress proliferation and its impact. For some caregivers, this scenario is undoubtedly overstated; for others, unfortunately, it describes that part of their caregiving careers entailing in-home assistance.

We turn now to some of the empirical evidence for the perspectives outlined above. In the analyses that follow, two time intervals are treated separately: the 1-year period between Time 1 and Time 2 and the 3 years separating Time 1 and

Time 4. These intervals provide both short- and long-term perspectives of the proliferation of caregiving stressors to other areas of life. The short-term cohort is composed of caregivers who persisted in providing in-home care at Time 2, and the long-term cohort consists of only those who continued to provide care through Time 4. Of course, the numbers of caregivers falling within these two groups are different. The ranks of caregivers who persisted in providing in-home care declined as time progressed. Thus, our short-term analysis is based on the largest longitudinal subsample ($n = 352$), whereas the long-term analysis is based on the smallest longitudinal subsample ($n = 137$). We focus on these groups of continuing caregivers because the care environment remains the home. This enables us to disregard the impact of transitions from in-home care to institutional placement or bereavement, issues addressed in later chapters. In looking at both short- and long-term caregivers, therefore, we preserve both the advantages of a large sample and those of longitudinal data.

Proliferation over the Short-Term

The Impact of Objective Primary Stressors on Subjective Primary Stressors

In this section, we examine the extent to which the objective demands of care generate subjective stressors over the course of 1 additional year of continued in-home care. Specifically, we explore the extent to which deteriorating objective conditions result in the exacerbation of subjective stressors. This will be recognized as the first component in our model of stress proliferation.

A brief description of the form of the analysis we employed is necessary for the interpretation of findings. Paralleling the cross-sectional analysis discussed in chapter 4, three subjective stressors were considered—role overload, role captivity, and loss of intimate exchange. In each instance, the Time 2 value of the subjective stressor was regressed on four types of independent variables: (1) sociodemographic characteristics; (2) subjective stressors assessed at baseline; (3) objective stressors assessed at baseline, as change scores, and as the interaction of these two terms; and (4) extraneous stressors assessed in the same manner as objective stressors. The sociodemographic characteristics included in these analyses are kin relationship between caregiver and patient (i.e., husband, wife, daughter caring for mother, and other), patient age, education, income, employment status, ethnicity, city, and the duration of caregiving at baseline. The inclusion of the baseline measures of subjective stressors as determinants of the same kinds of stress in the future means that these analyses are prospective (i.e., they concern change in subjective stressors over time).

The treatment of the objective primary stressors, finally, is somewhat more complicated. As you may recall, there are four such stressors: cognitive impairment, ADL dependencies, problematic behavior, and patient resistance. In the tables presenting results, each of these stressors is represented in the regression equations by multiple terms. One term is the *baseline measure* which, in conjunction with the other terms, captures the stable component of the intensity of the stressor that is present at both Time 1 and Time 2. The second term, the *change variable,* assesses the impact of the magnitude of change between these two time periods.[1] The last term is the *multiplicative interaction* of the previous two terms, which tests whether the impact of change varies according to the initial level of demand.[2] Because each of these regressions contains a large number of statistically insignificant terms, we present only those coefficients that attain significance in Table 6.1.

As may be seen, the three subjective stressors display moderate levels of stability over the course of 1 year. (Auto-regression coefficients are the variable at follow-up regressed upon its baseline value). The auto-regression coefficients range from .520 to .565 and account for roughly one-third to one-half of the variance in the subjective stressors over time. These coefficients, it should be noted, do not mean that caregivers maintained the same absolute scores across time, but rather that caregivers tended to maintain their relative ranking with one another with regard to these sources of stress. The multivariate analyses extend the bivariate analyses presented in the previous chapter (see Table 5.1) by showing that the self-sustaining quality of these stressors persists even when numerous other factors are taken into consideration. In addition, two subjective stressors have crossover effects upon other subjective stressors, as also shown in this table: Loss of intimate exchange tends to intensify subsequent role overload and role overload contributes to an increasing sense of being held captive by caregiving. These findings indicate that subjective primary stressors tend to perpetuate themselves over time.

At the same time, there is, nonetheless, considerable fluctuation in subjective stressors remaining once their initial values are taken into consideration. Table 6.1 illustrates that stressors and background characteristics explain about 10% of the change in subjective stressors over time. The extent to which subjective stressors intensify depends upon the exacerbation of the objective demands of care as time passes. Interestingly, too, there seems to be a clear specialization between particular objective and subjective stressors.

This specialization is apparent in the case of cognitive impairment, the objective stressor most indicative of disease progression. Impairment is significantly associated with loss of intimate exchange, but does not have an appreciable independent impact upon either role overload or role captivity. The absolute level of impairment and the pace of deterioration are both associated with an increased sense of loss of intimate exchange over time, the effects being of approximately equal magnitude. Progressive cognitive incapacitation, which erodes the persona of the patient, heightens the caregiver's sense of having lost the person he or she once knew, his or her husband, wife, mother, or father.

The impact of problematic behavior, in contrast, appears to be specific to role captivity. Both the intensity of disruptive problematic behaviors and increases in such behaviors contribute to increases in subsequent role captivity. These effects are of similar magnitude and comparable to that of role overload. Thus, behavior

Table 6.1 Change in Subjective Primary Stressors over 1 Year
as a Function of Objective Primary Stressors

Objective primary stressors and characteristics	Subjective primary stressors: Time 2[a]					
	Role overload		Role captivity		Loss of intimate exchange	
	b (SE)	β	b (SE)	β	b (SE)	β
Role overload: Time 1	**.565***** (**.045**)	**.572**	.122* (.050)	.114	—	—
Role captivity: Time 1	—	—	**.562***** (**.046**)	**.569**	—	—
Loss of intimate exchange: Time 1	.118* (.050)	.113	—	—	**.520***** (**.048**)	**.561**
ADL dependencies: Change Time 2–Time 1	*1.073**** (*.222*)	*.773*	—	—	*.121** (*.059*)	*.100*
ADL dependencies: Change × Time 1	*−.342**** (*.074*)	*−.705*	—	—	—	—
Problematic behavior: Time 1	—	—	*.197** (*.096*)	*.111*	—	—
Problematic behavior: Change Time 2–Time 1	—	—	*.234** (*.099*)	*.115*	—	—
Cognitive impairment: Time 1	—	—	—	—	*.120** (*.057*)	*.131*
Cognitive impairment: Change Time 2–Time 1	—	—	—	—	*.176*** (*.056*)	*.142*
San Francisco (/Los Angeles)	—	—	—	—	−.234** (.071)	−.144
Duration of care: Time 1	—	—	−.057** (.018)	−.136	—	—
Income (thousands of dollars)	—	—	−.005* (.002)	−.098	—	—
White (/other)	—	—	.374** (.115)	.138	—	—
R^2 Total	.562***		.532***		.480***	
R^2 Auto-regression	.445***		.447***		.380***	
R^2 Difference	.117***		.085***		.100***	

[a]Boldface numbers indicate auto-regression variables; italicized numbers indicate stress proliferation.
*$p \le .05$. **$p \le .01$. ***$p \le .001$.

that requires vigilance and control on the part of the caregiver, especially when it is escalating, leads caregivers to feel increasingly trapped in their roles as in-home care continues over time.

Finally, ADL dependencies are linked to role overload while having no discernible effect on role captivity or loss of intimate exchange. The form of this association differs from that found in the previous two analyses. Specifically, the coefficient for the baseline level of ADL dependencies does not attain statistical significance, but the interaction of this baseline value with the change score is significant, as is the change score itself. The individual and combined impact of ADL dependencies is substantial, exceeding that of the stability term. It should be noted that the sign of the interaction term is negative. This pattern means that increasing dependency upon the caregiver substantially exacerbates role overload, especially among those whose initial responsibilities were comparatively light. Thus, caregivers whose obligations rapidly change from limited to extensive also experience the greatest intensification in their sense of being overwhelmed by the demands of care. In contrast, those who start out with heavier loads are not quite as affected by further increases in their care-related responsibilities.

In sum, the exacerbation of subjective stressors from one year to the next depends, at least in part, upon the augmentation of objective primary stressors. The linkages between the objective and subjective aspects of primary stressors are specialized rather than general: role overload increases as the patient becomes more dependent upon the caregiver, role captivity intensifies when disruptive behaviors become even more troublesome, and loss of intimate exchange deepens as the dementia follows its inevitable degenerative course. Although three of the four objective primary stressors are linked to deterioration in one source of subjective stress, the fourth objective stressor, patient resistance, does not contribute independently to the explanation of subsequent states of subjective stress.

Turning now to the impact of background sociodemographic characteristics, Table 6.1 illustrates rather limited effects once care-related stressors are taken into consideration. The absence of a discernible impact is complete for role overload and almost so for loss of the patient. In contrast, role captivity decreases slightly over time among those with high incomes and among ethnic groups other than non-Hispanic whites. Curiously, the duration of care at baseline is negatively related to subsequent role captivity: Those who have been at the task longest have slightly declining levels of feeling trapped in their roles, whereas those who have recently taken up caregiving tend to feel increasingly forced to do one thing as they simultaneously prefer to do another.

> If I want to go anywhere, I go for 1–2 hours while he takes a nap. Otherwise I have to be an available person. I feel stuck.

Although the direct contributions of background and demographic characteristics appear to be limited, their importance should not be overlooked. The background characteristics, as you may recall, emerged as important correlates of primary stressors at baseline. Role overload, role captivity, and loss of intimate exchange, therefore, appear to be linked to caregiver characteristics by two mechanisms. First, these attributes are associated with baseline levels of subjective primary stressors (see chapter 4); their influence upon subsequent levels is transmitted via the stability of these stressors over time. Second, background characteristics are associated with objective primary stressors as well (see chapter 4); their influence on change in subjective stressors over time is conducted by means of change in the objective demands of care as time passes. Thus, the absence of substantial independent associations between sociodemographic characteristics and change in subjective stressors does not mean that these traits are unimportant, rather that their influence is carried by the internal workings of care-related stress processes.

The Impact of Primary Stressors on Secondary Role Strains

We turn now to the second stage in the proliferation model, the conversion of primary stressors into secondary sources of stress; specifically, role strains. As in the previous analysis, the dependent variable is assessed at follow-up (Time 2): in this instance, family conflict, work conflict, or income.[3] In addition to the full array of independent variables included in the previous analyses, the current analysis adds the outcomes of those analyses (i.e., change in subjective primary stressors between Time 1 and Time 2). The model also contains the entire set of secondary role strains assessed at baseline: family conflict, work strain, work reduction, unemployment, income, increased expenses, and insufficient money to meet monthly expenses. Thus, regression coefficients may be interpreted in terms of change produced in the secondary role strains over time. The statistically significant coefficients from these regressions appear in Table 6.2.

As may be seen, the secondary role strains, like the primary stressors, tend to be relatively stable over time. That is, problems experienced in the workplace tend to continue over time, as do strains within the family: Stability coefficients account for 20 to 30% of the variance in these strains at follow-up. Family income remains fairly constant from one year to the next: This auto-regression accounts for three-quarters of the variance in income a year later. In essence, these secondary stressors tend to perpetuate themselves. Each of the secondary role strains, however, also is influenced, at least in part, by the ebb and flow of primary stressors, especially those of a subjective nature. Stressors and background characteristics explain some of the change in income, but there is little change to explain. These variables do a better job of explaining change in the other two role strains: family conflict and work conflict.[4]

Family conflict is intensified when caregivers increasingly feel that care obligations obstruct other life goals. This is the sole stressor to contribute to escalating family conflict. A second factor contributing to changes in family conflict is demographic. Table 6.2 illustrates that compared to other caregivers, wives en-

Table 6.2 Change in Secondary Role Strains over 1 Year as a Function of Primary Stressors

Primary stressors and characteristics	Secondary role strains: Time 2[a]					
	Family conflict		Work conflict[b]		Income	
	b (SE)	β	b (SE)	β	b (SE)	β
Family conflict: Time 1	**.538***** **(.053)**	.526	—	—	—	—
Work conflict: Time 1	—	—	**.441***** **(.104)**	.439	—	—
Income: Time 1	—	—	—	—	**.814***** **(.033)**	.827
Not employed: Time 1	—	—	−.553* (.218)	−.275	—	—
Role captivity: Change Time 2–Time 1	*.120*** *(.044)*	*.154*	*.178** *(.081)*	*.245*	—	—
Role overload: Change Time 2–Time 1	—	—			−2.235* (.928)	−.080
Patient age	—	—	—	—	−.196* (.080)	−.085
Education	—	—	—	—	.546* (.239)	.072
Wife (/other)	−.244* (.119)	−.182	—	—	—	—
R^2 Total	.401***		.460**		.798***	
R^2 Auto-regression	.300***		.212***		.773***	
R^2 Difference	.101*		.248		.025	

[a]Boldface numbers indicate auto-regression variables; italicized numbers indicate stress proliferation.
[b]Limited to caregivers employed at Time 2, $n = 116$.
*$p \leq .05$. **$p \leq .01$. ***$p \leq .001$.

counter declining conflict over time. These two variables explain about 10% of the change in family conflict from one year to the next.

Role captivity is pivotal in linking caregiving to problems encountered at work. As shown in Table 6.2, the relative exacerbation of this state over time produces difficulties at the juncture of caregiving and work. That is, increases in work conflict may be anticipated when role captivity escalates as time passes. In addition, caregivers who entered the workforce between Time 1 and Time 2 have lower levels of work strain at Time 2 than those who were employed at both of these times. These effects are of similar magnitude, albeit of opposite signs, and account for one-quarter of the change over time in conflict between work and caregiving. Finally, although income is highly stable over time, increased levels of role overload are associated with decreased income (i.e., with an intensification of financial strain).

Earlier we saw that the linkages among objective and subjective primary stressors are quite specialized; by contrast, those between primary and secondary stressors seem to be less so. In particular, role captivity seems to be a critical juncture in the translation of care-related stressors into secondary role strains. Role overload, in contrast, appears especially pertinent to financial strains.

The Impact of Primary Stressors on Secondary Intrapsychic Strains

The second aspect of the conversion of primary stressors into secondary sources of stress concerns the genesis or exacerbation of intrapsychic strains. As in the previous analysis, the dependent variable is secondary strain assessed at Time 2: loss of self, lack of caregiver competence, and absence of caregiving gains. The baseline values of these variables are included as independent variables, allowing the regression coefficients to be interpreted as changes in intrapsychic strains over time. In addition to sociodemographic characteristics and extraneous stressors, the independent variables include the primary stressors at Time 1 and the change between Time 1 and Time 2.[5] The statistically significant coefficients from these regressions appear in Table 6.3.

As we have seen with most of the other elements of the stress process, intrapsychic strains tend to perpetuate themselves over time. Each of the auto-regressions accounts for a substantial amount of the variation in intrapsychic strains over time, about 30 to 40%, which may be attributed to the self-perpetuating character of these strains. Again, however, despite their stability, there is considerable room for change in these self-perceptions. Primary stressors and background characteristics make the smallest contribution to explaining changes in lack of caregiver competence and the greatest impact upon loss of self. As may be seen in Table 6.3, each of these strains depends, at least in part, upon changes occurring within the primary stressors over time. The types of primary stressors that sometimes generate intrapsychic strains are illustrated by the caregiver shown here as he moves his wife, gets her settled, and attends to her needs (see photographs 9–12).

This generalization applies least well to the case of lack of caregiver competence.[6] Change in this self-appraisal is influenced by only one of the stressors considered in this analysis, cognitive impairment. As the condition of the patient deteriorates, doubts about oneself as a caregiver abate somewhat. This relationship does not simply signify the impact of practice at performing the role because the duration of caregiving is controlled in the model (although it does not attain statistical significance). Instead, disease progression, as distinct from the mere passage of time, appears to enable caregivers to feel somewhat better about the adequacy of the care they provide. This finding invites speculation that declines

Table 6.3 Change in Secondary Intrapsychic Strains over 1 Year
as a Function of Primary Stressors

	Intrapsychic strains: Time 2[a]					
	Lack of caregiver competence		Absence of caregiving gains		Loss of self	
Primary stressors and characteristics	b (SE)	β	b (SE)	β	b (SE)	β
Lack of caregiver competence: Time 1	**.486***** (**.050**)	**.500**	—	—	.183* (.071)	.123
Absence of caregiving gains: Time 1	—	—	**.553***** (**.046**)	**.575**	—	—
Loss of self: Time 1	—	—	—	—	**.401***** (**.055**)	**.403**
Patient resistance: Time 1	—	—	.178* (.086)	.110	—	—
Cognitive impairment: Change Time 2–Time 1	−.085* (.042)	−.105	—	—	—	—
Role overload: Time 1	—	—	—	—	.143** (.053)	.163
Role overload: Change Time 2–Time 1	—	—	−.123* (.053)	−.115	.133* (.055)	.123
Role captivity: Time 1	—	—	—	—	.119* (.049)	.148
Role captivity: Change Time 2–Time 1	—	—	.101* (.050)	.103	.251*** (.051)	.251
Loss of intimate exchange: Time 1	—	—	—	—	.127* (.059)	.137
Loss of intimate exchange: Change Time 2–Time 1	—	—	−.126* (.057)	−.118	.164** (.058)	.151
ADL dependencies: Change Time 2–Time 1	—	—	−.148* (.060)	−.122	—	—
Education	—	—	.036* (.014)	.124	—	—
San Francisco (/Los Angeles)	—	—	−.271*** (.072)	−.170	—	—
R^2 Total	.384***		.484***		.476***	
R^2 Auto-regression	.324***		.379***		.283***	
R^2 Difference	.060		.105***		.193***	

[a]Boldface numbers indicate auto-regression variables; italicized numbers indicate stress proliferation.
*$p \leq .05$. **$p \leq .01$. ***$p \leq .001$.

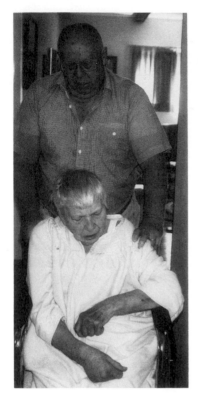
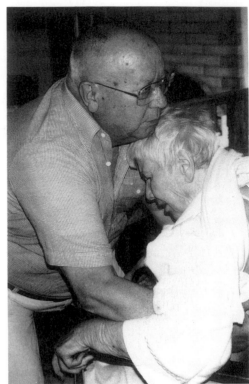

Photographs 9 and 10

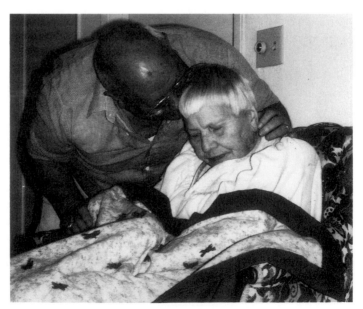

Photograph 11

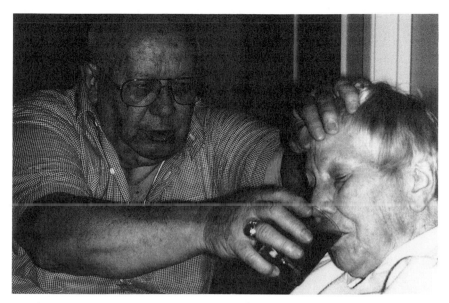

Photograph 12

in cognitive functioning may enable caregivers to attribute unsatisfactory aspects of caregiving to the disease rather than to themselves.

Frank

As we saw earlier, Frank was completely devoted to his wife Beth. When he was no longer able to care for her at home, Frank continued to care for her within a nursing home setting. Her death has left him bereft. In retrospect, he sums up the consequences of his caregiving career:

I didn't realize how far I'd slipped because I had been totally dedicated to taking care of Beth. My social life had gone to pot. I drive aimlessly around to fill the time. I spend too much time at home. My energy level is lower than it should be for the last couple of months. It was high when Beth was here and I had enough energy to do what I did. Funny feeling that I was drawing on reserves. When Beth finally died I began to ebb. I'm trying to recover.

Frank's advice to others who find themselves in the same type of caregiving situation highlights his own sense of depletion:

Try to be totally realistic and don't allow yourself to become a martyr. It will only destroy you and you are worth far less when destroyed. Can't be useful. Take care of the caregiver as fully and carefully as you can. It's like swimming upstream. Don't expect the stream to change directions to accommodate you.

Table 6.3 further reveals that the absence of perceived gains from caregiving is more closely tied to changes occurring within the constellation of primary stressors. The direction of these relationships, however, is the reverse of what one might expect: Deteriorating conditions enable caregivers to feel they have personally been enriched by their caregiving experiences. Thus, increases in ADL dependencies, estrangement from the care recipient, and intensified role overload lead caregivers to identify beneficial aspects of their experiences. In interpreting these coefficients, it should be noted that the baseline values of these primary stressors are also included in the model and, although they are not significant contributors to change in this dependent variable, they are of negative sign. The exceptions to this pattern are shown in Table 6.3: High levels of patient resistance are related to an increase in this source of stress over time, as is an augmented sense of role captivity. These variables exert roughly the same impact on a caregiver's sense of gaining something from being a caregiver. In general, then, the absolute value of these stressors is less important to the development of a sense of achievement than is the magnitude of change experienced from one year to the next. As caregivers provide increasing amounts of assistance to dementia patients from whom they feel more and more separate under conditions of escalating burden, they cultivate beliefs that something has been gained from their hardships; nonetheless, these sentiments are offset to the extent that caregivers feel they are held captive by recalcitrant patients.

I have no goals.

The intrapsychic strain that appears to be most sensitive to primary stressors is loss of self; the intensity and exacerbation of caregiving hardships diminishes a caregiver's sense of identity. As is also apparent in Table 6.3, the baseline and the change scores for three primary stressors are related to increases in self loss over time: role overload, role captivity, and loss of intimate exchange with the dementia patient. That is, when initially high levels of overload, captivity, and loss are coupled with further deterioration in these areas, caregivers are most likely to experience diminishment in their sense of personal identity. The strongest effect is for changes in role captivity. Whatever gains caregivers may experience as a result of the intensification of their caregiving obligations, therefore, apparently occur at some cost to their own self-concept.

The Impact of Primary and Secondary Stressors on Depression

The final component of the stress-proliferation model concerns the conversion of care-related stressors into symptoms of emotional distress, specifically, depression. Depression was assessed with a seven-item scale: "lack enthusiasm for doing anything, feel bored or have little interest in things, cry easily or feel like crying, feel downhearted or blue, feel slowed down or low in energy, have your feelings hurt easily, [and] feel that everything was an effort." Symptoms were rated for the week preceding the interview, with response categories ranging from *no days* (1) through *5 or more days* (4). This measure demonstrates strong internal consistency reliability ($\alpha = .86$).

> The whole thing hit me like a ton of bricks. I felt like all the strength I had had drained out through my heel.

Depression is a rather common experience among caregivers to spouses and parents suffering from dementia. At the time of the baseline interview, the overwhelming majority of caregivers had experienced at least one symptom on one or more days of the preceding week (87.4%). The average caregiver experienced three to four symptoms during that period. Many of these symptoms were ephemeral, however. Nonetheless, 3 in 10 caregivers experienced at least one symptom for most of the preceding week (i.e., for at least 5 days). Furthermore, of those who encountered frequent symptoms, most experienced more than one (71.2%). Overall, 7.9% of the sample reported a majority of depression symptoms (four or more) for most of the preceding week (5 or more days). Thus, most caregivers experienced ephemeral symptoms of depression, but a subgroup experienced numerous symptoms over lengthy periods of time.

Following a now familiar analytic strategy, in this analysis the dependent variable is depression at Time 2. As in preceding analyses, the inclusion of the Time 1 value of depression as an independent variable means that the regression coefficients may be interpreted as accounting for change in depression over 1 year. The independent variables consist of sociodemographic characteristics, as well as the following stressors assessed both at Time 1 and as change from Time 1 to Time 2: objective and subjective primary stressors, secondary role strains and intrapsychic strains, and extrinsic stressors. The significant coefficients from this regression are shown in Table 6.4.

As may be seen, change in depression is related to the progression of both primary and secondary stressors over time. Although depression tends to be relatively stable over time, primary and secondary stressors, along with background characteristics, explain about 20% of the change in depression from year to year.

The absolute amount of role overload and the rate at which overload worsens over time independently contribute to increases in depressive symptomatology among caregivers. The impact of the persistent amount of overload is somewhat more important than the rate at which it is increasing. Thus, feeling overwhelmed by the rigors of caregiving is depressive, especially when this sentiment continues over time and when it becomes more intense. In addition, an increasing sense of role captivity tends to exacerbate emotional distress.

None of the other primary stressors exert independent effects on changes in depression, but several have bivariate associations worth mentioning. Specifically, depression at Time 2 is positively correlated with baseline levels of problematic behavior, patient resistance, and loss of intimate exchange. The impact of

Table 6.4 Change in Depression over 1 Year as a Function of Primary and Secondary Stressors

Primary and secondary stressors, and characteristics	Depression: Time 2[a]	
	b (SE)	β
Depression: Time 1	**.375*** (.052)**	.377
Role overload: Time 1	*.128** (.045)*	*.165*
Role overload: Change Time 2–Time 1	*.094* (.046)*	*.098*
Role captivity: Change Time 2–Time 1	*.101* (.044)*	*.113*
Family conflict: Time 1	*.136* (.059)*	*.117*
Work conflict: Change Time 2–Time 1	*.232* (.090)*	*.124*
Loss of self: Time 1	*.194*** (.057)*	*.217*
Loss of self: Change Time 2–Time 1	*.168*** (.049)*	*.183*
Lack of caregiver competence: Change Time 2–Time 1	*.155* (.066)*	*.107*
Wife (/others)	.248* (.115)	.162
Education	−.023* (.012)	−.090
R^2 total	.616***	
R^2 auto-regression	.416***	
R^2 difference	.200***	

[a]Boldface numbers indicate auto-regression variables; italicized numbers indicate stress proliferation.
*$p \le .05$. **$p \le .01$. ***$p \le .001$.

these other primary stressors on changes in depression, therefore, appears to be transmitted via two pathways: the covariation of these stressors with role overload and role captivity, and their association via the stability of depression over time. The most notable feature of these bivariate results is the virtual independence between cognitive impairment, including its rate of decline over time, and changes in caregiver depression.

The secondary role strains with independent effects on depression concern the domains of work and family. Those who encounter increasing levels of conflict between the demands of work and the demands of care tend to become more depressed over time. Moreover, caregivers with consistently elevated levels of family conflict tend to become more depressed over time. Family and work problems make approximately the same contribution to worsening states of depression.

Although the remaining role strains do not independently contribute to changes in depression, most are related to the absolute level of depression at Time 2 in bivariate analysis. The impact of these role strains, especially economic strains, appears to be captured by the stability of depression over time and by other elements of the stress process.

In Table 6.4, it is apparent that secondary intrapsychic strains also contribute to the development of depression. The loss of self is particularly salient in this regard; concretely, caregivers whose sense of personal identity has been eroded by caregiving tend to become more depressed as time passes, especially when this loss of identity persists over time or is progressive. These coefficients are stronger than those for primary stressors and secondary role strains. It may be noted that like those who lose some of their personal sense of identity, caregivers who feel less proficient as caregiving extends over time also tend to become somewhat more depressed.

Parenthetically, the baseline values of all three intrapsychic strains are significantly correlated to the absolute level of depression at Time 2. The impact of the absence of caregiving gains, therefore, appears to be shared with loss of self and lack of self-appraised competence, as well as with the stability of depression over time.

In addition, wives are inclined to become somewhat more depressed over time, and education often alleviates these symptoms.

Like most other aspects of care-related stress processes, depression tends to be self-perpetuating, with baseline depression accounting for 41.6% of the variation in depression at Time 2. Nonetheless, primary and secondary stressors, both in their intensity and as they intensify, make substantial contributions to declines in emotional well-being.

A Synthesis of the Short Course of Care-Related Stress Proliferation

Figure 6.1 synthesizes the results presented in this section concerning the stress-proliferation process as it unfolds over a 1-year interval. Only major linkages among key constructs are depicted because the detailed results are tabulated in Tables 6.1 through 6.4.

The actual demands imposed by the tasks of providing care exert very specialized effects on the subjective stressors of caregiving. Cognitive impairment influences this process through one principal route: Deteriorating cognition lessens the bond between caregiver and patient which, in turn, is experienced as a loss of personal identity, a loss with depressive consequences. This pathway represents the contribution of the disease itself to the stressors impinging upon the caregiver and his or her emotional well-being. The actual tasks of caregiving, represented by

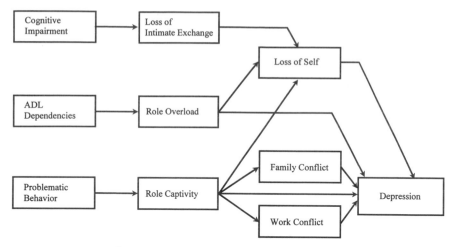

Figure 6.1   Pathways of short-term care-related stress proliferation.

ADL dependencies, also follow a singular route: As these dependencies intensify, caregivers experience an escalating sense of being overwhelmed, which is depressing in and of itself and because it often leads to a loss of personal identity. Disruptive patient behavior is consequential to proliferation because it contributes to the sense of being held captive by caregiving.

All of the subjective primary stressors have depressive effects via their impact upon loss of self. Estrangement from the patient, feeling drained by the burdens of care, and being enveloped by these demands combine to jeopardize the caregiver's sense of being the same person. Role captivity exerts a depressive effect via two secondary stressors as well: intensifying conflict with other relatives and exacerbating tension between the demands of care and the circumstances of paid employment.

Three secondary stressors influence emotional well-being directly, transmitting the effects of the primary stressors: loss of self, family conflict, and work conflict. In addition to their impact transmitted by way of secondary stressors, two primary stressors are depressive on their own: role overload and role captivity. Contrastingly, the impact of loss of intimate exchange is captured completely by the intrapsychic strain loss of self.

Proliferation over the Long-Term

We now turn our attention to the matter of how the elements of the stress process are manifest over a 3-year arc of the caregiving career. As in the preceding analyses, the sample is limited to those who continued to provide care in the home because the setting of care remains constant. Understandably, the number of in-home caregivers declines substantially in the interval between Time 1 and

Time 4, from 555 to 137 persons. Subsequent transitional events and phases of the caregiving career—the placement of relatives in institutional care (chapters 8 and 9), and death and bereavement (chapters 10 and 11)—are considered separately in later chapters.

The regression models are of the same form as those employed in the first part of this analysis with two exceptions: The dependent variables are evaluated at Time 4 and the change variables are calculated as the difference between Time 1 and Time 4.[7] The smaller sample size reduces statistical power, meaning that small effects are less likely to be detected than in the 1-year analysis, a technical problem exacerbated by the large number of variables being considered. Although the regression models contain the full array of independent variables (i.e., baseline and change variables for each stressor),[8] only those variables that attain statistical significance appear in Table 6.5.

There are elements of similarity between the short- and long-term results, as well as striking differences. On the one hand, like the short-term analyses, the long-term analyses suggest that subjective primary stressors are rooted in objective primary stressors (i.e., in the demands of care), and that the subjective states are important to the intensification of depression over lengthy periods of time. On the other hand, increments in secondary sources of stress that accrue over the long haul, with the exception of loss of self, appear to be rather independent of the primary stressors entailed in the provision of care. Furthermore, these secondary stressors generally are not directly tied to long-term changes in the depressive consequences of caregiving.

Rosemary

The protracted course of in-home caregiving can exact an enormous toll from even the most dedicated of caregivers. In the following excerpts, we see how Rosemary was too busy taking care of her husband to attend to her own health.

My hearing is very bad and my sight has deteriorated, especially after I had shingles. I got shingles and didn't realize what it was around my head. One morning I woke up and could hardly see and I went to the doctor. It was too late and it badly affected my eyes.

When she herself suffered a stroke, she "didn't know how to respond" and worried first about her husband:

It was in the morning and he was still upstairs in bed and I was trying to make coffee in the kitchen. With my left hand I was able to dial 911. I couldn't communicate: How was I to tell the people from 911 who came that my husband was upstairs and what to do with him? A neighbor came in, who's very intelligent and she helped them to find my son's phone number. By asking me questions and repeating numbers, to which I could nod a response, she got his phone number out of me. Steven got over here in half the time that it normally takes him to get here, and he took over completely. He abandoned his work and moved in to take care of Peter. His daughter from Detroit came and kept house for me. This was a big sacrifice for her. She was a student in the Ph.D. program at the University of Michigan and it was a real hardship for her, but she came. Steven got a housekeeper for me. Steven did everything. Suzanne stayed until Steven found a housekeeper.

Of her inability to talk after her stroke, Rosemary says:

It drove him wild. He couldn't understand why I didn't talk to him. He never realized that I'd had a stroke. He couldn't understand it, why I was a different person. I used to read out loud to him a lot and I couldn't do that anymore. He took it personally—that I didn't love him anymore.

Table 6.5   Change in Subjective Primary Stressors over 3 Years as a Function of Objective Primary Stressors

| Objective primary stressors and characteristics | Subjective primary stressors: Time 4[a] | | | | | |
| | Role overload | | Role captivity | | Loss of intimate exchange | |
	b (SE)	β	b (SE)	β	b (SE)	β
Role overload: Time 1	**.410*** (.093)**	**.387**	—	—	—	—
Role captivity: Time 1	—	—	**.545*** (.072)**	**.538**	—	—
Loss of intimate exchange: Time 1	—	—	—	—	**.397*** (.099)**	**.399**
Problematic behavior: Time 1	*.487*** (.170)*	*.284*	—	—	—	—
Problematic behavior: Change Time 4–Time 1	*.658*** (.165)*	*.386*	*.461** (.151)*	*.242*	—	—
Cognitive impairment: Change Time 4–Time 1	—	—	—	—	*.220* (.104)*	*.205*
Resistance: Change Time 4–Time 1	—	—	*.509** (.180)*	*.196*	—	—
Duration of care: Time 1	—	—	—	—	*−.107*** (.028)*	*−.340*
White (/other)	—	—	*.439* (.169)*	*.169*	—	—
R^2 total	.463***		.638***		.382***	
R^2 auto-regression	.266***		.454***		.125***	
R^2 difference	.197***		.184***		.257***	

[a]Boldface numbers indicate auto-regression variables; italicized numbers indicate stress proliferation.
*$p \le .05$. **$p \le .01$. ***$p \le .001$.

As may be seen in Table 6.5, each of the subjective stressors displays a substantial amount of stability over the 3-year interval separating Time 1 and Time 4. In addition, each of these stressors is exacerbated over time by intensified stress experienced within the objective conditions of caregiving.

The caregiver's sense of role overload is magnified by an escalation in problematic behaviors displayed by the dementia patient. As shown in the table, both the baseline and change variables for problematic behavior are statistically significant. Role overload, therefore, depends upon both the extent of such behavior and the rate at which it has deteriorated. It should be recalled that these troublesome behaviors tend to be rather stable over 3 years (see Table 5.1). Consequently, role overload is typically exacerbated when dementia patients consistently exhibit intense problematic behaviors over protracted intervals, as well as when their behavior deteriorates. Conversely, when patients consistently display little troublesome behavior or when these behaviors abate, the long-term trajectory improves for caregivers, at least with regard to their sense of being overwhelmed.

This long-term model differs from the short-term model (see Table 6.1) insofar as problematic behavior appears to replace ADL dependencies as the primary influence on role overload.[9] These two stressors, ADL dependencies and problematic behavior, are similar in that they pertain to the intensity of the caregiver's direct involvement in patient care. They differ, however, with regard to the nature of the tasks performed by the caregiver, for example, assisting with personal care and household maintenance versus controlling the patient when he or she acts in a troublesome or disruptive manner. Additionally, ADL dependencies and problematic behavior are incongruous with regard to their long-term trajectory: As reported in chapter 4, ADL dependencies increase progressively over time, whereas problematic behaviors are rather independent of illness duration (see Figure 4.3). These patterns invite speculation that over the long haul, caregivers are able to anticipate and adjust to expected increases in patient dependency, but that erratic behaviors pose more of a challenge precisely because their appearance cannot be anticipated with the same degree of certainty.

Problematic patient behavior also appears to be at the center of changes in role captivity, a pattern that is consistent with the short-term relationships discussed previously (compare Tables 6.1 and Table 6.5). The deterioration of behavior over time seems to be more important than the intensity of such problems per se. Table 6.5 shows a second patient behavior also contributes to increasing role captivity: patient resistance to the caregiver's efforts to help. Thus, two behavioral dimensions are implicated in the caregiver's sense of being held captive by a tightening web of care-related restraints: troublesome actions on the part of the dementia patient and his or her resistance to aid. In both cases, it is the worsening of conditions that intensifies role captivity.

The final subjective primary stressor, loss of intimate exchange, depends upon cognitive impairment, a relationship that emerged for the short-term analysis (compare Tables 6.1 and 6.5) too. Over the long-term, the absolute level of impairment appears to matter less than the rate at which cognitive abilities have deteriorated given that the change variable attains statistical significance, but the baseline measure does not (although it is included in the full regression model). In addition, this sense of loss appears to fade over time when caregiving itself is of lengthy duration. The impact of illness duration, it should be noted, is independent of the effects of cognitive impairment. Thus, the influence of cognitive decline on loss of intimate exchange appears to be mitigated somewhat by lengthy involvement in caregiving.

Perhaps the most striking difference between short- and long-term stress proliferation and their effects is reflected in the relatively minor part played by the secondary stressors over the 3-year span. Unlike what was observed for the 1-year interval, the results for the longer period do not reveal any prominent functions for secondary stressors, either role strains or intrapsychic strains. With the exception of loss of self, these strains do not significantly depend upon any of the primary stressors. Moreover, the contribution of secondary stressors to long-term changes in depressive symptomatology is immaterial, again with the exception of loss of self. Secondary stressors that contribute to depression in the short run, such as family and work conflict, do not appear to play major roles in the long-term escalation of the depressive consequences of caregiving. As a result, we present in Table 6.6 only the regression analyses pertaining to loss of self and to depressive symptoms.

As may be seen in the table, loss of self over a 3-year interval depends importantly upon the caregiver's experience of role captivity, a finding isomorphic to the results for the 1-year interval (see Table 6.3). Both the baseline and change terms for role captivity are statistically significant. Thus, the amount of role captivity, as well as the rate at which it is intensifying, produces a diminished sense of personal identity over a prolonged course of caregiving. As noted previously, role captivity itself tends to be moderately stable over time (see Table 5.1). Loss of self, therefore, often occurs when role captivity is consistently elevated or has increased appreciably over long periods.

Increments in depressive symptomatology over a protracted period of caregiving are associated with increments in role overload, role captivity, and increased expenses, as also illustrated in Table 6.6. In each instance, it is change in the stressor, as distinct from amount per se, that influences increased depressive symptomatology. Thus, difficult circumstances, in and of themselves, do not seem to intensify depression over lengthy intervals of caregiving, rather it is the magnification of these difficulties that ignites a worsening spiral of emotional distress. Once again, noticeably absent from the long-term results is a substantial contribution from secondary stressors. The sole independent effect is for increased expenses, which is associated with an exacerbation of depression.

Loss of self, which plays a pivotal role in mediating the short-term depressive consequences of primary stressors (see Table 6.4), does not emerge as an independent contributor in the long-term analysis. It should be noted, however, that loss of self is highly correlated with both role captivity ($r = .493, p \leq .001$) and role overload ($r = .375, p \leq .001$), two of the factors independently contributing to changes in depression. Moreover, loss of self is associated strongly with contemporaneous levels of depressive symptoms ($r = .451, p \leq .001$). This correlation is similar in magnitude to that observed between depression on the

Table 6.6 Change in Loss of Self and Depression over 3 Years
as a Function of Primary Stressors

Primary and secondary stressors, and characteristics	Loss of self: Time 4		Depression: Time 4[a]	
	b (SE)	β	b (SE)	β
Loss of self: Time 1	**.303***** (**.086**)	**.308**	—	—
Depression: Time 1	—	—	**.309**** (**.092**)	**.311**
Role overload: Change Time 4–Time 1	—	—	*.197** (*.083*)	*.232*
Role captivity: Time 1	*.349**** (*.082*)	*.427*	—	—
Role captivity: Change Time 4–Time 1	*.527**** (*.091*)	*.524*	*.243** (*.105*)	*.266*
Increased expenses: Time 4	—	—	*.258** (*.127*)	*.173*
Daughter caring for mother (/other)	−.449* (.208)	−.241	—	—
White (/other)	—	—	−.343* (.159)	−.182
R^2 total	.551***		.629***	
R^2 auto-regression	.195***		.264***	
R^2 difference	.356***		.365***	

[a]Boldface numbers indicate auto-regression variables; italicized numbers indicate stress proliferation.
*$p \leq .05$.   **$p \leq .01$.   ***$p \leq .001$.

one hand, and role captivity ($r = .454$, $p \leq .001$) and role overload ($r = .478$, $p \leq .001$) on the other; these two subjective stressors are themselves highly correlated ($r = .426$, $p \leq .001$).[10] This pattern suggests that multicollinearity is responsible for the lack of an observed independent depressive impact for loss of self. In essence, the impact of loss of identity on depression appears to be shared in common with the impact of role overload and role captivity. This interpretation is consistent with the short-term model portrayed in Figure 6.1, although in this instance, loss of self independently contributes to a worsening of depression.

I needed bypass surgery: I didn't realize that I was having major health problems. I thought it was depression.

Figure 6.2 summarizes the main factors contributing to increments in depressive symptomatology emerging over a protracted course of caregiving (i.e.,

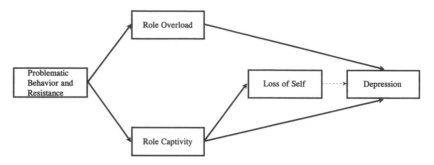

Figure 6.2   Long-term increments in depression.

over 3 years). This system is driven by the behavior of the dementia patient—troublesome and disruptive behavior, as well as resistance against the caregiver. As problematic behaviors persist and intensify, the subjective burdens experienced by the caregiver also escalate. These subjective stressors are specific to the role of caregiver, tapping sentiments of being overwhelmed and engulfed by this role. Increments in the stressors, in turn, are accompanied by a worsening of the caregiver's depressive symptomatology.

In addition, the caregiver's sense of personal identity is eroded by a continuing or intensifying sense of being held captive by caregiving. Although this loss of identity lacks a definitive linkage to increments in depression, the suggestive evidence indicates that loss of self mediates at least some of the depressive impact of care-related stress, especially that entailing the sense of being tied to caregiving while preferring to do otherwise. Finally, depressive symptomatology lessens when interactions with the dementia patient are relatively free of problematic behavior, or when these interactions become easier over time, an effect that is mediated by role overload and role captivity.

Summary

This chapter has demonstrated that the primary demands of caregiving generate problems in other areas of life and damage emotional well-being, a process we identify as stress proliferation. Some of the highlights of the findings include the following:

• Over a 1-year period, poor and deteriorating cognitive functioning leads to an increased sense of having lost one's relationship to the patient; behavior problems, especially those that escalate, produce an intensification of role captivity; and expanding patient dependency upon the caregiver generates role overload, particularly among those whose initial responsibilities were circumscribed.

• Increases in primary stressors are accompanied by increments in certain role strains and by an erosion of personal identity, secondary stressors with depressive consequences manifest across an interval of 1 year.

• As the primary conditions of care worsen over the course of 1 year, caregivers change their appraisals of themselves in relation to caregiving, generally for the better. They lessen doubts about their skills in performing care-related tasks and generate a sense of having gained something from these hardships.

• Over a longer arc of the caregiving career, 3 years, increases in objective stressors intensify subjective stressors which, in turn, exacerbate the depressive consequences of caregiving.

• Secondary stressors, however, appear rather separate from long-term increments in care-related stress and its depressive sequelae.

• Augmentations in depression over the long-term appear to be triggered by unmanageable patient behavior and mediated by role overload and role captivity.

• The impact of sociodemographic characteristics on subsequent exposure to care-related stressors appears to be indirect, transmitted via the stability of these stressors over time.

• The influence of sociodemographic characteristics on changes in depression as time passes is largely indirect, relayed by way of the stability of care-related stressors and the association of these stressors with depression.

Discussion

At this point, it is useful to recall that the analyses of stress proliferation described in this chapter pertain to changes in emotional distress over time as distinct from the amount of distress per se. In both the short- and long-term analyses, the inclusion of the baseline level of depression captures and conveys the cumulative impact of conditions generating distress in the first place.

Hence, it is worthwhile to note briefly the baseline correlates of depression. These correlates include most of the primary stressors entailed in the actual provision of care; secondary role strains in the areas of family, work, and finances; and all of the role-specific intrapsychic strains. Sociodemographic characteristics also are associated with baseline levels of depression: Husbands tend to be somewhat less distressed than other caregivers and these symptoms are inversely associated with income. These two factors mirror patterns repeatedly observed in the general population; namely, men tend to be less depressed than women, and depression is inversely related to socioeconomic status (SES).

Clearly, the conditions of care, their intrusion into other domains of life, role-specific self-perceptions, and depression are intertwined at the start of the study. These correlations represent the accumulation of prior care-related stress processes. The effects are perpetuated over time by the self-sustaining nature of care-related stressors.

In contrast, the longitudinal analyses reported in this chapter reveal how this system maintains itself in the short-term and over a protracted course of in-home caregiving. The historical accretion of care-related stress and its emotional costs are taken into consideration in the analyses with the inclusion of baseline levels of the conditions. In effect, then, the longitudinal analyses identify circumstances that alter the equilibrium of this system.

It is evident that the patient's impairment, its behavioral manifestations, and the resulting dependencies are a core catalyst in the stress-proliferation process, especially the *rate* of decline exhibited as time progresses. Waning cognitive abilities and the erosion of the patient's persona represent a persistent force upon caregivers. The patient's decline in these areas is inevitable and consequential for the caregiver's sense of self and his or her emotional well-being. The impact of these clinical considerations is most evident relatively quickly insofar as these effects emerge over 1 year.

The primary demands impinging upon the caregiver, however, do not necessarily intensify over time, and it is the ebb and flow of these conditions that contribute most forcefully to processes of stress proliferation. In particular, both ADL dependencies and problematic patient behavior, although somewhat stable over time, expand and contract over the short-term. These objective conditions stimulate changes in the caregiver's subjective evaluation of his or her situation, especially with regard to feeling restrained by caregiving and overwhelmed by its demands. These subjective states, in turn, generate increments in emotional distress over both short and long intervals of caregiving.

A striking aspect of the longitudinal results reported in this chapter concerns the role played by secondary stressors when considering short-term versus long-term stress proliferation. Over the 1-year interval, these stressors are linked to the primary stressors of caregiving and are consequential to the caregiver's emotional well-being. In contrast, these stressors appear to be largely disconnected from the conditions of caregiving and their emotional sequelae over the 3-year interval.

In this regard, it is important to recall that caregivers who continued to provide in-home care over the long haul became an increasingly select group. This pattern was described in the previous chapter in reference to the average course of various stressors over time (see Figures 5.1 and 5.2). Specifically, caregivers appeared to discontinue providing in-home care (i.e., institutionalize patient or experience bereavement) when cognitive impairment was severe, they became extensively engaged in the work of providing care, and caregiving conditions were experienced as burdensome. In contrast, no such selection effects were observed for the secondary stressors. Thus, compared to those who exited the in-home caregiving phase, the long-term continuing care subsample started the study caring for dementia patients with low levels of impairment who required circumscribed care and thus, limited hardship was imposed upon the caregiver. These two groups were comparable, however, in the extent to which they experienced secondary sources of stress. Furthermore, for in-home caregivers as a group, the amount of secondary stress remained at the same average level of intensity as time passed even though the amount of primary stress increased.

These patterns suggest that exits from in-home caregiving act as brakes for an otherwise runaway train of escalating care-related stress. In some sense, death of the dementia patient inherently halts stress proliferation because care is no longer required. Although bereavement poses its own adaptational challenges (see chapter 11), caregiving itself no longer possesses the potential to intrude into other areas of life (i.e., to generate secondary sources of stress). The admission of one's impaired relative to a nursing home, in contrast, is a purposive act. Thus, caregivers who are pushed to their limits may turn to institutional care, which has the effect of containing secondary stressors.

The extent to which institutionalization, death of the care recipient, or both of these career transitions acts to constrain stress proliferation is taken up in subsequent chapters (see chapters 9 and 11). At this point, we turn to the issue of how caregivers manage to contain this process while they remain in the in-home care phase of role enactment.

Notes

[1] Change scores are calculated as Time 2 minus Time 1. For patient resistance, which is dichotomous, the change score is a dummy variable scored as 1 for patients who started to resist between Time 1 and Time 2, and as 0 in all other instances.

[2] The interaction terms are calculated by multiplying the change score by the baseline score and are included in regression models only when statistically significant.

[3] The other indicators of secondary role strains are categorical and display too little change over time to permit meaningful multivariate analysis: unemployment, work reduction, insufficient money, and increased expenses.

[4] The difference between the complete model and the auto-regression is not statistically significant for income or for work conflict, even though the latter increment is quite large. Because this analysis is restricted to those working at Time 2, this anomaly may be attributed to the large number of variables added to the model and to the reduction in sample size.

[5] The interaction of baseline and change scores did not attain statistical significance in any instance and, therefore, is not included.

[6] The difference in R^2 is not significant for caregiver competence. Also, because the increment is small relative to the large number of variables added to the model, this coefficient should be viewed cautiously.

[7] A final difference is the deletion of extraneous stressors from the multivariate model. The baseline measure emerged as a statistically significant predictor of role overload, role captivity, and loss of intimate exchange in multivariate analysis; the change variable, however, did not independently contribute to any of these outcomes. The Time 1 and Time 4 extraneous stress measures are not associated at the bivariate level with the outcomes of interest, either within or across time. We regard the multivariate terms, therefore, as happenstance, especially because these extraneous stressors have proved to be unimportant to understanding care-related stress processes in the other analyses reported throughout this book. Nonetheless, it is possible that the baseline levels of extraneous stress represent a complex sleeper effect, with eventful stress in one's social network producing an increased sense of subjective stress several years later.

[8] The inclusion of both baseline and change variables simplifies the interpretation of significant coefficients even when only one of the two attains statistical significance.

[9] It should be emphasized that this difference is not an artifact of multicollinearity because ADL dependencies and problematic behavior are only modestly correlated with one another within and across time. Moreover, ADL dependencies lack significant bivariate association with role overload over the long-term interval.

[10] These correlations are for Time 4 values of the variables.

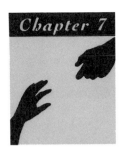

The Containment of Care-Related Stressors

In observing the proliferation of stressors, we are able to capture the changing realities faced by caregivers caught up in difficult circumstances, especially as these conditions continue over time. Stress proliferation also provides a partial answer to the question of why people exposed to seemingly similar stressors are affected by them in dissimilar ways. This variability may be due to the emergence of secondary stressors in that persons who are alike with regard to primary stressors may, nonetheless, be quite unalike with regard to their total exposure to care-related stressors. However, even if we were clever enough to identify and measure all of the stressors to which caregivers are exposed, there would remain considerable variability in observed outcomes.

An additional explanation for the differential impact of care-related stressors is that caregivers possess varying amounts and kinds of resources that mitigate the consequences of exposure to stress. These resources, which are the focus of this chapter, are made up of certain characteristics, dispositions, and relationships that have the capacity to protect caregivers from the full power of stressors. Correspondingly, those lacking resources are more susceptible to the impact of caregiving exigencies.

In addition to serving as a guide to the observation of emergent stressors, the stress process model is a useful framework for directing attention to the points at which the protective functions of resources may be detected. These resources may influence not only the ultimate outcome of care-related stressors, such as the level of depression, but also the intermediate outcomes located at the various junctures of the stress process. Elsewhere it has been argued that confining attention to the final outcome, the standard method for assessing the efficacy of psychosocial resources, is insufficient because it fails to attend to these inter-mediary links (Aneshensel, in press; Pearlin, 1989; Pearlin et al., 1990). Our model of proliferation suggests additional points at which resources may affect the unfolding of the stress process; namely, the degree to which they regulate the conversion of objective demands into subjective stressors and the degree to which these primary stressors lead to those that are secondary. The multiple points at which the functions of resources may be observed in the stress process model unavoidably and substantially complicate the analytic task. We believe, however, that this broad view of the functions of resources yields a more detailed and realistic picture of the strengths and vulnerabilities of caregivers immersed in situations of sustained hardship. In particular, it reveals that the entire stress process may be constrained by social and personal resources and, in this way, indirectly reduce the risk of deleterious outcomes.

The central task of the present chapter is to demonstrate the empirical basis for the above statement. Before moving to the data, it is first necessary to describe the ways in which resources are assessed and, following this, to consider the various mechanisms by which resources may constrain the stress process.

Psychosocial Resources: Social Support and Mastery

Our analysis focuses upon two types of coping resources, social assets in the form of *social support*, and personal assets in the form of a sense of *mastery* or *self-efficacy*.

Social Support

In general terms, social support refers to the satisfaction of a person's basic social needs—affection, esteem, approval, belonging, identity, and security—

through interaction with others (Cobb, 1976; Thoits, 1982). House and Kahn (1985) have identified three distinct dimensions of social support: (1) integration, the existence of social relations; (2) networks, the structure of social relations; and (3) support, the functional content of social relations, including socioemotional, instrumental, informational, and appraisal dimensions.

Our evaluation of social support emphasizes two functional components: instrumental and socioemotional support. There are two major categories of instrumental support: *informal,* provided by family or friends, and *formal,* provided by trained people who are paid for their help. We employ three indicators of instrumental support: informal hands-on assistance with the patient; informal assistance with household chores and logistics; and formal assistance in the way of social services performed by trained, paid personnel, such as an in-home attendant. We measured informal instrumental support by asking two questions: "Is there a friend or relative who helps you look after your (relative) on a *regular* basis, for example, who stays with (him/her) or who helps (him/her) do things like bathing or dressing?" and "Now think about the household chores or tasks that you have to do, things like shopping, cleaning, or laundry. In a typical month, do you ever get any help, from your friends or relatives, with these or other household chores?"

How many caregivers received informal help with the care they provided? At the start of the study, about one in three caregivers reported receiving regular help with the care of the patient. This aid was most often provided by daughters, sons, sisters, brothers, or friends. Although a diverse group of other relatives also helped regularly (e.g., in-laws and nieces), no one specific category predominated. Overall, one in five caregivers evaluated the total assistance received from family and friends as being far less than needed. Thus, most family caregivers did not receive regular help with the care of the dementia patient, and a substantial minority rated all help received from family and friends as insufficient compared to need.

Fewer caregivers received regular assistance with household chores: one in four. Daughters, sons, husbands, and siblings were the most common sources of regular help; other relatives and friends also contributed, but not as often as immediate family members. A substantial minority of caregivers (16.0%), however, reported not wanting help with domestic chores. Nonetheless, there was considerable unmet need in this area: In considering those without regular help, about half obtained no help at all or help that was far less than what they required. Overall, two out of three caregivers received less help than they needed with domestic chores, care of the patient, or both of these activities.

If you ask enough people, you can get help.

Formal instrumental assistance was measured by asking how often the caregiver used each of 16 services. Several of these services were used too infrequently to be of analytic value. Therefore, we focus upon the following: home health care or a visiting nurse, Alzheimer's day care, adult day care, out-of-home respite care, and in-home attendant or companion. Some analyses concentrate exclusively on the latter, which was used by 3 out of 10 caregivers. Among this group, two out of three had such help more than half of the time (i.e., at least four times a week). Although informal help with patient care and domestic chores are correlated with one another ($r = .36, p \leq .001$), neither is correlated with having an in-home attendant; that is, the formal and informal receipt of help appear to be relatively independent of one another.[1]

The socioemotional side of social support was assessed by asking how strongly the caregiver agreed or disagreed with eight statements about their friends and family (exclusive of the dementia patient). These items[2] evaluate the perceived availability of individuals who are understanding ("there is really no one who understands what you are going through"*), caring ("the people close to you let you know that they care about you, you have people around you that help you to keep your spirits up, [and] there are people in your life that make you feel good about yourself"), and familiar or trustworthy ("you have a friend or relative in whose opinions you have confidence, you have someone that you feel you can trust, you have at least one friend or relative you can really confide in, [and] you have at least one friend or relative you want to be with when you are feeling down or discouraged"). This scale has response categories ranging from *strongly disagree* (1) to *strongly agree* (4) and displays strong reliability ($\alpha = .87$). The average of the responses yields a mean of 3.23 ($SD = .51$), which indicates that the caregivers generally felt a strong connection to their social networks, although some were completely isolated, scoring at the lowest value on this measure.

If we were to describe the social support received by the typical caregiver, two dimensions would warrant emphasis. The average caregiver receives less informal assistance than needed with the tasks of caregiving and maintaining a household, and this shortage is not compensated for adequately by the use of an in-home attendant. On the other hand, despite this unmet need, caregivers generally feel cared for and connected to their friends and relatives. None of the instrumental support measures is significantly correlated with sentiments of emotional support. Clearly, therefore, this sentiment is fostered by factors other than the direct help received with instrumental tasks of caregiving. As suggested by this woman, who is caring for her mother, support may be derived from the mere presence of other family (see photographs 13–15).

Mastery

The second type of resource, mastery, is personal rather than social in nature: It is the control individuals feel they are able to exercise over forces importantly affecting their lives (Pearlin et al., 1981, 1990; Pearlin & Schooler, 1978). Mastery is a cognitive orientation attributing outcomes, such as success and failure, to personal characteristics like ability and effort (Pearlin & Schooler, 1978). Mirowsky and Ross (1984) equated the concepts of mastery, self-efficacy, internal

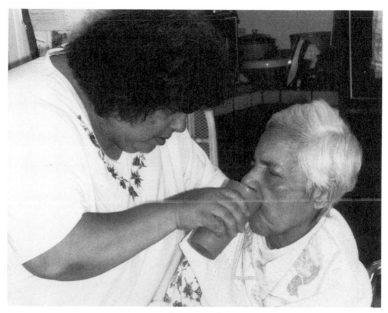

Photograph 13

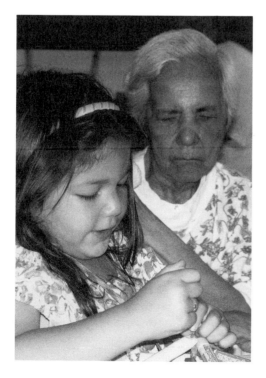

Photograph 14

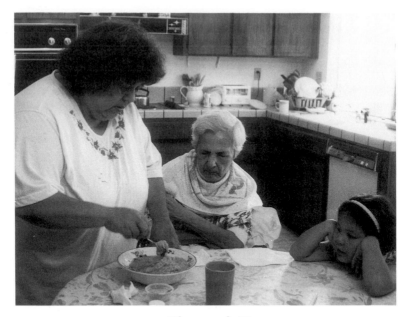

Photograph 15

locus of control, personal control, perceived control of the environment, and instrumentalism, concepts that are opposite in meaning to fatalism, external locus of control, powerlessness, and learned helplessness.

Our measure of mastery is the summation of seven items rated from *strongly disagree* (1) to *strongly agree* (4). These items include the following:[3]

> There is really no way I can solve some of the problems I have,* sometimes I feel that I'm being pushed around in life,* I have little control over the things that happen to me,* I can do just about anything I really set my mind to do, I often feel helpless in dealing with the problems of life,* what happens to me in the future mostly depends on me, [and] there is little I can do to change many of the important things in my life.*

The mastery scale displays strong internal consistency reliability ($\alpha = .75$). Its mean value of 2.81 ($SD = .50$) signifies that, on average, caregivers feel considerable control over their lives, although some feel virtually no control, scoring the lowest value on the measure.

Thus, despite the inexplicable occurrence of dementia and the intractable course of the disease, many of those who are caught up in caregiving maintain a sense of being in control of their lives. Mastery is not associated with any of the indicators of instrumental social support, informal or formal, but is positively correlated with socioemotional support ($r = .32, p \leq .001$): Caregivers who feel efficacious also tend to feel cared for by others.

Given that the stressors associated with caring for someone with dementia generally are not easily managed, a belief in personal control may appear counterproductive. Mastery, however, appears to exert pervasively positive effects on emotional well-being, challenging this inference. This contradiction has been considered with regard to the overall relationship between stress and emotional well-being. Wheaton (1980), for example, maintained that although external attributions may be beneficial in some specific circumstances, they are pervasively harmful because they make goals of social action seem less attainable, undermining motivation. Thoits (1987) similarly suggested that a sense of control lessens the emotional impact of uncontrollable events by encouraging active problem solving in their aftermath. Even in the context of the stubborn difficulties spawned by a progressive dementia, therefore, mastery should help to lessen their influence on emotional well-being.

The Ebb and Flow of Psychosocial Resources

In general, psychosocial resources tend to be stable over time, but at the individual level, some caregivers enjoy gains, whereas others suffer losses. Half of these caregivers (49.1%) had insufficient informal help with patient care at both Time 1 and Time 2, and less than a quarter had informal help at both times (22.4%); gains (15.2%) and losses (13.2%) over time tended to offset one another. This pattern is even more pronounced for informal help with chores: Nearly two out of three caregivers lacked such help at Time 1 and Time 2; the remainder were equally divided among the stable presence of help and its loss or gain over time. A somewhat different pattern emerges for the use of a formal in-home attendant. Again, the majority of caregivers (56.8%) lacked assistance at both times, and out of those who had this help, few (20.4%) had it consistently over time. Nonetheless, more caregivers (18.5%) acquired in-home attendants than lost them (4.3%). In sum, the total number of caregivers who received informal help with patient care or with household chores remains relatively constant across time, but there is a net gain in the use of formal attendants. Nevertheless, the modal pattern for all types of instrumental assistance is its continued absence.

Subjective resources also tend to be rather stable over the course of 1 year. Mean levels of socioemotional support and mastery are approximately the same at baseline and follow-up. Moreover, there is substantial correlation across these times for both socioemotional support ($r = .55$) and mastery ($r = .65$).

Sustained, Acquired, and Lapsed Resources

The long-term constellation of psychosocial resources to some extent resembles that observed over the short-term. Despite an additional 3 years of incumbency in the caregiver role, most caregivers lacked adequate hands-on assistance with patient care and household chores, but, nonetheless, felt cared for by others and believed they had substantial control over their lives.

Among those who continued to provide in-home care, there was an appreciable net loss from Time 1 to Time 4 of instrumental assistance from family and friends with patient care (39.9% vs. 28.6%), a steady state of assistance with household chores (24.1% vs. 27.7%), and a substantial net gain in the use of paid in-home attendants (21.9% vs. 44.5%). Very few of those caregivers who lacked regular instrumental assistance at Time 1 acquired this type of aid by Time 4. Such gains are least common with regard to help from family and friends with patient care (12.5%), modest for informal assistance with household chores (21.2%), and most common with regard to paid in-home attendants (33.6%). However, some caregivers who received support at Time 1 lost this aid by Time 4. These decreases are most marked for informal help with patient care (47.2%) and household chores (51.5%), and least common for paid in-home attendants (16.7%). The mean level of socioemotional support remains fairly stable from Time 1 to Time 4 (3.21 vs. 3.08), and the average level of self-efficacy is also similar at these two points in time (2.83 vs. 2.73).

In general, then, for help with patient care, caregivers come to rely increasingly on formal sources of assistance as the interval of in-home care grows longer and there is a concomitant decrease in access to and use of informal sources of help. These changes pertain to shifts in the average level of resources, but at the individual level, some caregivers gain while others lose.

Resources and Their Naturalistic Interventions

The analyses presented in this chapter are oriented to learning how social psychological resources influence the unfolding of the stress process and, therefore, help to account for differences in the effects of care-related stressors. This line of inquiry is not new as it has been followed in a substantial body of prior stress research. Most of this literature has examined the effects of resources in two ways. One means has been to explore what are referred to as buffering effects, which posit that the protective functions of resources become more pronounced as the level of the stressors to which people are exposed increases. This idea suggests a type of distributive justice in that people whose lives are the most difficult are thought to benefit most from the possession of psychosocial resources. Operationally, buffering effects are detected through the interactions of stressors and resources on various outcomes. The search for these buffering effects at the various junctures of the stress process is one of the major tasks of our analysis.

A second type of protective pathway that is also prominent in stress research is represented by what are referred to as the main effects of resources. Unlike those that are interactive, main effects are independent of exposure to stressors. In the case of caregiving, for example, the magnitude of the protective effect of the resource would have nothing to do with the magnitude of the stressors: Those under heavy demands and those under light demands would benefit equally. Again, the additive effects of resources will be closely examined below.

The analysis of buffering and main effects is surrounded by some complicating considerations that should be recognized. Concretely, the analysis of these functions typically assumes that the resources are acting upon the stress process and its outcomes without themselves being changed by the very process that they are affecting. Of course, the level of resources might remain stable over time, but it might also enhance or deplete over time partly as a result of exposure to the same stressors the resources are ameliorating (Ensel & Lin, 1991; Wheaton, 1985). Looked at in this way, resources are cast not solely as reactive elements in the stress process, but as active elements that shape the subsequent occurrence of care-related stressors.

Resources as Stress Mediators and Moderators

Mediating Processes

Stress mediators, like social support and mastery, must be associated not only with exposure to stress, but also with the outcome of interest. These conditions pertain to any intervening variable, which must depend upon the independent variable and affect the dependent variable. Thus, social support and mastery must be influenced by exposure to stress and, in turn, must influence well-being.

The first step in our analysis, therefore, evaluates the extent to which social support and mastery are influenced by the primary and secondary stressors of caregiving. In theory, these coping resources may be unchanged, enhanced, or depleted by exposure to stress (Ensel & Lin, 1991; Wheaton, 1985). The first possibility—care-related stress does not alter, positively or negatively, coping resources like social support and mastery—is referred to by Ensel and Lin (1991) as the *stress-deterrent model* because psychosocial resources act independently to enhance well-being, offsetting the impact of care-related stress.[4]

The second and third possibilities fall under Ensel and Lin's (1991) general classification of coping resource models, which cast psychosocial resources as reactive elements in the stress process, triggered by the occurrence of external stressors. The *stress-suppression model* posits that the emergence or intensification of stress mobilizes a resource, such as social support or self-efficacy, and then consequently, distress is alleviated. As life difficulties worsen, an individual may rely more heavily upon his or her internal strengths, receive more aid and succor from social ties, or experience both of these gains. In stark contrast, the third possibility is that stress depletes psychosocial resources. Those providing social support may tire of the task and turn away, or inner resolve may be eroded. Ensel and Lin (1991) referred to this alternative as the *deterioration model*: stressors reduce or weaken resources.

To assess mediational effects, psychosocial resources were added to the regression analyses reported in chapter 6. These results may be summarized quite briefly: No empirical evidence of stress mediation was found. In some instances (see below), the psychosocial resources themselves were related to the outcome.

However, in none of these analyses did the addition of the psychosocial resources appreciably alter the regression coefficients for the effect of a stressor on an outcome. Thus, these psychosocial resources do not appear to mediate the impact of care-related stressors on other care-related stressors or on the caregiver's emotional well-being.

As a part of this analysis, we also considered the question of whether the psychosocial resources available to caregivers are affected by the stressors they encounter. Although these associations do not serve a mediational function, we summarize them briefly because they are informative about who has access to resources and whether resources are aligned with need.

In cross-sectional analysis, caregiver attributes appear most important to informal social support, whereas stressful conditions encountered in providing care appear most important to formal support, socioemotional support, and mastery. The most predominant characteristic is kin relationship: Spousal caregivers, especially wives, are markedly more likely than adult children to receive help with the care of the patient and domestic chores, yet, husbands and wives are least likely to feel cared for by others and to believe they are in control of their lives. Also, income is an important contributor to socioemotional support and mastery: These sentiments are most pronounced among the prosperous. Only one care-related stressor is positively associated with resources: Problematic behavior prompts the use of an in-home attendant. In contrast, other associations are negative: The actual demands and constraints of caregiving are accompanied by a depletion of psychosocial resources.

The longitudinal results echo several of the themes present in the cross-sectional analyses. Specifically, change in informal instrumental assistance—help received from family and friends with patient care and household chores—is largely independent of the dynamics of care-related stress proliferation. Only two stressors attain statistical significance: Caregivers who consistently carry a heavy burden of ADL dependencies tend to gain help with patient care over time, and those who encounter increased problematic behavior typically acquire help with chores. Change in formal support—acquiring an in-home attendant—depends upon two critical factors: the state of patient impairment and family income. Several stressors are related to declines in mastery, socioemotional support, or both of these resources: lack of caregiver competence, role captivity, loss of identity, work strain, and lack of caregiving gains. Finally, characteristics of the caregiver have little to no impact on changes in psychosocial resources over time.

People get tired of hearing your tale of woe.

In sum, when care-related stress affects resources, the relationships are more often negative than positive. That is, stressors appear more likely to deplete resources than to enhance them, although in select instances need does indeed appear to elicit support.

Moderating Processes

Thus far, we have considered whether social psychological resources mediate the impact of care-related stressors. The social psychological resources considered here, however, do not appear to mediate the impact of care-related stressors to any appreciable extent. Mediation, nonetheless, represents only one means by which social psychological resources might affect the impact of care-related stressors. The other major route concerns *stress moderation* of these stressors. Such effect moderation entails a contingency among stress, resource, and outcome: The impact of stress is greater among those lacking resources than among those who receive assistance from social networks or formal helpers, feel cared for by their friends and family, or feel a sense of control over their lives.

We now turn to the question of whether psychosocial resources affect the impact of stressors on various outcomes. These resources were treated as intervening variables in the preceding analysis, the conduit through which stressors are linked to outcomes. Here, resources are treated as effect modifiers, as altering the magnitude of the relationship between stressor and outcome. Specifically, the effects of stressors are hypothesized to vary inversely with resources (i.e., to decrease in magnitude as resources increase). This configuration of stressor, outcome, and resource usually is referred to as stress buffering (see Wright et al., 1993, for a recent review of stress buffering among caregivers).[5] The form of the relationship is conditional: The impact of a stressor depends upon how much of the resource is present. This association typically is modeled as a statistical interaction, the stressor multiplied by the resource.

We examined these interactional terms in relation to all of the outcomes examined in chapter 6 (i.e., subjective primary stressors, secondary stressors, and depression). The explanatory efficacy of two models were compared to determine the importance of conditional effects. The first model contained the stressors and background variables previously determined to be related to changes in an element of the stress process over time (see Tables 6.1 through 6.4), the resource, and its change between Time 1 and Time 2. The alternative model added the interaction of the resource with all of the stressors from the preceding model. An F test was used to analyze the statistical significance of the increment in explained variance that was obtained with the addition of the stress-buffering terms. To reduce problems of multicollinearity, separate models were estimated for each of the five resources: informal instrumental help with the patient, informal instrumental help with household chores, the presence of an in-home attendant, socioemotional support, and mastery.

The results are straightforward: The inclusion of the stress-buffering interaction terms did not improve the explanatory efficacy of any of the outcomes examined. The addition of the interaction terms does not produce a significant increment in the R^2 value of the model relative to its degrees of freedom. This finding is consistent across all five resources and the various outcomes: subjective primary stressors, secondary role strains, secondary intrapsychic strains, and depressive symptomatology. Thus, there is no detectable evidence that these resources modify the effect of care-related stressors on the process of stress proliferation or its emotional sequela.[6]

The Independent Effects of Psychosocial Resources

To this point, our examination of psychosocial resources has focused exclusively upon their role in conjunction with care-related stressors. Specifically, we have considered whether these resources mediate and modify the effects of stressors. The results indicate that neither of these functions is served by the resources we are considering.

Psychosocial resources need not be entwined with stressors, however, to be consequential to caregiving outcomes. Instead, they may exert independent effects on the outcomes (i.e., be beneficial to caregivers irrespective of the magnitude of their exposure to care-related stressors). Our analyses indicate that this, indeed, is the case: Resources independently affect various outcomes of the stress-proliferation process.

Rosemary

Looking back after her husband's death, Rosemary reflects on how she coped and offers some advice:

Don't try to do the things you cannot do. I tried for too long to look after Steven alone in the house. Don't be too heroic. It doesn't pay in the end. Didn't pay for Steven or me. But I don't think I'd have taken this advice myself.

I never considered myself ill-used at all or that fate was unkind. Never felt sorry for myself at any time. But now, looking back, I realize that it was really something to deal with. It came gradually and I dealt with it as I could as things went along. Now, looking back, I realize that that was quite something.

Another advice, I would say, is don't let yourself be utterly consumed by this. You have to live your own life, at least a little. Even if you just save time to read. Be very firm that you are not in that situation — you are refreshing yourself with a wider exposure to something else, at least a little bit.

The analysis of the independent influences of resources builds upon the proliferation results reported in chapter 6, adding resources to the models containing stressors and background characteristics. The five resources we have been considering were again included as both baseline values and as change over time: informal instrumental help with the patient, informal instrumental help with household chores, the presence of an in-home attendant, socioemotional support, and mastery. Four types of outcomes, which were assessed at follow-up, were considered: subjective primary stressors, secondary role strains, secondary intrapsychic strains, and emotional distress. The baseline values of these outcomes were included as independent variables, meaning that the analyses reported here pertain to change in outcomes over time. The other independent variables are those that attained statistical significance in the earlier analyses (see Tables 6.1 through 6.4).

Resources and Subjective Primary Stressors

As may be seen in Table 7.1, two resources influence the proliferation of the subjective primary stressors: informal instrumental help with the patient and mastery. The magnitude of help received with the patient, not its change over time, is associated with increases in two subjective stressors: role overload and role captivity. The direction of this association is the reverse of what we would expect theoretically, given that social support is thought to alleviate stress. Instead, when caregivers receive instrumental help with the patient, they tend to experience increasing amounts of role overload and role captivity over time. To understand this perplexing result, it should be noted that the receipt of help connotes not only that assistance is available and utilized, but also that help is needed. It may well be that needing help, as distinct from obtaining help when it is needed, is the active element in this association.

The resource that matters most to the subjective stressors is the caregiver's sense of mastery. A consistently strong belief that one has control over important aspects of one's life leads to a reduction in stress associated with role overload, role captivity, and loss of intimate exchange. Moreover, increments in this sense of control over the course of caregiving pervasively contain the subsequent proliferation of two subjective primary stressors, role captivity and loss of intimate exchange.

As in the earlier analysis of stress proliferation, several stressors retain independent effects on these outcomes as well (compare with Table 6.1). In the previous analysis, we found that cognitive impairment, the objective stressor most indicative of disease progression, is significantly associated with loss of intimate exchange. It is apparent in Table 7.1 that this relationship persists when resources are taken into consideration. The absolute level of impairment and the pace of deterioration are both associated with an increased sense of loss over time. Thus, the scope of cognitive impairment and the rate at which cognitive abilities deteriorate as time passes heighten the caregiver's sense of having already lost one's husband, wife, mother, or father.

Table 7.1 illustrates that for role captivity, the most important primary stressor is problematic behavior, an association that is maintained when psychosocial resources also are taken into consideration. In the earlier analysis, both the intensity of problematic behavior and change in these disruptions contributed to subsequent role captivity. In the current analysis, only change over time retains

Table 7.1   Change in Subjective Primary Stressors over 1 Year as a Function of Psychosocial Resources

Resources, stressors, and characteristics	Subjective primary stressors: Time 2[a]					
	Role overload		Role captivity		Loss of intimate exchange	
	b (SE)	β	b (SE)	β	b (SE)	β
Role overload: Time 1	**.620*** (.042)**	**.625**	.111* (.047)	.103	—	—
Role captivity: Time 1	—	—	**.583*** (.043)**	**.586**	—	—
Loss of intimate exchange: Time 1	.136** (.046)	.130	—	—	**.532*** (.044)**	**.575**
ADL dependencies: Change Time 2–Time 1	*1.065*** (.211)*	*.775*	—	—	—	—
ADL dependencies: Change × Time 1	*−.310*** (.072)*	*−.649*	—	—	—	—
Problematic behavior: Time 2– Time 1	—	—	.207* (.091)	.100	—	—
Cognitive impairment: Time 1	—	—	—	—	*.132* (.055)*	*.144*
Cognitive impairment: Change Time 2–Time 1	—	—	—	—	*.202*** (.055)*	*.163*
San Francisco (/Los Angeles)	—	—	—	—	*−.226** (.069)*	*−.138*
Non-Hispanic white (/other)	—	—	.274* (.111)	.101	—	—
Informal support: Patient, Time 1	.225* (.103)	.118	.306** (.108)	.147	—	—
Mastery: Time 1	−.210* (.089)	−.115	−.331** (.103)	−.166	−.214** (.081)	−.132
Mastery: Change Time 2–Time 1	—	—	−.483*** (.109)	−.198	−.298** (.096)	−.150
R^2 Total	.532***		.552***		.476***	
R^2 Auto-regression	.437***		.452***		.388***	
R^2 Difference	.095***		.100***		.088***	

[a]Boldface numbers indicate auto-regression variables; italicized numbers indicate stress proliferation.
*$p \leq .05$.   **$p \leq .01$.   ***$p \leq .001$.

its statistical significance.[7] Thus, as in-home care continues over time, escalating troublesome behavior leads caregivers to feel increasingly trapped in their roles, irrespective of the resources they possess.

Finally, ADL dependencies continue to be linked to increments in role overload even when psychosocial resources are taken into consideration. As in the previous analysis, increasing dependency upon the caregiver substantially exacerbates role overload, especially among those whose initial responsibilities are comparatively light. The inclusion of psychosocial resources does not alter appreciably the impact of these dependencies.

The persistence of these independent effects on the subjective aspects of primary stressors should not obscure the functions of resources. Mastery, in particular, serves to blunt these effects, and the assistance provided by family and friends in caring for the patient appears to be a response to the severity of the patient's debility.

Resources and Secondary Stressors

The next step in the analysis considers the second stage in the proliferation model: The conversion of primary stressors into secondary sources of stress. We look first at the function of psychosocial resources in inhibiting or enhancing the emergence of secondary role strains over time. The two role strains analyzed here are family conflict and work strain.[8] Again, psychosocial resources are added to the statistically significant conditions obtained in the earlier analysis of proliferation (compare with Table 6.2), as shown in Table 7.2.

As may be seen, the impact of psychosocial resources on changes in role strains are quite specific. Of the five resources considered in the analysis, two contribute significantly to changes over time, each affecting one role strain. Specifically, high levels of emotional support, especially when it is maintained over time, is related to subsequent decreases in family conflict. In addition, a strong sense of mastery, particularly when it becomes stronger over time, is associated with declines in conflict between the demands of caregiving and those of paid employment.

We find that psychosocial resources, although effective, do not necessarily eliminate proliferation. For example, family conflict is still likely to be intensified over time by any increase in feelings of role captivity. The exacerbation of role captivity as time passes similarly contributes to increments in work strain.

The second aspect of the conversion of primary stressors into secondary sources of stress concerns the genesis or exacerbation of intrapsychic strains. As may be seen in Table 7.3, socioemotional support and mastery play central parts in the changes in these strains over time, just as they did in the case of role strains. Loss of self, absence of caregiver competence, and lack of caregiving gains are related to both baseline levels and changes in socioemotional support as time elapses. These strains also are related to baseline levels and changes in mastery over 1 year, with the exception of lack of caregiving gains. Thus, intrapsychic strains are lessened among caregivers who consistently feel cared

Table 7.2 Change in Secondary Role Strains over 1 Year as a Function of Psychosocial Resources

	Secondary role strains: Time 2[a]					
	Family conflict		Work conflict[b]		Financial strain	
Resources stressors, and characteristics	b (*SE*)	β	b (*SE*)	β	b (*SE*)	β
Family conflict: Time 1	**.517***** **(.051)**	**.503**	—	—	—	—
Work conflict: Time 1	—	—	**.408***** **(.086)**	**.415**	—	—
Income: Time 1	—	—	—	—	**.867***** **(.026)**	**.876**
Not employed: Time 1	—	—	−.362* (.165)	−.179	—	—
Role captivity: Change Time 2–Time 1	*.092** *(.040)*	*.121*	*.160** *(.066)*	*.224*	—	—
Role overload: Change Time 2–Time 1	—	—	—	—	*−1.990** *(.800)*	*−.072*
Husband (/other)	−.213* (.107)	−.151	—	—	—	—
Socioemotional support: Time 1	−.173** (.066)	−.145	—	—	—	—
Mastery: Time 1	—	—	−.293.* (.117)	−.258	—	—
Mastery: Change Time 2–Time 1	—	—	−.267* (.127)	−.193	—	—
R^2 Total	.358***		.444***		.776***	
R^2 Auto-regression	.298***		.195***		.770***	
R^2 Difference	.060*		.249***		.006	

[a]Boldface numbers indicate auto-regression variables; italicized numbers indicate stress proliferation.
[b]Limited to caregivers employed at Time 2, $n = 120$.
*$p \leq .05$. **$p \leq .01$. ***$p \leq .001$.

for by others and those who experience an increase in this sentiment over the course of caregiving. Caregivers who consistently feel control over their lives and those who develop this perspective as time passes have an enhanced sense of personal identity and see themselves as increasingly good at the job of caregiver.

The addition of psychosocial resources does not alter appreciably the impact of care-related stressors described previously in regard to proliferation (compare with Table 6.3).[9] Thus, we may conclude that these resources counterbalance the effects of care-related stressors, as distinct from eliminating their effects. Finally, loss of self is exacerbated by the rates of increase in role overload, role captivity,

Table 7.3 Change in Secondary Intrapsychic Strains over 1 Year as a Function of Psychosocial Resources

	Intrapsychic strains: Time 2[a]					
	Lack of caregiver competence		Absence of caregiving gains		Loss of self	
Resources, stressors, and characteristics	b (SE)	β	b (SE)	β	b (SE)	β
Lack of caregiver competence: Time 1	**.438*** (.044)**	**.460**	—	—	.139* (.065)	.096
Absence of caregiving gains: Time 1	—	—	**.543*** (.043)**	**.563**	—	—
Loss of self: Time 1	—	—	—	—	**.353*** (.053)**	**.354**
Cognitive impairment: Time 1	−.062* (.029)	−.107	—	—	—	—
Cognitive impairment: Change Time 2–Time 1	−.083* (.036)	−.104	—	—	—	—
Role overload: Change Time 2–Time 1	—	—	−.123* (.053)	−.115	.128* (.051)	.120
Role captivity: Change Time 2–Time 1	—	—	—	—	.201*** (.048)	.206
Loss of intimate exchange: Change Time 2–Time 1	—	—	—	—	.151** (.053)	.140
ADL dependencies: Time 1	—	—	−.129* (.057)	−.124	—	—
ADL dependencies: Change Time 2–Time 1	—	—	−.160* (.056)	−.134	—	—
Education	—	—	.041** (.013)	.139	—	—
San Francisco (/Los Angeles)	—	—	−.166* (.071)	−.104	—	—
Socioemotional support: Time 1	−.128* (.052)	−.129	−.292*** (.077)	−.193	−.181* (.077)	−.121
Socioemotional support: Change Time 2–Time 1	−.167** (.056)	−.148	−.197* (.083)	−.115	−.168* (.082)	−.098
Mastery: Time 1	−.251*** (.056)	−.239	—	—	−.316*** (.091)	−.199
Mastery: Change Time 2–Time 1	−.197** (.064)	−.154	—	—	−.261** (.099)	−.134
R^2 Total	.421***		.479***		.469***	
R^2 Auto-regression	.326***		.376***		.266***	
R^2 Difference	.095***		.103***		.203***	

[a]Boldface numbers indicate auto-regression variables; italicized numbers indicate stress proliferation.
*$p \leq .05$. **$p \leq .01$. ***$p \leq .001$.

and loss of intimate exchange with the patient. Therefore, the influence of primary stressors on secondary intrapsychic strains remains intact when psychosocial resources also are taken into consideration.

Resources and Depression

The final component of the stress-proliferation model concerns the conversion of care-related stressors into symptoms of emotional distress (i.e., depression). It is evident in Table 7.4 that two resources contribute to decreases in depression over time: informal help with the patient and mastery. Specifically, caregivers who enjoy an expansion of assistance from family and friends with the tasks directly entailed in taking care of the dementia patient have, on average, declining levels of depression over time. Depression also decreases as time passes

Table 7.4   Change in Depression over 1 Year as a Function of Psychosocial Resources

Resources, stressors, and, characteristics	Depression: Time 2[a] b (SE)	β
Depression: Time 1	**.373*** (.050)**	**.375**
Role overload: Time 1	*.128** (.040)*	*.165*
Role overload: Change Time 2–Time 1	*.096* (.041)*	*.100*
Loss of self: Time 1	*.179*** (.050)*	*.199*
Loss of self: Change Time 2–Time 1	*.162*** (.044)*	*.177*
Mastery: Time 1	−.262** (.084)	−.183
Mastery: Change Time 2–Time 1	−.342*** (.082)	−.194
Gain informal support: Patient, change Time 2–Time 1	−.219** (.082)	−.108
R^2 Total	.603***	
R^2 Auto-regression	.400***	
R^2 Difference	.203***	

[a]Boldface numbers indicate auto-regression variables; italicized numbers indicate stress proliferation.
*$p < .05$. **$p < .01$. ***$p < .001$.

among caregivers who maintain a belief in their capacity to control important forces in their lives, as well as among those whose sense of control increases over the course of caregiving.

Although we have been emphasizing the function of resources, it may be observed that support and mastery do not eliminate stress proliferation. As in the preceding analyses, the inclusion of psychosocial resources does not alter appreciably the impact of care-related stressors in regard to depression (compare with Table 6.4). Thus, resources do not alter the impact of care-related stressors, but instead, tend to offset their effects.

The Impact of Psychosocial Resources over 1 Year

Figure 7.1 synthesizes the results presented in this section concerning the impact of psychosocial resources on the stress-proliferation process as it unfolds over the course of 1 year. Only major linkages among key constructs are depicted because the detailed results are tabled (Tables 7.1 through 7.4). This figure portrays two types of influence: Psychosocial resources affect elements in the stress-proliferation process that ultimately impact emotional well-being, and psychosocial resources influence stressors that have no direct impact upon depression.

Mastery and instrumental assistance with the patient emerge as the key contributors to stressors that, in turn, influence the course of depression as time passes. Mastery itself directly affects depression: A consistently strong sense of self-efficacy, or one that grows stronger over time, tends to reduce emotional

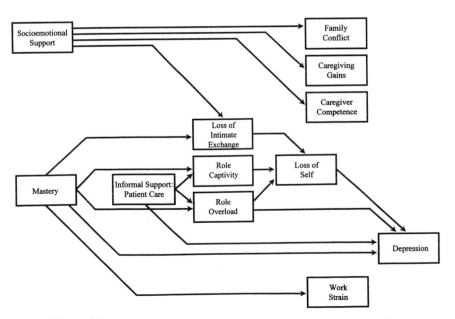

Figure 7.1 Impact of psychosocial resources on stress proliferation over 1 year.

distress. In addition, mastery exerts indirect effects upon depression through its impact on several stressors. A strong sense of control tends to decrease three subjective primary stressors: loss of intimate exchange with the patient, role captivity, and role overload. This reduction in stress then leads to better emotional well-being, either directly or because reducing these stressors lessens damage to the caregiver's sense of personal identity.

Constance

Caregivers often find comfort in the belief that they have benefited from the care they provide, as described by Constance:

But it gives you some things too — a lot of confidence that I can handle this and that I'm doing something that I always told myself I would do. Made me feel good about myself even though it imposed some restrictions. More positives than negatives. It has changed my outlook on the world. My approach to the world is more confident. I used to find my mother terribly embarrassing — you overcome that. I lived through it. I wasn't hit by a bolt of lightning and made to disappear.

She also shares some of her own strategies for survival:

Laugh at it. It may seem cruel but if you didn't see the humor, it would drive you crazy. Understand that the behavior is not voluntary, that they have no control.

While her mother lived at home, Constance took her to day care to obtain respite for herself and time to be with her husband:

Sometimes I just came home and sat. We would tend to have company in for lunch rather than in the evening when we could, so that she was not there. I'd go shopping, hit the malls, or use that time for a dentist appointment, something like that. Anything that we wanted to do together we'd do between 10 and 3. Our life revolved around those times.

Informal help with patient care has rather complex ties to depression. When family and friends assist with patient care, the caregiver tends to become increasingly burdened in terms of the subjective stressors of role captivity and role overload, stressors that then magnify distress directly or via damage to the caregiver's sense of personal integrity. The receipt of assistance, then, indirectly *elevates* depressive symptomatology. As discussed earlier in this chapter, these links may be the result of the need for care, which is embodied in the receipt of care, and as such, reflect a deteriorating care situation rather than the impact of help per se. On the other hand, informal assistance directly decreases depressive symptomatology over time. Therefore, its direct and indirect effects on depression are in opposite directions. When the indirect adverse impact is taken into consideration, the main effect of informal assistance is beneficial to emotional well-being.

Socioemotional support is consequential to elements in the stress-proliferation process, but its influence is felt most in domains separate from the exacerbation of depression. Only one indirect pathway is shown for socioemotional support and depression: Caregivers who feel cared for by others feel the loss of intimacy with the patient somewhat less than those lacking in support, which enables them to maintain a stronger sense of personal identity, thus, exerting a beneficial impact upon their emotional well-being.

However, socioemotional support has other consequences beyond this indirect link to depression. As may be seen in Figure 7.1, feeling cared for by others tends to reduce family conflict, lead to the perception that one has benefited from being a caregiver, and enhance self-assessment of competence as a caregiver. In a similar manner, mastery is linked to reduced conflict between the demands of work and caregiving.

The lack of an independent contribution to explaining depression does not mean that the linkage of psychosocial resources to elements in the stress process are unimportant. Clearly, these resources, socioemotional support in particular, tend to constrain the proliferation of care-related stressors. Depression represents only one of the potential outcomes of stress proliferation. As we have argued throughout this volume, the significance of various components of the stress process should not be judged by a single criterion, such as depression, but should encompass multiple outcomes. The impact of socioemotional support on family conflict, caregiving gains, and caregiver competence may well manifest in outcomes other than depression. This possibility is examined in subsequent chapters.

Thus far, we have considered relationships among psychosocial resources, care-related stressors, and emotional distress as these dynamics unfold over an interval of 1 year. From this vantage point, psychosocial resources are seen as exerting a substantial independent or main effect on the expansion and contraction of stressors over time and on their emotional sequelae. In contrast, there is no detectable evidence that these resources affect caregivers via processes of stress mediation or stress moderation. Thus, resources appear to matter in and of themselves, irrespective of concurrent levels of exposure to various stressors. We turn now to the impact of psychosocial resources over a longer interval, the 3 years separating Time 1 and Time 4.[10]

The Long-Term Impact of Psychosocial Resources

Earlier in this chapter we evaluated three types of relationships involving psychosocial resources: stress mediation, stress moderation, and the independent effects of resources on outcomes. The analysis of the 1-year interval only provided evidence for a direct association between resources and outcomes.

For the analysis of the 3-year interval, we limit our presentation to these independent effects for two reasons. First, in order to mediate the impact of stressors, resources must vary according to exposure to the very same stressors that affect outcomes. Although socioemotional support and mastery are affected by exposure to various stressors, they are not the stressors that prompt stress proliferation over the long-term (see Tables 6.5 and 6.6). The resources, therefore, cannot mediate the impact of those stressors that are consequential to stress proliferation. Second, the decline in the sample size from the 1-year to the 3-year interval means that the statistical power to detect contingent effects is diminished. Because effect modification was not detected in the more powerful analysis, it is doubtful that this type of effect could be detected with the reduced power available for the longer interval.

The analysis of the independent effects of psychosocial resources builds upon the long-term stress-proliferation results presented in the previous chapter. Thus, the outcomes we examine are three subjective primary stressors, role overload, role captivity, and loss of intimate exchange; one secondary intrapsychic strain, loss of self;[11] and emotional distress in the form of depressive symptomatology. The regression models contain the full array of independent variables previously found to produce change in the subjective stressors. The models also include both baseline and change variables for each psychosocial resource: informal instrumental assistance with patient care and household chores, use of an in-home attendant, socioemotional support, and mastery. The baseline value for each outcome of interest also is included as an independent variable, meaning that the coefficients reported in Table 7.5 may be interpreted in terms of change over time; only those variables that attain statistical significance are tabled.

It is apparent that two psychosocial resources, socioemotional support and mastery, emerge as important contributors to two of the three subjective stressors, role captivity and loss of intimate exchange with the dementia patient. In contrast, none of the psychosocial resources contribute significantly to accounting for changes in the third subjective stressor, role overload (model not presented). The remaining psychosocial resources, the three indicators of instrumental support, do not emerge as significant explanatory factors with regard to the conversion of objective primary stressors into subjective primary stressors.

Caregivers who consistently receive socioemotional support typically feel less captive in their roles as caregivers as time progresses. In addition, those whose sense of mastery increases during the course of caregiving also tend to experience less role captivity over time. Earlier in this chapter, we saw that mastery was related to the containment of role captivity over the 1-year interval; the previously observed effect of informal help with patient care on changes in role captivity over 1 year, however, is not observed over 3 years (see Table 7.3). Role captivity continues to be influenced by problematic behavior and patient resistance, as reported here and in the earlier analysis of proliferation (see Table 6.5).[12]

The impacts of socioemotional support and mastery on the long-term loss of intimate exchange with the dementia patient are in opposing directions, as is apparent in Table 7.5. Caregivers who consistently and increasingly feel sup-

Table 7.5   Change in Subjective Primary Stressors over 3 Years
as a Function of Psychosocial Resources

Resources, stressors, and characteristics	Subjective primary stressors: Time 4[a]			
	Role captivity		Loss of intimate exchange	
	b (SE)	β	b (SE)	β
Role captivity: Time 1	**.616*** (.065)**	**.608**	—	—
Loss of intimate exchange: Time 1	—	—	**.359*** (.081)**	**.358**
Socioemotional support: Time 1	−.300* (.145)	−.162	.365* (.151)	.238
Socioemotional support: Change Time 4–Time 1	—	—	.378* (.166)	.220
Mastery: Time 1	—	—	−.522** (.186)	−.303
Mastery: Change Time 4–Time 1	−.499** (.188)	−.213	−.707*** (.194)	−.360
Problematic behavior: Change Time 4–Time 1	*.421*** (.137)*	*.222*	—	—
Patient resistance: Change Time 4–Time 1	*.378** (.166)*	*.146*	—	—
Duration of care: Time 1	—	—	−.120*** (.025)	−.374
R^2	.652***		.429***	

[a]Boldface numbers indicate auto-regression variables; italic numbers indicate stress proliferation.
*$p \leq .05$. **$p \leq .01$. ***$p \leq .001$.

ported by others feel distant from the care recipient. In contrast, caregivers with a consistently strong sense of mastery and those whose possession of this resource increases over time tend to feel less estranged from the dementia patient as caregiving extends over lengthy intervals. Thus, the receipt of socioemotional support is linked to an increasing sense of being separate from the dementia patient, whereas a strong sense of self-efficacy tends to maintain the caregiver's connection to the patient. The mastery effect replicates the pattern observed for the 1-year interval, but the socioemotional support effect emerges only over the longer 3-year interval (compare with Table 7.1). Although the statistically significant impact of cognitive impairment previously reported in the proliferation model (see Table 6.5) does not attain statistical significance in the present containment model, this decline itself is not significant.[13]

In contrast, Table 7.6 illustrates that both mastery and socioemotional support exert beneficial effects with regard to the caregiver's sense of personal identity, the only secondary stressor modeled in this analysis (see endnote 11). Caregivers who consistently experience high levels of socioemotional support tend to retain a strong sense of self, as do those who gain such support over time, although the impact of change in support is marginally nonsignificant (b = -.241, SE = .181, β = -.143, $p \le$ .12). Both the baseline and change variables for mastery attain statistical significance, nonetheless, meaning that a consistently strong sense of

Table 7.6   Change in Loss of Self and Depression over 3 Years
as a Function of Psychosocial Resources

Resources, stressors, and characteristics	Loss of self: Time 4			Depression: Time 4[a]		
	b (SE)		β	b (SE)		β
Loss of self: Time 1	**.313*** (.074)**		**.319**	—		—
Depression: Time 1	—		—	**.343*** (.075)**		**.345**
Socioemotional support: Time 1	−.336* (.141)		−.224	—		—
Socioemotional support: Change Time 4–Time 1	—		—	—		—
Mastery: Time 1	−.407* (.180)		−.241	—		—
Mastery: Change Time 4–Time 1	−.512** (.181)		−.269	−.353* (.159)		−.204
Informal support: Patient, Time 1	—		—	−.287* (.142)		−.189
Informal support: Patient, change Time 4–Time 1	—		—	.444* (.184)		.156
Role captivity: Time 1	*.264**** (.078)		*.321*	*.150** (.062)		*.200*
Role captivity: Change Time 4–Time 1	*.296**** (.083)		*.288*	*.221*** (.072)		*.236*
Daughter caring for mother (/other)	−.373* (.183)		−.201	—		—
Non-Hispanic white (/other)	—		—	−.336* (.128)		−.176
R^2	.528***			.584***		

[a]Boldface numbers indicate auto-regression variables; italicized numbers indicate stress proliferation.
*$p \le$ .05.   **$p \le$ .01.   ***$p \le$ .001.

self-efficacy, or one that intensifies over time, is protective of personal identity. When these resources are taken into consideration, role captivity continues to exacerbate loss of self (compare with Table 6.6). The long-term effects mirror those reported earlier in this chapter for the 1-year interval (see Table 7.3).

Although mastery matters to changes in depression over 3 years, socioemotional support falls out of the picture, as also is apparent in Table 7.6. Informal instrumental help with patient care, which arose as an important factor in the analysis of variations in depression over 1 year (see Table 7.2), emerges as well with regard to changes in depression over 3 years. The two coefficients for instrumental support, however, are of opposite signs: negative for the baseline variable and positive for the change variable. This combination means that caregivers who consistently receive help from family and friends tend to be less depressed over time, whereas caregivers who acquire such help over the course of the 3-year interval are typically more depressed over this time span. The latter association, as we have emphasized in earlier analyses, may well represent the emergence of the need for help with patient care as distinct from the receipt of help (i.e., this effect may signify a deterioration in the caregiving situation). Depression continues to be affected by role captivity, but the influences of role overload and increased expenses on changes in depression over 3 years become statistically nonsignificant (compare with Table 6.6).[14]

> Every failure contributes to the possibility of success—the result of cumulative experiences.

In summary, socioemotional support and mastery emerge as important contributors to the containment of care-related stressors over lengthy intervals of time. Although the effects of mastery are uniformly beneficial, this may not be the case for socioemotional support insofar as it is related to intensified feelings of separateness from the dementia patient. The instrumental support variables do not emerge as important contributors to the long-term containment of stress proliferation, but informal help with patient care is important to understanding changes in depression over time.

The Impact of Psychosocial Resources over 3 Years

The major routes by which psychosocial resources act to contain the proliferation of care-related stressors is illustrated in Figure 7.2, which summarizes the more detailed results appearing in Tables 7.5 and 7.6. Socioemotional support and mastery are both associated with three outcomes—loss of intimate exchange, loss of self, and role captivity. For mastery, these effects appear to be beneficial, leading to reductions in each of these sources of stress. These effects are not uniformly beneficial with regard to socioemotional support, however, insofar as this resource leads to increased estrangement from the care recipient over protracted periods of time. The remaining relationships involving this type of sup-

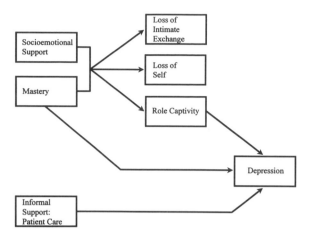

Figure 7.2   Impact of psychosocial resources on stress proliferation over 3 years.

port are advantageous, with socioemotional support enhancing personal identity and diminishing role captivity.

The impacts of socioemotional support and mastery on role captivity are additionally important because this stressor contributes to increased levels of depression over time. That is, these two resources exert indirect effects upon depression via their influences on role captivity. In addition, self-efficacy is directly associated with long-term improvements in emotional well-being.

The role of hands-on help with patient care is complex. Caregivers who received help from family and friends both initially and at follow-up tended to improve in their emotional well-being over time. Increasing emotional distress, however, characterizes caregivers who acquired support that they previously lacked. Although not statistically significant, those who lose aid over time also tend to be slightly more depressed as time passes. The comparison group consists of those who lacked aid at baseline and at follow-up. Relative to this group, those who acquire help and those who lose it are somewhat elevated in subsequent levels of depression, whereas those who retain help over time have the lowest levels of depression. These patterns appear to reflect the confounding of the need for help with the receipt of help.

Figure 7.2 also illustrates two yardsticks that may be used to measure the importance of psychosocial resources. One of these standards is the impact of these resources, direct or indirect, on symptoms of depression. The second criterion is outcomes that do not necessarily influence emotional well-being (e.g., loss of intimate exchange and loss of self). These stressors may not have long-term detectable effects upon depression, but may be influential nonetheless. For example, as we shall see in chapter 11, loss of intimate exchange is consequential to the course of grief.

Summary

This chapter has examined the ways in which social psychological resources constrain the proliferation of care-related stressors and their emotional consequences. Three types of effects were examined: stress mediation, stress moderation, and the independent impact of psychosocial resources.

• Two out of three caregivers receive less instrumental assistance than needed from family and friends, and only 3 in 10 caregivers have paid in-home attendants. This pattern reveals substantial unmet need for assistance in this population, unmet need that persists over time.
• Despite insufficient help with patient care and household chores, caregivers as a group tend to feel supported, cared for, and understood by friends and family; some caregivers, however, are isolated.
• Caregivers are inclined to feel substantial control over important aspects of their lives even though they confront an illness that is irreversible, progressive, and unpredictable.
• In general, changes in care-related stressors neither mobilize nor deplete resources to any appreciable extent over time. Nonetheless, there are some important exceptions, such as self-perceived deficits as a caregiver, which tend to deplete socioemotional support and erode mastery, especially when this sense of inadequacy persists or intensifies over time.
• Psychosocial resources neither mediate the impact of care-related stressors, nor moderate the effects of these stressors.
• Socioemotional support and mastery contain the proliferation of care-related stressors as time passes, including subjective primary stressors and some secondary stressors.
• Mastery or self-efficacy, especially when it is consistently strong or intensifying over time, improves emotional well-being.

Discussion

Care-related stressors are associated with several psychosocial resources that were present at the start of the study; specifically, having an in-home attendant, socioemotional support, and mastery; the exceptions are informal instrumental assistance with patient care and household chores. As we have discussed previously, these baseline associations are important because they capture the accrual of care-related stress processes prior to the beginning of the study (i.e., the accumulation of these processes over time). Clearly, then, stressors and resources are not entirely independent of one another.

We find, however, that resources generally do not depend importantly upon shifts in care-related stressors over time. These longitudinal analyses provide the most rigorous test of the premise that changes in the stressors of caregiving produce corresponding changes in the resources that may be brought to bear upon these stressors. Few effects of these types were observed.

In order to mediate the impact of care-related stressors, social psychological resources must be responsive to the ebb and flow of these stressors. Moreover, these resources should account for some of the overall association between stressors and outcomes. In this direct test of mediation, we found no reductions in the impact of stressors on outcomes with the addition of resources to the explanatory model. Likewise, resources do not appear to modify the effects of care-related stressors. Consequently, to the extent that these resources matter to stress proliferation, they appear to do so via mechanisms other than mediation or moderation.

Instead, resources are important to stress proliferation because they exert independent effects on various outcomes. Thus, we have seen that socioemotional support, mastery, and the use of informal help with patient care tend to directly alleviate emotional distress over time. However, a second type of outcome merits emphasis: These psychosocial resources also influence exposure to care-related stressors. The linkages describe pathways through which resources indirectly influence emotional distress: Resources alter stressors which, in turn, generate emotional distress.

The key point we wish to make is that psychosocial resources appear to be antecedent to at least some care-related stressors, rather than consequences of these stressors. This distinction is pivotal to understanding the functions of psychosocial resources in the stress-proliferation process. The other models examined in this chapter treat stressors as the active causal agent: Stressors influence the occurrence of resources in the mediation model, and resources modify the impact of these stressors in the moderation model. Again, neither model was supported by our analyses.

Thus, psychosocial resources matter to stress proliferation because they contribute to the expansion and contraction of care-related stressors over time. In particular, socioemotional support, mastery, and receiving informal assistance with patient care influence the course of subjective primary stressors, secondary role strains, and secondary intrapsychic strains. For mastery and socioemotional support, these effects are generally beneficial: When these resources are consistently high or are becoming stronger, care-related stressors tend to diminish over time. Receiving help from family and friends with patient care, however, tends to exacerbate role overload and role captivity, the reverse of the expected relationship. This counterintuitive finding probably reflects the fact that caregivers need such assistance most when they are least able to maintain and control their relatives.

In essence, psychosocial resources appear to play an active, rather than reactive, role in the care-related stress process. These resources shape the development of stressors instead of being shaped themselves by the stressors.

In general, instrumental support does not appear to play a major role in the containment of care-related stressors, a surprising and rather disappointing set of results. These findings are attributable, at least in part, to the measures of instrumental support used in these analyses. Each measure is a single-item dichotomy, the individual receives such help or does not. These measures may not be powerful enough to detect existing relationships for several reasons. First, their dichotomous nature does not permit differentiation among caregivers in the amount of help they receive, lumping together those who receive extensive support and those who receive very little; this technique would tend to attenuate observed associations. Similarly, caregivers who do not receive support comprise two groups: those who need assistance, but do without it; and those who do not need assistance. The impact in these instances, again, would be to attenuate observed associations, which would further detract from the statistical power to detect interaction effects when they are indeed present. Thus, these disappointing results may be methodological artifacts of our measurement strategy.

Another possibility should be considered as well; namely, that the level of assistance provided may be insufficient. We refer here not to the maximum assistance obtained by any one caregiver, but to the average amount of help provided to caregivers who received any help at all. To the extent that aid is less than needed and the caregivers in this study rate all help received as far less than needed, it may not be possible to observe an effect of support because too few caregivers obtained enough to matter. In other words, instrumental support may, indeed, be important to the containment of care-related stressors, but we may fail to observe such effects because the average "dose" of support is inadequate to produce the desired "response."

Also, the receipt of instrumental support is more or less a matter of chance: It does not depend importantly upon the need for help. That is, the primary and secondary stressors entailed in caregiving generally exert only limited effects upon change in resources over time. The most notable exception to this generalization occurs for use of a paid in-home attendant, which becomes more likely as the patient's cognitive state declines. Nonetheless, instrumental support, especially informal support, is driven more by the characteristics of the caregiver than by the circumstances of care. Instrumental support may not contain the impact of care-related stressors, therefore, because many of those who need it most do without it.

Caregiver characteristics, in turn, help to shape these psychosocial resources demonstrated by cross-sectional associations at the start of the study. In particular, generation (spouse vs. adult child) matters importantly to how much informal instrumental assistance is received: Spousal caregivers receive more help from family and friends than do adult-child caregivers. On the other hand, wives and husbands report less socioemotional support and mastery than daughters and sons. As we saw previously with exposure to care-related stressors, generational differences are not simply a matter of more or less, but are a mix of benefit with regard to some resources and deficit with regard to others. Thus, it is also the type of resources that varies by kin relationship, rather than simply the total amount of resources.

Furthermore, income and financial strain matter importantly to the distribution of psychosocial resources in this population, especially with regard to the use of paid in-home help. Therefore, location in the social system influences not only the amount of exposure to various stressors, but also the type of resources that may be brought to bear on these stressors.

Notes

[1] It is also the case that neither type of informal support is significantly associated with a complete measure reflecting the *number* of services regularly used by the caregiver.

[2] Asterisk signifies an item whose scoring is reversed.

[3] Asterisk signifies an item whose scoring is reversed.

[4] Wheaton (1985) used the term *stress deterrent* to refer to the instances in which resources obstruct the occurrence of stressors.

[5] Wheaton (1985) identified a second type of stress buffering, one of the mediational models described earlier in this chapter, Ensel and Lin's (1991) stress-suppression model: Stressors mobilize resources, which then alleviate adverse outcomes, thereby reducing the total causal effect of stress. There was no evidence for this type of stress buffering in the stress mediation analyses. Wheaton (1985) argued cogently that the other mediational model, stress deterioration, explains how stress affects outcomes; it is not an instance of stress buffering, though, because the total causal impact of stress is explicated, but not reduced.

[6] Because the inclusion of interaction terms may produce problems of multicollinearity, we also operationalized the buffering model as a stratified analysis. Specifically, the impact of care-related stressors was examined in two strata: those in the top third of the distribution of the resource at Time 1 and those in the bottom third. Substantial change between Time 1 and Time 2 in the resource (more than one standard deviation) was included as an independent variable. In the stratified analysis, buffering effects are represented by a smaller regression coefficient for the stressor in the high resource model than in the low model. However, these coefficients did not differ significantly between strata.

[7] The difference in the magnitude of the coefficient for problematic behavior at Time 1 does not differ significantly between the regressions that include or exclude resources. Thus there is some slight evidence that mastery buffers the impact of problematic behavior on role captivity, but this finding is quite tenuous.

[8] Income is excluded because the addition of psychosocial resources did not produce a statistically significant increment in the explanatory efficacy of the model. The other indicators of secondary role strains are categorical and display too little change over time to permit meaningful multivariate analysis: becoming unemployed, decreasing work hours, having not enough money, and having increased expenses.

[9] For the analysis of these outcomes, variables previously found to be inconsequential were omitted to simplify the model. As a result of these deletions, some previously significant variables dropped below the criterion. We retained these variables in the model, however, due to their earlier importance in explaining the various outcomes considered here. The decline in the impact of these stressors occurs in the trimmed model and, hence, is not attributable to the subsequent inclusion of psychosocial resources.

[10] These analyses are limited to the 137 caregivers who continued to provide in-home care throughout this interval.

[11] The other secondary stressors were not analyzed for several reasons: insufficient change on dichotomous variables and on family income, too few subjects (work conflict), and nonsignificant proliferation results (family conflict and the other secondary intrapsychic strains).

[12]In the earlier analysis, both the baseline and change variables attained statistical significance, which is not the case when psychosocial resources are added to the model. However, the 95% confidence intervals overlap for the coefficients for identical variables in the two models, meaning that the apparent reduction in the impact of these stressors is not statistically meaningful.

[13]The 95% confidence intervals overlap for the cognitive impairment coefficient in the two models, meaning that the apparent reduction in the influence of cognitive impairment is not statistically meaningful.

[14]The 95% confidence intervals overlap for the coefficients for identical variables in the two models, meaning that the apparent reduction in the impacts of these stressors on changes in depression is not statistically meaningful.

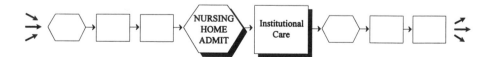

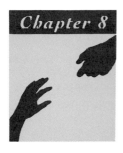

The Transition to Institutional Care

Given that caregiving is so arduous, why do so many people persist at this task year after year? The economics of long-term care impose constraints, of course: Many families simply cannot afford nursing home care, and at a societal level there are insufficient public funds and too few nursing home beds to provide for all those who require assistance. Yet, even when institutionalization is financially and logistically feasible, only some caregivers pursue this alternative; others do not, even though they face seemingly similar difficult circumstances. Moreover, when nursing home placement becomes inevitable, many caregivers accept it reluctantly, only as a last resort.

Table 8.1   Percent Distribution of Attitude
towards Placement and Rate of Institutionalization

Thinking about placement makes the caregiver	N	%	Rate of institutionalization[a]
Very upset	282	51.3	39.4%
Fairly upset	105	19.1	54.3
Just a little upset	77	14.0	39.0
Not at all upset	86	15.6	41.9

[a]Percent institutionalized prior to Time 4, including those who subsequently died or were lost-at-follow-up.

Negative sentiments about nursing home placement are widely evident among the caregivers participating in this study. At baseline, when all of the caregivers were providing in-home care, we asked them how upsetting it was to think about the possibility of placing their relatives in nursing homes or other facilities. Their responses are illustrated in Table 8.1. Over 70% of the caregivers said the prospect of admitting their parents or spouses made them either *very upset*, the most intense response choice among the alternatives, or *fairly upset*. The remainder indicated that the thought of placement creates little or no upset. Thus, although most caregivers face extremely demanding conditions, a substantial majority is reluctant to relinquish their care responsibilities to institutions. Some, however, are left untroubled by this prospect.

Most caregivers, then, abhor the very idea of admitting their spouses or parents to nursing homes, but most of them also ultimately accede to the forces pressuring them to do so. As described previously, 237 caregivers, or 42.5% of the original sample, turned to institutional care at some point over the ensuing 3 years.

Admission of a parent or spouse to a nursing home is *not* strongly related to the caregiver's preexisting sentiment about placement, as also shown in Table 8.1. The difference in the percent institutionalized across the four attitudinal categories approaches statistical significance ($\chi^2 = 7.511$, $df = 3$, $p \leq .06$), but this test does not reflect a systematic association between attitudes and behavior. Instead, only one group, those who are *fairly upset* at the prospect of institutionalization, have an exceptionally high rate of subsequent nursing home admission. The remaining three groups have lower and similar rates of institutionalization. Particularly striking is the comparability between the two most extreme groups— *very upset* and *not at all upset*: Those who are most discrepant in their initial attitudes about placement are indistinguishable in their subsequent behavior.[1]

Thus, many caregivers ultimately act contrary to their earlier preferences. This pattern suggests that placement comes about as the end result of an intense struggle to balance the enormous demands of active in-home care with the resources available to sustain in-home care and the resources necessary to obtain institutional care.

> Never. As long as I live.

Perhaps, prior dispositions become inconsequential to placement decisions because these dispositions eventually are swamped by the unrelenting degenerative course of dementia. As the demands of care swell, or remain continuously unabated, they might overwhelm the capacities of virtually any caregiver. For example, waning cognitive abilities render many patients immobile; acts of cleaning, feeding, and clothing the patient may come to require more physical exertion than may be maintained by an aging spouse, especially if caring simultaneously depletes the caregiver's own strength, vitality, and stamina. Caregivers who initially refuse even to think about nursing home admission may subsequently confront a situation in which admission is the *only* viable course of action.

The Average Course of In-Home Care

All of the dementia patients in this study eventually will die, but will they die at home or in an institution? As time marches on, the patients are increasingly likely to be institutionalized *and* increasingly likely to die. How often, then, does institutionalization arrive before death? Alternately, as in-home care extends over time, how likely is it to continue for yet one more year, or one more week, or one more day? How long does the typical caregiver endure?

The duration of in-home care—time from the start of care to the admission of the dementia patient to a long-term care facility—is displayed as a survival distribution in Figure 8.1. In this analysis, survival refers to the continuance of in-home assistance. Time begins to accrue when the caregiver first has to start helping the impaired relative do things that he or she is no longer able to do for him or herself (i.e., the duration of care reported at the baseline interview). This value is then incremented by the time from the baseline interview until admission to a nursing home.

As described earlier, many caregivers started to help their spouses and parents long before they realized that this assistance had become imperative. Thus, these dates are best viewed as approximations. Also, the actual onset of the disease and the initial recognition of the illness usually preceded the start of caregiving, as did diagnosis, or the formal labeling by the medical profession of the problematic behavior as an illness.[2] The duration of in-home care prior to institutionalization, therefore, typically is shorter than the duration of the disease or the illness prior to institutionalization.

What about those patients who were living at home at Time 4, or those who died at home? There is obviously no date of admission to an institution for these

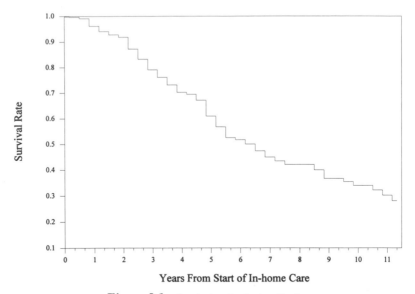

Figure 8.1   Survival to institutionalization.

care recipients or for those who were lost-to-follow-up while living at home. On the other hand, we do know that these individuals remained at home until their death, or, alternately, at least as long as the last interview. This information should not be discarded because it captures the experience of those who received the *longest* in-home care. Omitting these cases, therefore, would bias estimates of the duration of in-home care. Consequently, we treat patients who were not institutionalized as *censored* at their last observation or upon their death. The term *censored,* then, refers to those who died at home, continued to receive in-home care at Time 4, or were lost-at-follow-up without having been institutionalized.

   The distribution of survival times is cumulative, a running tally of those who have been institutionalized. Its initial value is 1, reflecting the fact that all of these dementia patients received in-home care at time 0, the point at which their spouses and children started to provide help. This proportion declines as the need for care continued across time and as more and more caregivers admitted their relatives to nursing homes. The distribution eventually will dip to 0, the point at which all care recipients have been institutionalized or have died.

   As may be seen in Figure 8.1, a plateau develops across the early years of in-home care, when the vast majority of patients continued to be cared for at home. At the end of 2 years, 96.1% remained at home.[3] This static interval is followed by a steady erosion of the ranks of in-home caregivers. The rate of decline over the next 10 years is relatively constant. By 3.5 years, roughly one in four caregivers have institutionalized their parents or partners; by 6.5 years, one in two have done so.[4] The mean duration of in-home care is 6.75 years. In-home caregiving, therefore, tends to be a long-term commitment.

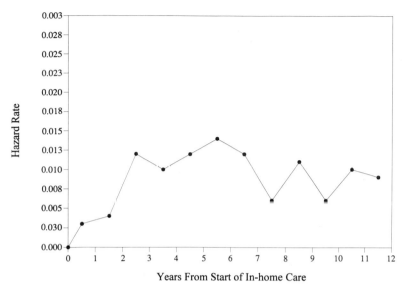

Figure 8.2   Hazard rates for admission to a nursing home.

Peak Periods of Risk

In Figure 8.2 we present hazard rates for institutionalization: The risk of admission to a nursing home at a specific point in time given that the patient still resides at home until that time. Whereas the survival distribution reflects cumulative outcomes over time, the hazard rate captures the moment. In essence, the hazard rate is a conditional probability, akin to an incidence rate.

The most notable feature of this plot is the deviation in risk for the early years of care as compared to the years that follow. The risk of admission to a nursing home is quite low for each of the first 2 years of in-home care. These low hazard rates generate the plateau in the survival distribution seen previously. Thereafter, the hazard rate increases sharply and then levels off. The fluctuation in rates over the ensuing years does not reflect statistically significant variation, meaning that there is no detectable difference in rates over these years.

Aside from the first 2 years when one is unlikely to make the transition from in-home to institutional care, the level of annual risk does not vary appreciably across time. For example, the risk of going from in-home to institutional care in Year 4 of in-home care is not significantly different from Year 7 as long as the patient is still living at home at the beginning of Year 7. The last phrase is an important distinction, emphasizing that these probabilities are conditional. The *cumulative* probability of placement, of course, necessarily increases with time, until placement or death becomes a virtual certainty (the obverse of the survival distribution in Figure 8.1).

Generation and Gender

How accurately does this descriptive picture portray different types of caregivers? Given that normative family roles are shaped, at least in part, by gender and generation, we expected to find marked differences in the duration of in-home care by the nature of the kin relationship between the giver and the recipient of care (Moen et al., 1994). Wives should provide substantially longer care than husbands, we reasoned, because they have a lifetime of greater experience in performing domestic tasks and taking care of sick family members (i.e., wives are better prepared to care for impaired husbands than vice versa). Compared to daughters, however, wives are more likely to be in frail health due to their older age and consequently, may be more likely than daughters to relinquish caregiving. On the other hand, daughters are more likely to have competing demands between caregiving and their own marriages, parenting roles, and work. Thus, we anticipated that wives and daughters would resemble one another, but differ from husbands, who would tend to give up the caregiver role early.

As shown in Figure 8.3, however, the typical duration of in-home care across these subgroups is quite similar. When tested statistically, there are no significant differences in the survival distributions between husbands, wives, daughters of mothers, and other caregivers ($\chi^2 = 1.568$, $df = 3$, $p > .65$).

The contrast between husbands and daughters of mothers is especially instructive because both are caring for a female dementia patient, but differ from one another in their own gender and generation. Because there are large gender differences in life expectancy, holding patient gender constant permits a strong test of the impact of type of family relationship. Yet, men and women are more similar than divergent from one another in how long they provide in-home care. The overall comparability seen between daughters and husbands and between

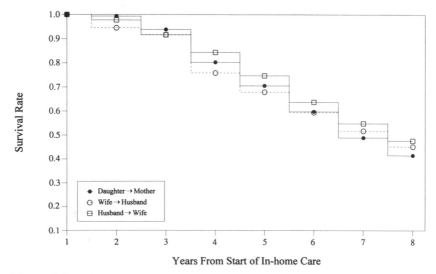

Figure 8.3   Survival distribution for duration of in-home care by relationship to the patient.

husbands and wives suggests that the gender stratification of family roles is less salient to the continuation of care than other considerations.

The Timing of Institutionalization

What other considerations? To the extent that institutionalization results from the deteriorating cognitive faculties and functional capabilities of the care recipient, these patient characteristics should be a dominant force regulating the timing of admission. Patient characteristics are unlikely to be the sole consideration, however, because continued in-home care depends upon the presence of someone who is willing and able to provide care. Also, no matter how urgent the caregiver's need for relief, institutional placement can occur only when facilities are available, affordable, and acceptable. Consequently, the risk of placement depends on multiple conditions, including the patient's health, characteristics of the caregiver, and the situational context.

Preliminary analyses of these data revealed some association between placement, background, and contextual factors, as well as degree of patient impairment. The impact of several dimensions of caregiver stress also was found to be pronounced in this association; particularly, economic strain and role captivity (Aneshensel et al., 1993). However, this earlier analysis was limited to only the first 3 waves of data; we extend it now to include outcomes through Time 4.

Patient characteristics often are presumed to be the prime force driving nursing home placement. Previous research has identified dementia itself as a key risk factor for placement among the general population of older persons (Branch & Jette, 1982; Greene & Ondrich, 1990). Among dementia patients, the following behaviors appear to precipitate institutionalization: extreme forgetfulness (Pruchno, Michaels, & Potashnik, 1990), incontinence, excessive irritability, inability to walk, wandering, hyperactivity, nighttime misbehavior (Knopman, Kitto, Deinard, & Heiring, 1988), and combativeness or angry outbursts (Chenoweth & Spencer, 1986). The risk of institutional placement has been found to be positively associated with other patient characteristics, such as advanced age (Branch & Jette, 1982; Cohen, Tell, & Wallack, 1986; Dolinsky & Rosenwaike, 1988; Greene & Ondrich, 1990; McCoy & Edwards, 1981; Vicente, Wiley, & Carrington, 1979), functional impairment (Branch & Jette, 1982; Cohen et al., 1986; Greenberg & Ginn, 1979; Greene & Ondrich, 1990; McCoy & Edwards, 1981), level of patient need for assistance with instrumental activities (Branch & Jette, 1982), and use of formal in-home help (Miller & McFall, 1991).

> I know it would be his knowing me. If he ceases to recognize me, no matter what his physical condition, he'd be an "other" and if he's an "other" I'd do what I have to do to save myself.

Although poor health may elevate the risk of placement in general, our initial analyses of these data suggested an interaction between health, cognitive impairment, and placement: Cognitive impairment increases the risk of placement, but the cognitively impaired who are in exceptionally good physical health are most likely to be placed (Aneshensel et al., 1993). Caregivers may find robust dementia patients especially difficult to manage, whereas nursing homes may be unenthusiastic about admitting patients whose medical management is complicated by dementia. These findings emphasize the need to consider the multiple influences that converge upon placement decisions.

The numerous potentially overlapping or offsetting influences are best captured in a multivariate analytic model, to which we now turn. The problem of censored cases persists in this shift from a descriptive to an explanatory model, so we employ the hazard model. Some explanatory variables are fixed, such as gender, but others, like declining cognitive status, change over time. These dynamic variables are treated as time-varying: Their initial value is that which is observed at baseline; this value is updated to the succeeding assessment until either placement takes place or the case is censored. As a result, these variables have values that are temporally close to the transitional event. Regression coefficients in this technique are calibrated to the log odds, which have no intuitive analog. Consequently, we present the exponential of the regression coefficient in order to simplify interpretation. This value is equivalent to a partial odds ratio (i.e., the multiplicative effect of a unit change in the explanatory variable on the odds of admission, other factors remaining the same).

Patient Health and the Risk of Placement

First, we consider the patient's health status as a selective factor influencing the risk of institutionalization. Given our preliminary findings concerning health status, we anticipated that dementia patients in especially good health would continue to display the counterintuitive pattern of early admission. In addition to the caregiver's rating of the patient's health status, we evaluated the impact of recent hospitalization, which may expedite the actual transfer of the patient from home to a long-term care facility. Advanced age is treated as a global sign of frailty and decline in health attributable to the aging process. The final indicator of patient health status is cognitive impairment, which represents the progression of the underlying dementia.

As shown in Table 8.2, Model 1, two of the four patient characteristics are significantly related to institutionalization in multivariate analysis. Hospitalization during the past year increases the risk of admission to a nursing home by about 50%. Excellent physical health also *increases* the odds of admission slightly. This counterintuitive finding reproduces the results from our preliminary analysis discussed above. As may also be seen in the table, the cognitive status of the patient per se is not independently related to the risk of placement.

The Impact of Primary Stressors

The second step of this analysis incorporates the remaining measures of objective primary stressors: problematic patient behavior, ADL dependencies,

Table 8.2   Relative Risk of Admission to a Nursing Home for Patient Characteristics, Primary Stressors, and Caregiver Characteristics

Patient and caregiver characteristics, and primary stressors	Model				Stepwise model
	1	2	3	4	
Patient age (in years)[a]	1.00	1.00	1.00	1.01	—
Patient physical health status (poor [1] to excellent [4])[a]	1.16*	1.17*	1.20*	1.19*	1.21**
Recent hospitalization (/no)[a]	1.55**	1.53**	1.53**	1.42*	1.54**
Cognitive impairment (0–4)[a]	1.01	1.06	1.03	.98	—
Problematic behavior (1–4)[a]	—	1.33*	1.14	1.15	—
ADL dependencies (1–4)[a]	—	.94	.93	1.01	—
Patient resists (/no)[a]	—	1.15	1.01	1.05	—
Role overload (1–4)[a]	—	—	1.06	1.17	—
Role captivity (1–4)[a]	—	—	1.35***	1.40***	1.44***
Loss of intimate exchange (1–4)[a]	—	—	1.18	1.13	—
Relationship to AD Patient[b]					
Husband	—	—	—	1.23	—
Wife	—	—	—	1.24	—
Daughter to mother	—	—	—	.95	—
Non-Hispanic white (/others)[b]	—	—	—	1.02	—
Family income (thousands of dollars)[a]	—	—	—	1.01**	—
Caregiver education (in years)[b]	—	—	—	.93*	—
Caregiver unemployed (/employed)[a]	—	—	—	1.24	—
Caregiver physical health status (poor [1] to excellent [4])[a]	—	—	—	1.28**	—
Site: San Francisco (/Los Angeles)[b]	—	—	—	.75*	—

[a]Time-varying covariate.
[b]Fixed covariate.
*$p \leq .05$.   **$p \leq .01$.   ***$p \leq .001$.

and patient resistance. It is apparent in Table 8.2, Model 2, that the objective demands imposed by dementia elevate risk, at least insofar as troublesome behaviors are concerned. Problematic behavior is assessed on a 4-point scale; an increase of one unit elevates the risk of placement by a third. In contrast, ADL dependencies and patient resistance do not independently contribute to placement. The indicators of the progression of the disease, therefore, appear to be far less pertinent to admission than are disruptive behavior.

In this context, it is important to recall that behavioral problems are independent of illness duration, whereas cognitive impairment and ADL dependencies increase as illness duration increases (see Figure 4.3). Recall as well that the hazard model statistically takes into account the passage of time, in this case, the length of time an individual has been at risk of institutional placement. That is, the joint dependency of both placement and impairment on the passage of time is taken into account. Severity of impairment, to the extent it may be distinguished from disease progression, therefore, appears to be rather unimportant to the risk of placement.

The next step in the analysis adds the subjective side of caregiving stress: role overload, role captivity, and loss of intimate exchange (Table 8.2, Model 3). Role captivity is the sole subjective stressor with a statistically significant independent relationship to placement; the other two variables, role overload and loss of intimate exchange, are significant only in bivariate analysis. Thus, the role captivity coefficient appears to represent that part of entrapment shared in common with overload and loss. The coefficient for problematic behavior becomes statistically nonsignificant with the addition of this set of variables. Apparently, troublesome patient behavior increases the odds of placement to the extent that this behavior engenders a sense of being held captive by the responsibilities of being a caregiver.

Rosemary

The deteriorating condition of the person suffering from dementia often makes nursing home placement the only viable course of action, as described here by Rosemary:

Three years before his death I finally couldn't manage it any more and gave it up. His disorientation became so severe that it led to violent verbal assaults on his part. I understood but it was too much to deal with. His behavior was like a 2-year-old child, but a 2-year-old you can control. No one could control Peter. He did what he wanted!

I wasn't getting any sleep. I couldn't get Peter in bed. He'd get very irritated and upset. He'd push and shove. He never hit out at me, never. I had to be very careful sometimes because he was strong. The situation got out of hand at night. We knew we'd have to do something.

So before we did that, Steven and I and a friend, took Peter to Big Sur for a last trip.

Characteristics of the Caregiver

The impact on placement of caregiver attributes—health status and sociodemographic characteristics—is considered next (Table 8.2, Model 4). As anticipated by the preliminary analysis reported earlier in this chapter (see Figure 8.3), the relationship of the caregiver to the patient appears to be immaterial to the duration of in-home care. Other things being equal, care recipients reside at home longer in San Francisco than Los Angeles, a differential that may be due to differences between sites in recruitment. The mean duration of care at Time 1 is significantly shorter for Los Angeles than San Francisco respondents (2.54 vs.

3.35 years, $t = 4.20, p < .001$). Because more caregivers were recruited early in their careers in Los Angeles than San Francisco, the Los Angeles caregivers had more opportunity to place their relatives early.

Both income and education are associated significantly with the odds of placement, although these effects are in opposite directions. Increasing income is associated with an increased likelihood of placing one's relative in a nursing home, whereas education is negatively associated with placement. This pattern is perplexing because income and education are positively associated with one another; that is, high income tends to accompany advanced education. At the bivariate level of analysis, the income coefficient is statistically significant, but the education coefficient is not. The part of education that translates into high income would appear to be redundant with the income coefficient, leading us to interpret the education coefficient as the impact of education that is separate from earnings. Specifically, at equal levels of income, advanced education appears to enable caregivers to maintain their impaired relatives at home for longer periods of time than their counterparts with fewer years of education. It may be that education enables caregivers to make somewhat more effective use of their resources, financial and otherwise, and, thus, persevere at caregiving.

Finally, when all other factors are considered, the odds of placement are highest for caregivers in excellent health and lowest for those in poor health. This finding, which also appears counterintuitive, seems to be an artifact of some of the other factors that are controlled statistically in this analysis. The coefficient for caregiver health is not significant in bivariate analysis and does not enter the equation in a subsequent stepwise analysis.

We conducted the stepwise analysis (final column of Table 8.2) because of the large number of nonsignificant covariates in the previous analyses. As may be seen, only three variables maintain their impact upon placement in this more parsimonious model: patient physical health status, recent hospitalization, and role captivity. Once these variables are taken into consideration, no other variables meet the entry criterion set at the equivalent of a .05 level of significance. Thus, several variables that attained statistical significance in the larger model (Model 4) do not remain in the stepwise model: family income, caregiver education, caregiver physical health status, and site. Consequently, the impact of these variables on the risk of placement appears marginal and redundant.

In sum, two patient characteristics and one primary stressor are independently related to an increased risk of nursing home admission. Both patient characteristics implicate physical health, revealing a rather complex set of contingencies. Hospitalization substantially increases the risk of subsequent placement in a nursing home. Aside from hospitalization, better patient health status also increases the risk of placement. This pattern suggests two pathways to placement: (1) serious health problems requiring hospitalization lead to nursing home admission, otherwise (2) poor patient health tends to inhibit admission. The hospitalization effect may reflect not only the poor health status of those who are hospitalized, but the impact of the formal health-care system in facilitating the transfer of patients from their own homes to nursing homes. For example, hospitalization may trigger placement because it separates the patient from the home, acting as a midway stop, or because it provides access to formal assistance in implementing the transfer.

Role captivity emerges as the sole primary stressor to exert an independent impact upon placement. Several other stressors are associated with placement at the bivariate level: an objective stressor, problematic patient behavior, and two subjective stressors: role overload and loss of intimacy. The impact of these other dimensions of stress appears to overlap with that of role captivity. In other words, troublesome patient behavior, being overwhelmed by the demands of care and feeling that one's parent or spouse has become a stranger apparently affect placement decisions to the extent that these experiences are also associated with feeling that being a caregiver obstructs the attainment of other life goals.

The Contribution of Secondary Stressors

We return now to one of our core questions: Can variation in the impact of caregiving be attributed to differences in exposure to secondary stressors? In this instance, the impact of caregiving is gauged by how long the caregiver endures; that is, by whether the caregiver continues to provide care or yields these responsibilities to an institution. Duration of in-home care is a decidedly different yardstick than those we employed in chapters 6 and 7. In these chapters, we calibrated the impact of caregiving by its consequences for the emotional well-being of the person providing care. The decision to institutionalize represents, we submit, an alternate outcome, an additional vantage point for surveying the consequences of care-related stress.

Although decisions about institutionalization are often phrased in terms of the patient's deteriorating health status, we have already seen that disease status is not the sole force shaping these decisions. By and large, the objective demands imposed by the patient's cognitive impairment matter insofar as these demands evoke stressful subjective states among caregivers. Specifically, the decision to institutionalize is shaped by both patient characteristics and the responses of caregivers to these characteristics. We now expand this focus to include the context of the patient–caregiver dyad; that is, the extent to which caregiving is embedded in secondary sources of stress.

This analysis utilizes the measures of secondary role strains and intrapsychic strains introduced in chapter 4. At the bivariate level, two role strains—not enough money to meet monthly expenses and a reduction in employment—significantly *reduce* the likelihood of placement; the remaining indicators of financial, work, and familial strain do not attain statistical significance. One intrapsychic strain, loss of identity, elevates risk at the bivariate level; caregiver competence and caregiving gains are not statistically important. The full complement of secondary stressors were considered in an extension of the previous stepwise model.

It is apparent in Table 8.3 that two secondary role strains emerge as statis-

Table 8.3   Relative Risk of Admission to a Nursing Home with the Stepwise Addition of Secondary Stressors and Potential Mediators

Patient characteristics, primary and secondary stressors, and potential mediators	Adding	
	Stressors	Mediators
Patient physical health status (poor [1] to excellent [4])[a]	1.17*	—
Recent hospitalization (/no)[a]	1.64***	—
Role captivity (1–4)[a]	1.55***	1.54***
Not enough money (some money left over [1] to not enough to make ends meet [3])[a]	.74**	.76**
Reduced employment (/no)[a]	.45***	.45***
Number of formal services (0–3)[a]	—	1.38***

[a]Tme-varying covariate.
*$p \leq .05$.   **$p \leq .01$.   ***$p \leq .001$

tically significant contributors to placement in multivariate analysis Insufficient money to pay monthly bills decreases the risk of placement by a quarter relative to having just enough money, and by 50% relative to having money left over. When a caregiver leaves the workforce or reduces the number of hours worked, the risk of placement is cut in half. As also shown in the table, the factors held constant in this analysis are patient physical health status, recent hospitalization, and the caregiver's sense of being held captive by his or her status as caregiver.

A more stringent test considered the importance of secondary stressors in the context of all of the patient characteristics, caregiver characteristics, and primary stressors considered previously. Because this model contains a large number of statistically insignificant coefficients, it is not reproduced here. Instead, we note only that insufficient financial resources and reduced employment continue to be associated with a substantial and significant reduction in the risk of admission to a nursing home when all other influences are taken into account. Furthermore, none of the remaining secondary stressors attain statistical significance in this large model. Consequently, it appears that these two role strains independently reduce the risk of placement and that these effects capture the overall impact of the secondary stressors assessed in this inquiry.

Finally, we consider the impact of stressors occurring outside the realm of caregiving, those we refer to as extrinsic stressors. As described previously, these stressors arise independent of the demands of care and the proliferation of care-related stress into other areas of life. Extrinsic stressors are events that are just as likely to erupt in the lives of persons who are caregivers as in the lives of those who are not. As disruptive as they may be to the caregiver, however, they do *not* independently contribute to the risk of institutionalization.

The Impact of Mental and Emotional Distress

We have already seen that one of the consequences of care-related stress is the creation and exacerbation of symptoms of psychological distress, for example, depressed mood. When caregiving results in oppressive internal states, caregivers may find themselves unable to perform the tasks associated with in-home care. In these instances, nursing home admission often looms as the only course of action. Similarly, caregivers may turn to institutional care in order to alleviate this internal distress. In this context, nursing home admission may be thought of as a coping behavior, an action taken to alleviate manifestations of stress (Pearlin & Aneshensel, 1986; Pearlin & Schooler, 1978).

Although we have emphasized dysphoric mood in earlier chapters, other dimensions of psychological distress also are pertinent to the outcome of institutional placement. These spheres include symptoms of anxiety and severe anger.[5] Each aspect of psychological distress might be examined for its unique contribution to nursing home admissions, but these measures are highly intercorrelated, posing problems of multicollinearity when included simultaneously as independent variables. Consequently, we employ a composite measure of nonspecific psychological distress. Analyses were repeated for each type of impairment considered separately. Irrespective of the measure used, the finding is the same: Psychological distress among caregivers does not independently contribute to the odds of admitting the care recipient to a nursing home once patient characteristics and care-related stressors are taken into account.

The Efficacy of Social Psychological Resources

If caregivers resort to institutional placement as a result of being overwhelmed by escalating demands, then assistance from others should prevent or delay nursing home admission. We considered this possibility by entering informal help into the models just considered (see Figure 8.3). Two specific time-varying factors were evaluated: whether the caregiver received help from family members or friends with (1) caring for the patient or (2) household tasks. Neither of these variables contributed independently to the risk of placement, nor did either have significant bivariate associations with placement.

Perhaps it is not so much practical assistance that matters to whether a caregiver can endure, but whether he or she feels cared for by friends and family members. This sense of socioemotional support may be influenced by the concrete care-related tasks performed by members of one's social network. Nonetheless, it is rooted more firmly in the basic, ongoing nature of these social ties: the history of the relationship and its mutuality, shared experiences and emotions, and the intangibles of interpersonal relationships that bond one person to another. The sense of being cared for by others, therefore, is not the consequence of a single action by a single person, but the synthesis of many actions by numerous persons. Because socioemotional support may ebb and flow over time, it was treated here as a time-varying covariate with regard to institutional placement.

Like practical support, however, emotional support does not independently add to the explanation of nursing home admissions.

Caregivers do not rely solely on informal help, of course, but often turn to formal services to supplement the informal assistance they receive or to compensate for its absence. With regard to the risk of placement, the most relevant types of help concern assistance with caring for the dementia patient. This factor was measured by whether the caregiver used any of the following services on a regular basis: home health care or a visiting nurse, Alzheimer's or adult day care, in-home attendant or companion, out-of-home respite care, or short-term board and care. Because the use of such services may fluctuate over time, formal help was treated analytically as a time-varying covariate. As is seen in Table 8.3, the use of formal services alters the risk of institutionalization, but in the opposite direction as might be expected; service use increases the risk of subsequent admission to a nursing home. It is also evident that the inclusion of this variable does not alter appreciably the impact on placement of the stressors included in the model.

The final resource considered here is the individual's sense of mastery. This sentiment, however, does not independently alter the odds of placing one's spouse or parent in a nursing home.

In sum, of the five social psychological resources considered as additions to the basic stress model of placement, only one attained statistical significance: use of formal health and social services. Moreover, rather than sustaining caregivers in their provision of in-home care, the use of these forms of assistance makes it more likely that caregivers will turn to institutional care.

Thus far, we have considered whether social psychological resources *mediate* the impact of care-related stressors. Mediation involves offsetting or counterbalancing those problematic conditions that motivate nursing home placement. The social psychological resources considered here, however, do not significantly decrease the risk of placement and, consequently, do not diminish the influence of those care-related stressors that prompt nursing home admission. Thus, these social psychological resources do not appear to mediate the impact of care-related stressors.

Mediation, however, represents only one means by which social psychological resources might affect the impact of care-related stressors on the risk of institutional placement. The other major route concerns the moderation of these stressors. Such effect moderation entails a contingency among stress, resource, and placement: The impact of stress upon placement is greater among those lacking resources than among those who receive assistance from their social networks or from formal helpers, feel cared for by their friends and family, or feel a sense of mastery over their lives.

Moderation effects are operationalized in this analysis as an interaction between stress and resource. The specific form of this interaction is multiplicative, Stress × Resource. The practical assistance indicators of support are dichotomous: Support is present or not, coded as 1 or 0. Consequently, there are two values of the interaction term: When support is present, this value is identical to the value of the stressor; when support is absent, this value is 0. If moderation occurs, the interaction term should be statistically significant and negative in sign: Stress exerts less of an impact upon placement among those with social support than among those who lack this support. The socioemotional support, social services, and mastery variables are ordinal, but the same basic logic as that just described is applied when interpreting their interaction with other variables.[6] Because the component variables are time-varying, the interaction terms are time-varying as well. Interaction terms were estimated between all five indicators of social psychological resources and those conditions that have an independent association with placement: patient health status, recent hospitalization, role captivity, not enough money to meet monthly expenses, and reduction in employment.[7]

As with the mediation analysis, however, the results of the moderation analysis fail to reveal any appreciable impact of these resources on the risk of institutional placement. The addition of the interaction terms does not produce a significant increment in the χ^2 value of the model relative to its degrees of freedom. This finding is consistent across all five resources. Thus, there is no detectable evidence that these resources modify the effect of care-related stressors on the duration of in-home care.

In sum, the social psychological resources examined here do not appear to reduce the risk of institutional placement, nor do they diminish the impact of care-related stressors in prompting placement. Instead, the sole significant relationship involving these resources is in the opposite direction: The use of formal services increases the risk of subsequently placing one's spouse or parent in a nursing home.

Catalysts for Institutionalization

What induces caregivers to admit their spouses or parents to nursing homes instead of continuing to provide in-home care? As we have just seen, this decision is influenced by the convergence of the actual demands of caregiving and the implications of these demands on other aspects of the caregiver's life. It has also been illustrated that the act of institutionalization often runs counter to the caregiver's personal sentiments about placement. Specifically, many of those who yield caregiving to an institution previously abhorred the very idea of doing so. Indeed, of those who admitted their relatives, almost half (47.4%) previously stated this prospect made them *very upset*. Thus, caregivers face competing pressures to alleviate their care-related burdens and to adhere to personal convictions and social norms regarding the care of one's mother, father, husband, or wife.

I knew that I needed a vacation. I put her in "temporarily." . . . She's never been out.

Caregivers who resolve this dilemma in favor of institutionalization interpret their actions within this discordant context. The act of institutionalization may be seen as the violation of potent social norms regarding family responsibilities. Yet, violation of these norms—internalized as personal conviction, dedication, and obligation—is socially sanctioned when extenuating circumstances absolve the caregiver of responsibility. Socially acceptable reasons for institutionalization, therefore, emphasize conditions that make it impossible for the caregiver to continue to provide care. For example, excessive or escalating care-related burdens, inadequate or declining resources, or shifts in patient or caregiver health status justify relinquishing in-home care. By contrast, personal distaste for the tasks of caregiving is likely to be viewed by others as dereliction of duty.

Consequently, it is not surprising that those who yield caregiving to an institution tend to express legitimate reasons for doing so. At the first postplacement interview, we asked caregivers why they moved their relatives into care facilities; specifically, whether any of 10 conditions motivated their decision. Caregivers could endorse multiple reasons or reject all of the options. These choices in descending order of endorsement are as follows:

- patient in danger of falling down and injuring self (50.6%)
- patient's loss of bowel and/or bladder control (50.2%)
- caregiver could not get the help needed to care for the relative at home (50.2%)
- caregiver too exhausted to carry on (48.7%)
- patient became physically ill (44.4%)
- too difficult to lift and move the patient (43.4%)
- difficulty controlling problem behaviors such as wandering or dangerous use of appliances (40.6%)
- patient too aggressive to handle (32.3%)
- patient no longer recognized family members (25.1%)
- caregiver became too ill to carry on (21.7%)

Each of these reasons was endorsed by about a quarter to a half of those caregivers who had recently institutionalized their relatives.

Clearly, most caregivers cited multiple reasons for their decision, averaging four per caregiver. Only seven caregivers did not endorse any item and about 10% gave only one reason. In all, the 237 caregivers who admitted their relatives to nursing homes gave 956 reasons for their actions. Obviously, there is no problem in finding justification for nursing home admissions.

Turning now to the reasons themselves (as distinct from the persons who cited them), Figure 8.4 illustrates that two themes predominate. About a third of the motives reflect concern that the dementia patient is potentially harmful to himself, herself, or others, the most common cluster of stimuli prompting relocation. Almost as common, however, is the caregiver's admission that he or she can no longer perform the tasks of caregiving: poor physical health, exhaustion, and inability to physically move the patient bespeak a level of burden that exceeds the caregiver's capacity to respond. The remaining third of the reasons are about

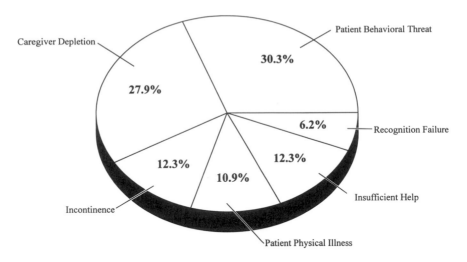

Figure 8.4   Distribution* of reasons for admission to a nursing home. (* Percent of all reasons given, *N* = 956.).

equally divided among poor patient health, incontinence, and insufficient social resources to balance these deteriorating conditions. In contrast, the patient's inability to recognize family members does not appear to contribute importantly to placement decisions.

We also asked caregivers if there were any other reasons for moving their relatives to long-term care facilities.[8] Numerous caregivers took this opportunity to describe the specific circumstances that prompted their action. These detailed explanations often echoed the themes implicit in our list of reasons. For example, several caregivers mentioned that others in the family did not help them sufficiently. Others commented that the patient was distressed or spent a lot of time alone, conditions potentially posing a threat to the well-being of the care recipient or others.

The information volunteered by caregivers also identified reasons for institutionalization not captured by our list. Some caregivers said they acted upon the advice of a physician. Their actions, therefore, were in some sense legitimated by an authority, having been given an official stamp of approval. Similarly, one caregiver cited the patient's own preference as a factor contributing to admission. Here, the permission to act contrary to social norms comes from within the family.

Constance

Because the decision to institutionalize runs counter to societal norms, caregivers sometimes need permission to take this action. Constance, who had made a commitment to herself to always take care of her mother was helped by her physician:

One day the doctor said that she shouldn't be alone anymore. She would leave the door unlocked and be alone in the house, or leave a pot boiling in the stove. I was aware that she was gradually slipping. I'd hoped to leave her as independent as possible. The number one trait of hers is "independence!" This was a very difficult adjustment for everyone. At the time the doctor said it was no surprise to me. It was getting obvious that she shouldn't be left alone.

There is scant evidence that yielding caregiving to an institution is a completely voluntary action. Only three caregivers stated outright that they were unwilling to continue to provide in-home care. Thus, almost without exception, caregivers see themselves as being compelled to act contrary to social norms mandating continued in-home care and often contrary to their own wishes to provide such care.

To what extent are the explanations provided by caregivers accurate reflections of the circumstances prior to institutionalization versus postadmission rationalization? Some tendency towards self-justification might be anticipated precisely because nursing homes carry such negative social stereotypes. Conditions encountered during the in-home phase of caregiving, therefore, might be reinterpreted in light of the subsequent decision to institutionalize.

We explored this possibility by comparing the explanations given *after* placement to the conditions existing *before* placement. Each category depicted in Figure 8.4 was treated as a dichotomous dependent variable: The reason was endorsed or not. These reasons were recorded at the first postplacement interview. Independent variables included the full set of explanatory variables considered in the earlier analysis of nursing home admission: patient characteristics, caregiver characteristics, primary and secondary stressors, nonspecific psychological distress, social support, service use, and mastery. These variables were set equal to the responses obtained at the interview immediately preceding placement. Stepwise logistic regression was used to generate a multivariate model of preadmission conditions contributing to postadmission accounts of these conditions. These results are displayed in Table 8.4.

The findings reveal quite clearly that the accounts given by caregivers are rooted in their actual experiences during the final months of in-home care. The first four columns represent motives that are ascribed to patient characteristics: physical illness, recognition failure, incontinence, and behavioral threat. These responses depict institutionalization as resulting from the declining functional status of the patient. The antecedent conditions that are associated with endorsing these reasons are, by and large, characteristics of the dementia patient. For example, the odds of citing poor health as an impetus to nursing home admission are increased for older patients, those who are in poor health or who have been hospitalized recently, and relatives who require considerable assistance with activities of daily living (ADL).

Table 8.4 Partial Odds Ratios for Effects of Preadmission Conditions on Postadmission Reasons for Placement[a]

Physical illness	Patient-centered reasons			Other reasons	
	Recognition failure	Incontinence	Behavioral threat	Caregiver depletion	Insufficient help
Patient age[b] 1.07**					
Patient physical health status[c] .52***					
Recent hospitalization 2.66**					
ADL dependencies 1.49*	ADL dependencies 1.70**	ADL dependencies 1.52**	Cognitive impairment .54** Problematic behavior 2.26**		

Role overload
1.63**

Role overload
1.65**

Income
.98*

Husband
3.32**

Wife
5.47***

Wife
4.10***

Education
.89*

Nonspecific
psychological distress
1.89*

$^a N = 224.$
^{b} In years.
^{c} Range from poor (1) to excellent (4).
$*p \leq .05.$ $**p \leq .01.$ $***p \leq .001.$

Only one factor outside of the realm of patient characteristics is associated with making this attribution: symptoms of nonspecific psychological distress—depression, anxiety, and anger—among caregivers. Thus, aside from psychological distress, conditions not indicative of patient health status have little, if anything, to do with subsequently citing health status as a reason for placement, whereas indicators of poor health and advanced age influence this attribution importantly.

A similar pattern emerges for other explanations relying upon patient characteristics. Thus, ADL dependencies contribute to attributions of incontinence and recognition failure, whereas cognitive impairment and problematic behavior play a role in explanations citing behavioral threats. Again, conditions not directly pertaining to the patient have little or no impact on the likelihood of giving these explanations. Two demographic characteristics make modest contributions: Wives are most likely to cite behavioral threats and the highly educated are least likely to cite incontinence.

The final two columns of Table 8.4 consider whether institutionalization is attributed to characteristics of the caregiver or to help received from other persons, as distinct from characteristics of the patient. Role overload during the in-home care period contributes significantly to citing both personal depletion and insufficient help as causes of institutionalization. In addition, spouses are most likely to cite poor health, fatigue, or difficulty lifting the patient—additional indicators of burnout. Apparently, husbands and wives are inclined to see themselves as resorting to institutionalization because of their own waning ability to provide care. Income tends to decrease the odds of selecting this explanation. In all likelihood, this association reflects the presence of resources that ease some of the burdens of care, such as use of an attendant.

Whereas patient characteristics and objective primary stressors were important contributors to patient-centered explanations, these characteristics have no appreciable association with explanations that focus upon the attributes of the caregiver or other helpers. One subjective primary stressor, role overload, however, figures prominently in admissions explained in terms of caregiver depletion or inadequate assistance.

Informal help from friends or family did not emerge as an important influence upon the specific reasons cited for placement. This negative finding is especially noteworthy with regard to caregivers who cited insufficient help as a reason for placement. Whether caregivers received help from family or friends directly with caring for the patient or with household chores was not significantly associated with citing lack of help as a reason for placement. Similarly, the use of health and social services does not contribute to this attribution. In this regard, it is useful to recall that informal and formal assistance did not emerge as important contributors to the risk of nursing home admission. Lack of assistance or support from others, therefore, appears to be an explanation that emerges after the fact.

In sum, the conditions encountered within the home immediately prior to institutionalization shape the caregiver's understanding of the transition into the institutional care phase of the caregiving career. Caregivers see their actions as motivated by three sets of deteriorating conditions: the patient's declining functional capabilities, the caregiver's own waning ability to provide care, and the contraction of assistance from other persons. In other words, the demands of caregiving eventually come to be seen as exceeding the caregiver's resources, providing the impetus to institutionalization.

The Family Context of Institutionalization

Although we have focused on the motivations of primary caregivers for placement of dementia patients, these individuals do not act within a social vacuum. Instead, most caregiver–patient pairs are embedded within larger family systems. For spousal caregivers, these systems typically include their adult children, their own siblings, and the siblings of the care recipient. Caregivers to parents, on the other hand, often have siblings who stand in the same familial relationship to the impaired person (i.e., parent–child). The siblings of the impaired parent—aunts and uncles to the caregiver—frequently form part of the familial context of caregiving as well. Moreover, many adult children have nuclear families of their own, spouses and children to whom they have responsibilities.

Because primary caregivers carry most of the burden of providing care, their ability and willingness to continue to do so establishes boundaries on the duration of in-home care. The actions of other family members, however, can affect the balance between the demands of care and the resources available to meet these demands. For example, tasks that become too physically demanding for a frail spouse, such as lifting and moving the patient, might be taken over by a son or daughter, thereby enabling the impaired parent to continue living at home. As the progressive course of dementia alters the requirements of care, the actions of other family members often determine the degree to which in-home care may be maintained. To what extent, then, are these other family members involved in the decision to cease in-home care?

Most caregivers consult other family members about this decision. At the first reinterview, we asked those who were continuing to provide in-home care whether they talked to various people about the possibility of moving the dementia patient to a care facility. Almost two-thirds (61.9%) reported having talked to relatives, whereas somewhat less than half had talked to friends (45.1%) or professionals (46.7%). Most of those who consulted family members also consulted friends, professionals, or both (80.6%). On the other hand, caregivers who did not discuss the possibility of placement with relatives also were unlikely to discuss this matter with friends or professionals. Thus, caregivers are more likely to consult others in the family than persons outside of the family about the decision to institutionalize. Moreover, when friends or professionals are consulted, it is most often within the context of family consultations. However, a sizable minority of those providing in-home care (26.9%) did not discuss the alternative of institutional care with anyone.

These consultations appear to be both exploratory and directive. We asked whether anyone had suggested moving the dementia patient into a care facility and if so, who had made this suggestion. When considering the caregivers who were continuing to provide care at follow-up, 4 out of 10 (40.3%) reported that someone had suggested moving the patient out of the home. This advice most often came from other family members, followed by physicians and then friends. A broad spectrum of relations offered this advice, but the most common mentions were the closest family relations: husbands, wives, sisters, brothers, sons, and daughters. In general then, many caregivers received the impetus for placement, or at least some support in this direction, from other family members.

How is the family viewed after the decision to place has been made and implemented? At the first interview following admission to a nursing home, caregivers were asked how helpful other family members were in making the decision to move the care recipient.[9] More than half (57.0%) rated their relatives as *very helpful* in making this decision, the most positive response option provided to respondents. In contrast, about one in five (18.4%) said their relatives were *not at all helpful*, the most negative response option, or that they had made the decision entirely on their own. Once again, in regard to family contributions to decision making on institutionalizing relatives, we find both a heavy tilt toward the positive and an appreciable number of quite negative feelings.

However, outright conflict over placement is uncommon. We asked caregivers whether they had any disagreement with family members over moving the patients to care facilities. Very few ($n = 20$) mentioned any conflict.

When asked who had been most helpful, the most commonly mentioned persons were those having the most immediate family ties: husbands, wives, daughters, sons, brothers, and sisters. In-laws also appear to assist in making the decision to institutionalize; frequently these individuals are married to sons, daughters, brothers, or sisters who are also named as being helpful. Aunts, uncles, grandchildren, and more distant relatives were mentioned only occasionally.

Institutionalization as a Stressor

Thus far, we have approached nursing home placement as the juncture between in-home care and institutionalized care: A transitional marker separating two phases of the role enactment stage of the caregiver career. In examining the duration of the in-home care phase, we have emphasized the impact of care-related stressors and the inner responses of caregivers to these demands. This orientation implicitly treats institutionalization as a coping response to abiding stressors: An action undertaken to alleviate at least some of the stress and distress associated with taking care of a cognitively impaired relative.

On the other hand, we have also portrayed institutionalization as a potentially stressful action in and of itself. It may be seen both as a betrayal of trust and of powerful emotional ties, as well as a violation of potent social norms, those governing obligations of caring for family members in times of serious, sometimes desperate, need. This perspective is echoed in the reasons caregivers give for institutionalization, which emphasize conditions that legitimize their actions, portraying nursing home admission as a necessary, but not willful, action. In addition to its inherent ability to evoke stress, however, nursing home admission also becomes stressful because it is a difficult transition to navigate. We turn now to difficulties experienced in association with the admission of a relative to a nursing home.

Anticipatory Stress

Some of the problems might well be labeled anticipatory stressors because they arise before concrete preparations for admission have begun. When family members contemplate moving their spouses or parents to nursing homes, they face a host of uncertainties. Most are unfamiliar with the options available, the steps necessary to locate suitable facilities, and the best ways to evaluate potential placement sites. Also, they can only guess about the impact of placement on their parent or spouse. Accepting current "wisdom" about care facilities and their effects, many caregivers expect adverse emotional responses from their relatives, such as anger or depression, or anticipate feeling disloyal or guilty themselves. Financial worries also arise: The length of time the impaired relative will reside in the care facility cannot be anticipated accurately so that cost estimates are uncertain. These ambiguities and uncertainties surrounding the transition understandably may generate misgivings and apprehension.

What anticipatory concerns surface most often for caregivers? At the first reinterview, we asked those who were continuing to provide in-home care about the prospect of moving their parent or spouse into a care facility. Specifically, we asked how concerned they were about six aspects of such a move with response options ranging from *not at all concerned* (1) through *very concerned* (4). A few caregivers (5%) declined to respond to these questions, rejecting outright any consideration of a nursing home. The responses are presented in Figure 8.5 in two forms: the *presence* of concern (all response options except *not at all concerned*) and the *intensity* of concern (*very concerned* versus all other response options).

Some worries arise for almost all caregivers as they contemplate a potential nursing home move, especially misgivings about the welfare of their parents and spouses. As may be seen in the figure, 9 out of 10 caregivers are concerned about the quality of care their relatives would receive, whether their relatives would be upset in a care facility, and the safety of their relatives. These considerations are also the areas in which caregivers have the most intense apprehension. Approximately two out of three caregivers selected the most extreme response category (i.e., *very concerned*) to describe their sentiments about aspects of institutional care that directly pertain to patient welfare. Thus, when caregivers harbor these concerns, they are not faintly entertained, rather they are likely to be intense. The woman shown in these photographs clearly demonstrates that concern for the patient's welfare and close affectional ties persist after the transition to institutional care as well (see photographs 16–18).

Instrumental worries also are extremely prevalent, but somewhat less in-

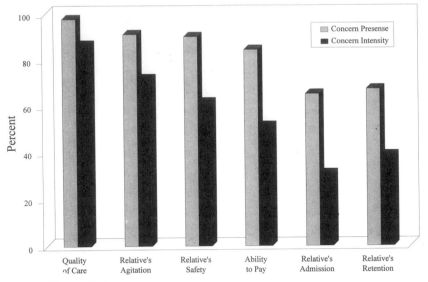

Figure 8.5   Percent distribution of anticipatory concerns about placement.

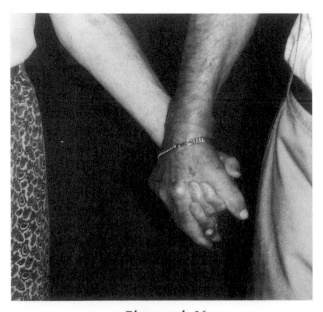

Photograph 16

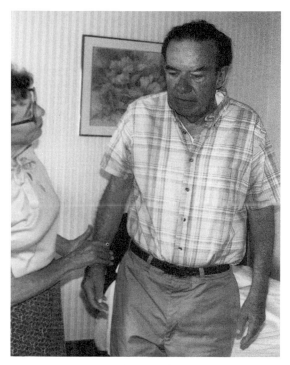

Photograph 17

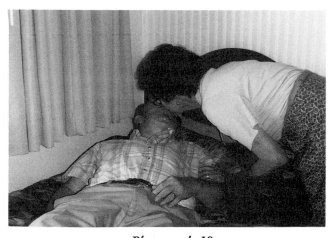

Photograph 18

tensely felt than worries about patient well-being. At least two-thirds of the caregivers cite some anxiety with their ability to pay for this type of care, whether their relatives would be accepted into a care facility, and whether their relatives could remain in the care facility if necessary. About one-third have intense concerns about these instrumental matters; that is, about half of those who have this reluctance are *very concerned*. Thus, these issues matter considerably to caregivers who are providing in-home care, but are lacking in gravity when compared to issues directly concerning the welfare of their parents or spouses.

In absolute terms, the level of anticipatory worry experienced by caregivers represents a substantial load, especially when added to the stressors simultaneously encountered while providing in-home care. The prospect of placement has a pervasive presence in the consciousness of caregivers, one that is most intense when it is most personal and most directly tied to the care recipient. One component of the in-home phase of caregiving, therefore, is worry about the future course of care.

> If she gets too sick and goes into a nursing home,
> I wouldn't want to see her again—too painful.

Indeed, these anticipatory misgivings flow, at least in part, from conditions encountered during the period of in-home care. In general, caregivers who are most taxed by caregiving, paradoxically, are also those who tend to develop the most severe apprehensions about their ability to situate their relatives in nursing homes that safeguard patient well-being.

This conclusion is based on an analysis of the association between care-related stressors and subsequent concerns about placement. The dependent variable of placement worries is a summated scale of the items displayed in Figure 8.5, weighted by the intensity of concern (response categories 1 through 4); this composite measure is adequately reliable ($\alpha = .68$). The mean value of 3.1 reflects a considerable burden of anticipatory worry. The independent variables are care-related stressors assessed at the baseline interview, social psychological resources, and characteristics of the patient and the caregiver. The results of this stepwise regression analysis appear in Table 8.5.

As may be seen, some of the factors that ultimately prompt placement also tend to generate anticipatory worries about this change. Patients who exhibit numerous problematic behavior have caregivers who worry about locating a suitable nursing home and about the patient's welfare within that facility. Role overload is the only other primary stressor to contribute independently to the development of placement worries. Two secondary stressors also elevate uneasiness: having insufficient funds to meet monthly expenses and not feeling particularly good about how one performs the role of caregiver. One caregiver characteristic independently contributes to these worries—education—which has an inverse relationship to apprehension (i.e., those with the least formal education worry the most about the potential admission of their spouses or parents to

Table 8.5   Regression of Anticipatory Worries about Placement at Time 2
upon Prior Care-Related Stressors, Resources, and Background Characteristics

Stressors, resources, and characteristics at Time 1	Regression coefficients ($N = 334$)	
	Unstandardized (*SE*)	Standardized
Problematic behavior (1–4)	.144* (.064)	.122
Role overload (1–4)	.093* (.040)	.129
Not enough money (some money left over [1] to not enough to make ends meet [3])	.156** (.054)	.156
Caregiver competence (1–4)	−.137* (.062)	−.113
Caregiver education (in years)	−.043*** (.012)	−.178
Intercept	3.445*** (.330)	
R^2	.148***	

*$p \leq .05$.   **$p \leq .01$.   ***$p \leq .001$.

nursing homes). These five variables collectively explain a modest amount of the variation in anticipatory concerns about placement. Uneasiness about placement, therefore, is rooted in the experience of in-home caregiving, but is influenced by other factors as well.

Not appearing on the list of independent predictors of placement concerns are several factors that logically should be implicated in these worries. For example, income would appear to be pertinent to the prospect of placement because residence in a nursing home typically imposes substantial financial hardship. Stepwise regression techniques can obscure the impact of some factors, especially factors that are highly associated with other predictor variables. For instance, financial strain may eclipse income in multivariate analysis because low income contributes to financial strain. In this regard, we note that some variables are significantly associated with placement concerns, but only at the bivariate level: loss of intimate exchange, loss of self, family conflict, poor caregiver health, low income, being non-Hispanic white, nonspecific psychological distress, emotional support, use of community-based services, and being the wife of the dementia patient. These factors do not emerge as independent predictors of placement worries because they are redundant with the variables identified in Table 8.5.

We would like to call attention, however, to some factors that lack even a bivariate association with placement worries, especially indicators of the primary demands of caregiving: cognitive impairment, patient resistance, recent hospitalizations, patient health. Certain secondary stressors appear to be empirically unimportant to placement, although they might reasonably be hypothesized as contributing to anticipatory concerns. These include role captivity, work strain, reduction in employment, and increased expenses. Informal social support in the form of help with the patient or help with chores similarly lacks significant association with these concerns.

In sum, placement worries are more prevalent against the background of some in-home care conditions than others. One set of conditions involves inadequate financial resources that exacerbate concerns about the future of the care recipient: low income, low education, and running out of money each month. A second set centers on the demands of care: Caregivers worry most about the admission of their spouses or parents to nursing homes when they act in troublesome and inappropriate ways and when the provision of in-home care seems overwhelming. A third cluster revolves around the notion of loss: Worry about nursing home admission is especially pronounced among caregivers who feel they have already lost their relatives to the ravages of dementia and whose own sense of self has been eroded over the course of caregiving.

Transitional Stress

The anticipatory concerns of in-home caregivers are well justified insofar as numerous problems indeed emerge during the transition to institutional care. We asked caregivers whose relatives were receiving institutional care at follow-up whether they had encountered any of nine specific problems while they were searching for a care facility. By far, the most commonly cited difficulty was finding suitable facilities to choose from, a problem encountered by roughly one in three caregivers (37.0%). About one in five caregivers also experienced problems with obtaining financial assistance or routing through the obstacles of insurance programs (25.1%), finding care facilities in a hurry (21.7%), and encountering long waiting lists to get into care facilities (20.4%). Although the remaining problems were confronted less frequently, they are by no means uncommon, occurring for about 1 in 10 persons who go on to place their relatives. These difficulties include locating someone who could answer questions (14.9%), finding someone to stay with the patient while the caregiver looked at facilities (12.8%), managing the paperwork required on applications (11.6%), being refused admission because of the patient's memory and behavior problems (17.1%), and various other problems (16.6%).

It should be recognized that these retrospective reports underestimate the problems encountered by caregivers in seeking nursing home placements because they were obtained only from those persons who successfully resolved these problems (i.e., those who placed their relatives in nursing homes). Those who found these problems insurmountable do not appear in these tallies. Also, these reports were obtained only when the patient still resided in a nursing home at follow-up; those whose relatives died shortly after admission are not represented. Given the difference in the outcome of admission—patient survival versus death (see chapter 10)—we can assume that only some of the problems encountered in the transition to institutional care are captured in this analysis.

At the first postplacement interview, approximately one-third of the caregivers reported not facing *any* of these specific problems. Additionally, the median number of problems is one. Concrete problems, therefore, tend to be less common than anticipatory problems. Lest we mistakenly conclude that these individuals navigated this transition without difficulty, it should be noted that they may well have encountered other problems that were not included on our list. This possibility should be taken seriously given that we asked an abbreviated inventory. Still, the list samples a wide spectrum of problems, and caregivers had the option of responding to an open-ended probe. The high density of caregivers at the low end of this distribution means that a substantial subgroup of caregivers experience few or no practical difficulties in implementing the transition to institutional care.

On the other hand, the frequency of reported problems covers the full range from 0 to 9, indicating considerable variation in the extent to which the implementation of this transition is problematic. Indeed, almost half have run up against two or more problems. A second subgroup of caregivers, therefore, may be described as confronting multiple problems. Thus, two major pathways emerge: relatively clear sailing and being battered by a relentless storm.

Another indication that anticipatory concerns about placement are well justified for some caregivers may be found in the overall assessments of those who have made this transition. Caregivers who mentioned any problems encountered while searching for care facilities were asked how difficult these problems were to deal with overall. The modal response category was the most extreme one, *very difficult* (43.9%). In contrast, less than 1 in 10 selected the response option of *not at all difficult* (7.3%). In essence, some caregivers encounter a fair number of problems in searching for care facilities, and these difficulties tend to be of notable severity.

These problems flow, at least in part, from the conditions existing just prior to admission. The number of problems reported at the first postplacement interview was regressed upon a set of independent variables assessed at the interview immediately preceding placement: characteristics of the dementia patient, the caregiver, and their relationship to one another; primary stressors associated with the demands of care; secondary stressors present in other areas of life; and social psychological resources.[10] The results of this stepwise analysis appear in Table 8.6.

In multivariate analysis, four variables emerge as independent contributors to the number of problems encountered during the transition to institutional care. Caregivers who are in poor health, especially those caring for patients who also are in poor health, tend to have more difficulty arranging for nursing home admission than healthier caregivers caring for relatively healthy patients. Also, those who are beset by conflict with other family members, as well as those who are short of money, appear to experience problems in maneuvering through the

Table 8.6 Regression of Problems Encountered during Placement upon Prior
Care-Related Stressors, Resources, and Background Characteristics

Stressors, resources, and characteristics at interview preceding placement	Regression coefficients ($N = 171$)		
	Unstandardized	(SE)	Standardized
Patient physical health status (poor [1] to excellent [4])	−.315*	(.153)	−.149
Caregiver health (poor [1] to excellent [4])	−.434*	(.189)	−.166
Family conflict (no disagreement [0] to quite a bit [3])	.565**	(.199)	.201
Not enough money (some money left over [1] to not enough to make ends meet [3])	.483*	(.216)	.164
Intercept	2.49**	(.836)	
R^2	.158***		

*$p \le .05$.   **$p \le .01$.   ***$p \le .001$.

maze of paperwork, logistics, and costs entailed in relocating their spouses or parents from home to nursing home. In contrast, then, caregivers with harmonious ties to the larger family circle, those who are financially secure, and those in robust health, especially those caring for healthy relations, tend to experience the fewest problems in relocating their husbands, wives, fathers, and mothers. These four variables in combination explain a modest amount of the variation in placement problems.

Several other variables also are associated with the number of problems encountered in bivariate analyses, but their impact appears to overlap with the four variables listed in Table 8.6. These additional variables include role overload, loss of self, and not feeling especially competent as a caregiver. These attributes help regulate the occurrence of problems to the extent that they coexist with poor caregiver patient health, financial strain, and family conflict. Finally, anticipatory worries are associated slightly with the number of problems subsequently encountered ($r = .27, p \le .05, n = 77$).[11]

We would like to call attention, additionally, to factors that lack even a bivariate association with placement problems, especially indicators of the primary demands of caregiving: severe cognitive impairment, patient resistance, and recent hospitalizations. Secondary stressors that appear unimportant to placement problems include role captivity, work strain, reduction in employment, and increased expenses. Also, social psychological resources, along with the caregiver's own emotional functioning, are not associated with the number of problems encountered in the transition from in-home care to institutional care.

In sum, placement problems are more common under some conditions than others. In general, these conditions point to the presence of one or more *other* problems in the caregiver's life: money, family, or health. Most noteworthy, the extent to which problems emerge is more directly related to dimensions of the caregiver's life than to the state of cognitive or functional impairment of the patient.

Summary

This chapter has described the average course of in-home care and identified conditions that accelerate the admission of one's spouse or parent to a nursing home. In particular, we have focused upon the role of care-related stress and on social psychological resources that might diminish the impact of these stressors. The transitional event of institutional placement also has been examined as a source of stress in and of itself. Major findings from these analyses are:

• Preexisting dispositions towards institutional care do not have an appreciable impact on whether the caregiver subsequently admits his or her relative to a nursing home.

• During the early years of in-home care, the risk of nursing home admission is quite low, but this plateau is followed by a steady decline in the percentage of caregivers who continue to provide in-home care.

• The annual risk of admission to a nursing home is fairly constant from year to year, with the exception of the first 2 years when admissions are uncommon.

• In-home care is long-term care with an average duration of almost 7 years.

• Husbands, wives, daughters of mothers, and other caregivers follow similar in-home care trajectories, with no detectable difference in the duration of this career stage.

• Having been hospitalized during the past year increases the risk of admission to a nursing home by about 50%.

• The progression of the underlying dementia appears to be far less important to institutionalization than disruptive behavior on the part of the patient.

• Troublesome patient behavior appears to elevate the risk of institutionalization because these behaviors engender a sense of being held captive by caregiving responsibilities.

• Several secondary role strains emerge as significant, independent factors in delaying institutional placement: having insufficient money to pay monthly bills and leaving the workforce or reducing the number of hours worked.

• Caregiver's psychological distress does not independently contribute to the odds of admitting the patient to a nursing home.

• The social psychological resources examined here—social support, service use, and mastery—do not appear to reduce the risk of institutional placement, nor do they diminish the impact of care-related stressors on prompting placement.

• The use of formal services, however, increases the risk of subsequently placing one's spouse or parent in a nursing home.

• Caregivers see the decision to institutionalize as motivated by three sets of deteriorating conditions: the patient's declining functional capabilities, the caregiver's own waning ability to provide care, and the contraction of assistance from other persons.

• Primary caregivers tend to consult family members about whether the dementia patient should be institutionalized. In general, they tend to find these consultations helpful, although one in four caregivers have not discussed the possibility of institutionalizing their relatives with anyone.

• Almost all in-home caregivers experience anticipatory stress about institutionalization in the form of concern about the welfare of their relatives and worry about concrete matters such as finances.

• These anticipatory worries are directly tied to the conditions of in-home care, including inadequate financial resources, troublesome patient behavior, role overload, and feelings of inadequacy as a caregiver.

• The anticipation of institutionalization appears to be more problematic for many caregivers than the actual transition itself.

• Although some caregivers navigate this career transition with little difficulty, others confront numerous problems.

• Complications in the transition to nursing home care depend, at least in part, on the preexisting conditions of in-home care, including caregiver health, family conflict, and financial strain.

Discussion

These results demonstrate the orderly nature of the processes that lead caregivers to admit their spouses and parents to nursing homes. The forces converging upon this transitional event represent, on the one hand, the sheer passage of time and, on the other hand, the impact of care-related stress processes.

For dementia patients and their families, time means the inevitable and progressive decline in cognitive abilities characteristic of dementia and, ultimately, the death of the patient. The passage of time, therefore, necessarily connotes, on average and over the long-term, disease progression. Time and disease progression are difficult to evaluate independently precisely because they are inextricably connected.

Several of our findings, however, lead to the conclusion that time, rather than disease progression, leads caregivers to institutionalize. First, the likelihood of placement does not depend upon the caregiver's attitudes about placement; many caregivers ultimately act contrary to their personal sentiments. This deviation between attitudes and behavior, although by no means uncharacteristic of human conduct, suggests the presence of pressures that ultimately overwhelm, or, in other words, an accumulation of burden.

Second, given that the patient still resides at home, the risk of admission does not vary appreciably from year to year (except for the first few years when this risk is virtually nil). Specifically, this risk does not increase as time progresses, the pattern that one would anticipate if disease progression in and of itself played a pivotal role in admission. Third, the severity of cognitive impairment is not associated with institutionalization when illness duration is taken into consideration.

The transitional event of nursing home admission, therefore, may be seen as a normative occurrence in the caregiving career, as something to be expected by all caregivers unless death intervenes. The cessation of in-home caregiving should be viewed not as a failure to master the tasks required by this situation, but as the inescapable conclusion of one phase of caring for one's relative and the beginning of another.

At any specific point in time, however, some caregivers are more likely than others to place their relatives. The physical health of the patient matters to this variation in risk; this influence, nonetheless, appears to have at least as much to do with access to health and social services as with health status per se. In this regard, we note that the coefficients for indicators of physical functioning become statistically nonsignificant when such service use is taken into consideration (see Table 8.3). Thus, the physical health of the patient appears to matter because it contributes to the use of services, and service use increases the risk of subsequently being admitted to a nursing home. The key to this set of relationships appears to be that supplemental assistance to in-home caregivers facilitates the transition to institutional care.

Institutionalization also is regulated by the exposure of the caregiver to both primary and secondary sources of stress. Caregivers who feel trapped by their responsibilities are particularly likely to turn to institutional care. This sense of role captivity arises from the objective burdens of care. In this instance, care-related stress results in institutionalization, perhaps as a direct attempt to alleviate these burdens, as an effort to cope.

Care-related stressors also serve to deter institutionalization, however, as evidenced by the two secondary stressors that are predictive of placement. Specifically, financial strains and reduced involvement in the workplace inhibit institutionalization. These stressors arise outside of the context of the direct provision of in-home care, yet influence whether one continues to provide that care.

Financial strain and reduced work involvement, it will be recalled, are associated with the primary demands of care. As we have just seen, these primary demands often lead to institutionalization, at least insofar as these hardships are translated into a sense of being held captive by caregiving. The pressures that elevate these secondary stressors, therefore, tend to prompt placement, but the secondary stressors themselves act to suppress placement. Reduced work involvement increases the time and energy that can be allocated to caregiving, perhaps reducing its attendant strains and delaying institutionalization. Although escalating burdens may prompt a desire to admit one's relative to a nursing home, institutional care is costly and often out of reach for those who are already financially strapped. As the pressures to institutionalize grow, therefore, one may be increasingly unable to act on those pressures because reductions in work and finances make this course of action impossible.

In conclusion, the process of stress proliferation set in motion by long-term caregiving gives an accelerating impetus to place one's relative in a nursing home, but the overflow of caregiving in other domains of life often impedes this institutional resolution of care-related stress.

Notes

[1]The analysis was repeated using a hazard model to take into account the length of time an individual had been at risk of placement. Even in this new analysis, caregivers' sentiments about placement were not associated with the risk of placement in the original analysis.

[2]The difficulty of obtaining a precise date for the onset of care is readily evident. Often, the mutual exchange of assistance in everyday family life gives way gradually to unilateral care, a transition that may be noticed only in retrospect. Difficulties in recalling when this transition occurred may be particularly pronounced when it took place long before our first interview. Consequently, the estimates of the duration of in-home care provided here should be regarded as approximations. Errors in the dating of the initiation of caregiving, however, are not likely to be systematic with regard to the timing of the termination of caregiving—the other element used to calculate the duration of care—because initiation reports were obtained at the baseline interview, whereas placement always occurred after the baseline interview. Thus, recall error in the timing of initial events undoubtedly occurs, but is unlikely to bias estimates of the factors affecting the duration of in-home care.

[3]The distribution probably underestimates placement during the early stages of caregiving because our sampling design is more likely to result in the selection of long-term than short-term caregivers. When the duration of a condition is variable, the probability of selection is greatest for those with the longest duration because they are "at-risk" of being sampled for a long time; those with short durations, however, are less likely to be identified while "in episode." The same principle applies to durations of caregiving. The relatives with dementia who have been cared for over a long time de facto were not institutionalized early on. To the extent that long-term caregivers are oversampled, then, the risk of placement early in the caregiving career is underestimated by these data.

[4]The proportion of patients living at home at the end of 13 years is higher than the proportion of caregivers providing continuing care at Time 4 because the survival analysis takes into account those who died or who were lost-at-follow-up while living at home.

[5]The symptoms of anxiety are "feel nervous or shaky inside, feel tense or keyed up, feel afraid or fearful, [and] worry about everything." The symptoms of severe anger include the following: "feel very critical of others, become easily annoyed or irritated, have temper outbursts that you couldn't control, [and] get angry over things that are not important." The depressive symptoms are: "lack enthusiasm for doing anything, feel bored or have little interest in things, cry easily or feel like crying, feel downhearted or blue, feel slowed down or low in energy, blame yourself for everything, have your feelings hurt easily, feel that everything was an effort, [and] have trouble getting to sleep or staying asleep." The response categories are: *no days* (1), *1 or 2 days* (2), *3 or 4 days* (3), and *5 or more days* (4). This summated measure of nonspecific psychological distress displays excellent internal consistency reliability ($\alpha = .94$).

[6]In order to lessen multicollinearity in this analysis, the stress and emotional support measures are demeaned (Belsley, 1984).

[7]To reduce problems associated with multicollinearity, five interaction-term models were estimated: one model for each of the resources. The explanatory efficacy of the moderation effects was assessed as an increment in χ^2 relative to the model without these interaction terms.

[8]Caregivers were not asked this question when the dementia patient was admitted to a nursing home and died prior to the next scheduled interview. These open-ended responses, therefore, reflect only the attitudes of caregivers whose relatives survived admission (see chapter 10).

[9]Questions about the process of admission to a nursing home were not asked of caregivers whose relatives died within the interval between placement and the next interview.

[10]The prospective data is, therefore, extracted from the Time 1, Time 2, or Time 3 interview depending upon whether placement occurred between Times 1 and 2, Times 2 and 3, or Times 3 and 4, respectively.

[11]Assessment of this association is limited to those caregivers who placed their relatives after Time 2 because anticipatory worries were not measured until that interview, and to those who participated in at least one institutional care interview, the point at which problems were ascertained. For the latter subgroup, anticipatory problems attain statistical significance in the multivariate model as well.

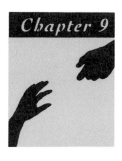

Adaptation Following Institutionalization

Institutional placement marks a major transition in the caregiving career. It signifies the end of around-the-clock involvement in patient care and leads to a major restructuring of the caregiver role. The decision to institutionalize, as we saw in the previous chapter, may be painfully challenging and difficult. The same may be said for the period following the actual admission of one's relative into a nursing home.

Many people, professionals and family members alike, encourage primary caregivers to admit their relatives into nursing homes, believing that placement will put an end to the burdens associated with caregiving. However, caregiving typically continues after placement. Thus, placement alters, rather than eliminates, the stressors of caregiving. No longer responsible for the day-to-day hands-on care of their relatives, caregivers must now redefine and restructure their involvement in caregiving. Emergent challenges include issues of how often to visit the nursing home, how to interact with the patient and staff in the new setting, how much supplemental assistance to provide, redefining relationships with family and friends, and, in a larger sense, redefining one's own identity as the spouse or child of someone who is institutionalized.

Rosenthal and Dawson (1991) have described the situation of women who institutionalize their husbands as "quasi-widowhood": no longer having the companionship of a married person, yet retaining the formal status of wife. In this situation, wives may experience contradictory pressures, being encouraged by others to move on with their lives *and* to maintain their obligations to their husbands. They may consider taking on new commitments, such as work or social relationships, but experience guilt about doing so. Husbands who place their wives no doubt experience similar contradictory pressures and emotions.

This chapter describes the postadmission phase of the caregiving career, identifying the principal ways in which caregivers enact an institutional caregiver role. It focuses as well upon one of the core questions guiding this entire inquiry: "What accounts for variation in the responses of caregivers to seemingly similar circumstances?" In this chapter, these circumstances refer to the act of institutionalization. As we have previously seen, understanding the concrete demands and tasks of providing care is necessary, but not sufficient, for understanding how caregivers fare over time. Individual variability in adaptation emerges from the personal, social, and economic contexts of caregiving.

In the following sections, we first consider continuity and change in the caregiver role following admission of the dementia patient to a nursing home, describing patterns of visiting and caring for relatives within the facility. Also, we describe stressors specifically associated with institutional care. We then compare caregivers who place their relatives with those providing continuing care in the home in order to identify dimensions of the stress process that are altered by placement. Next, we look at the factors differentiating caregivers who make effective adjustments following placement from those who adapt poorly. Finally, we describe long-term trajectories of psychological adaptation following placement.

Continuity and Change in the Caregiver Role

Contrary to prevailing social stereotypes, most caregivers do not abandon their relatives after placement (Pratt, Schmall, Wright, & Hare, 1987; Smith & Bengston, 1979). Instead, they often remain involved with the patient in a variety of ways, providing some of the very same care that they previously provided at

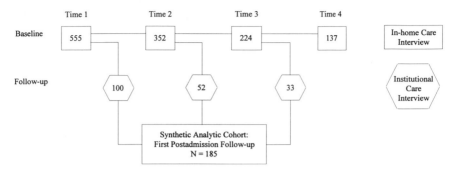

Figure 9.1   Creation of the short-term postadmission cohort.

home (Chenoweth & Spencer, 1986; Rosenthal & Dawson, 1992; Rosenthal, Sulman, & Marshall, 1993).

Our description is based upon data collected at the first institutional care interview following admission of the patient to a nursing home. As reported previously, a total of 237 dementia patients were institutionalized prior to Time 4. In some instances caregivers did not participate in a postadmission interview because the patient died before this interview could take place ($n = 52$).[1] The remaining 185 caregivers participated in at least one institutional care interview. Of these persons, 52 were wives, 43 were husbands, 67 were daughters caring for mothers, and 23 were other caregivers (i.e., daughters caring for fathers and caregiving sons). The interval between admission and the first postplacement interview ranges from 0 to 16 months, with an average of 6.5 months ($SD = 3.8$).

As shown in Figure 9.1, nursing home admission occurred throughout the course of the study. Consequently, we found it necessary to reformat the data so they are centered around the transitional event of admission rather than the time of data collection. Thus, information about the immediate aftermath of admission is derived from Time 2 ($n = 100$), Time 3 ($n = 52$), or Time 4 ($n = 33$), depending upon whether admission occurred after Time 1, Time 2, or Time 3. These three sets of cases are stacked upon one another to form a synthetic institutional care cohort ($N = 185$).

Similarities in Caregiving

In general, caregivers remained invested in the care of their parent or spouse to a much greater extent than they withdrew. For example, most caregivers visited regularly, slightly more than an average of 3 days per week: About one in four visited daily and one in three visited at least three times a week. Less than 10% did not visit their institutionalized relatives on a regular basis.

> Sometimes it's pretty hard to go to the hospital but I go.
> I force myself to go. She looks forward to having me there.

The amount of time caregivers spent at the nursing home during weekdays ranged from 0 to 30 hours. On average, caregivers visited their relatives for 5 hours per week. On weekends, these times ranged from 0 to 12 hr, with an average of 2.5 hr. These figures do not include the time it takes to travel to and from the facility, which in some cases was considerable. Although over half (56.7%) of the caregivers traveled between 15 and 45 min to the care facility, 1 in 10 traveled more than 1 hr. Thus, visitation tended to be both a frequent and time-consuming activity.

When visiting the nursing home, caregivers assisted their relatives with many of the same personal care activities that they had helped them with at home. For each of 10 activities of daily living (ADLs), caregivers were asked, "During a usual visit, do you *regularly* help your (relative) with any of the following things?"[2] On average, caregivers routinely helped with two to three activities; less than a third provided no assistance. The most commonly reported activities are assistance getting around inside the facility (52.3%) and its outside grounds (45.1%). Other common activities are help with eating (44.9%), brushing hair or teeth (30.7%), going to the bathroom (20.5%), getting going in an activity (20.5%), and dressing (17.6%). The least common activities are assistance with changing diapers or pads; bathing, showering, or washing hair; and taking medications. Some of the more taxing activities, then, tend to be delegated to institutional staff. Yet, one-third of the caregivers remain involved even in these more demanding activities, performing one or more of these tasks regularly. These two women, one caring for her mother and the other caring for her husband, are seen as they go about providing supplemental care within nursing homes (photographs 19–25).

Frank

Frank admitted Beth to a nursing home immediately after he struck her once out of frustration. Here he describes his daily visits with her.

I'd be there for an hour or hour and a half, walk with her. I'd sit across the table from her. She enjoyed touch. Tactile experience became most important in her awareness. Gave her the opportunity to reach out. I embraced her, kissed her.

In sum, withdrawal from caregiving upon admission to a nursing home appears to be a career path followed by a small group. The majority of caregivers continued to help their spouses and parents throughout their tenure as institutional denizens. As such, many care-related burdens persisted from the in-home to the institutional care phase of role enactment, albeit alleviated to a considerable extent by the services provided by nursing home staff.

New Sources of Stress

Providing supplemental assistance is not the only activity that commands the attention of caregivers. They also must deal with the facility, adapting to its

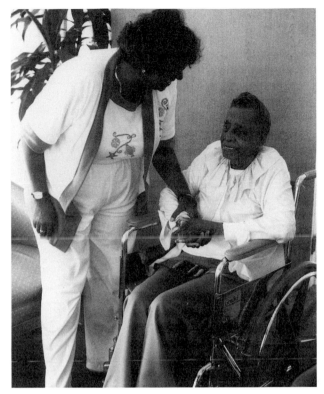

Photograph 19

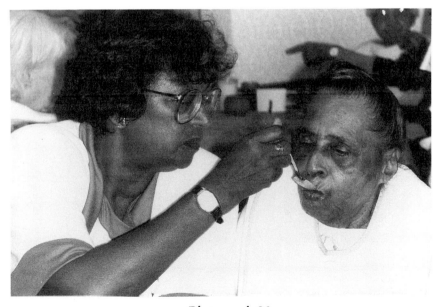

Photograph 20

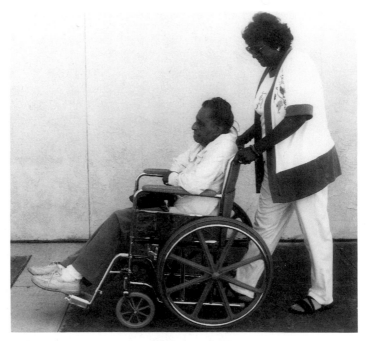

Photograph 21

staff, standards, procedures, and requirements. In this manner, institutional care can introduce entirely new sources of stress into the lives of caregivers. These stressors were assessed by asking caregivers how often they encountered various problems with the nursing home or its staff. Large numbers of caregivers report-ed *never* experiencing the following difficulties: the patient being given too much or the wrong kind of medication (84.2%), inability to find people in charge to discuss concerns (77.1%), unexpected charges (71.2%); the feeling that staff do not like to answer questions (72.6%); or frequent staff changes (66.1%). The

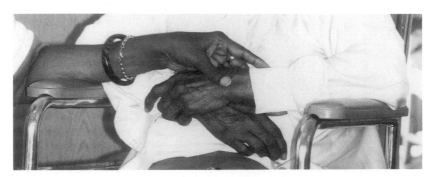

Photograph 22

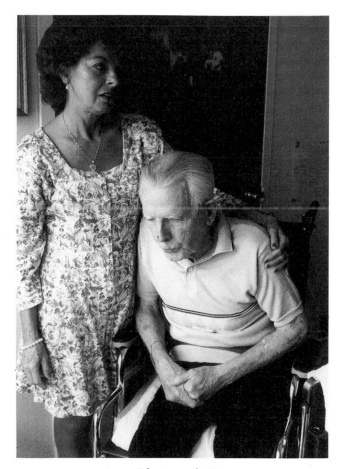

Photograph 23

most common concern relates to frequent staff changes, and only 18.1% rated themselves as frequently concerned about this issue. In combination, 56.2% of caregivers mentioned no more than one problem with the facility, 26.0% had two to three problems, and the remaining 17.8% had four to six problems. Thus, a substantial minority of caregivers encountered multiple problems with regard to the nursing home and its staff, whereas most caregivers reported only a small number of difficulties.

You don't solve the problem. Just trade one problem for another when you put her in a nursing home.

For the most part, caregivers were generally comfortable with the institutional care their relatives received. The majority of caregivers described themselves as

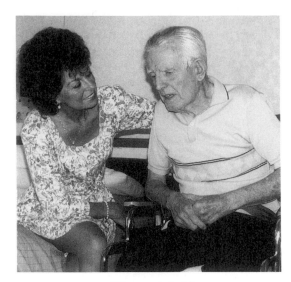

Photograph 24

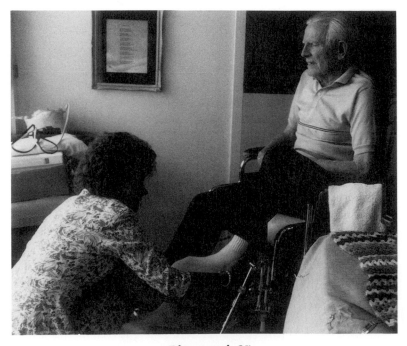

Photograph 25

very satisfied with the facility's visiting hours (92.8%), cleanliness (73.1%), safety (70.7%), smell (66.5%), food (59.0%), recreational activities (53.2%), the pleasantness of their relatives' rooms (55.8%), the contact they have with their relatives' doctor (48.0%), the quality of care provided by the facilities nurses (55.8%) and physicians (52.1%), the number of staff (52.2%), and the protection of their relatives' property (51.4%). Overall, 43.4% felt *very satisfied* with the care facility, 49.3% were *fairly satisfied,* and 7.3% felt *just a little satisfied* or *not at all satisfied* with the facility.

These reports belie negative social stereotypes of nursing homes. On the whole, nursing homes and their staff were described by caregivers as being above average to excellent. These high marks included the level of care the facilities provided the patient. Nonetheless, a small subgroup of caregivers found their relatives' situation problematic and were quite dissatisfied with their living arrangements. Thus, the generally positive experiences of large numbers of caregivers does not negate the presence of other circumstances that are unacceptable.

The chances are quite good, then, that caregivers will enjoy a reasonable level of satisfaction with the institutions in which they have placed their relatives and the care provided by these facilities. Indeed, the anticipation of placement and the problems encountered in finding an appropriate facility (see chapter 8) were generally much more difficult than the postadmission experience. No doubt, these primarily positive experiences attest to the painstaking effort taken in selecting suitable nursing homes. Moreover, caregivers who sought, but could not locate, suitable nursing homes are not part of this picture because they continued to provide in-home care.

The Impact of Institutionalization

Although it is reasonable to expect that caregivers gain relief from the strains directly associated with providing around-the-clock hands-on care when their relatives are institutionalized, our stress-proliferation model posits that caregivers will continue to encounter care-related stressors in ways that reflect the continuity of their roles as caregivers. For example, we may anticipate that paying for institutionalized care will be difficult for most caregivers and that the effort required to visit the facility will tax the energies of many, especially caregivers who are themselves in frail health. Thus, although we expect the transition to institutional care to reduce the subjective primary stressors associated with caregiving and the secondary role strains that develop in response to the demands of in-home caregiving, we do not expect that they will be completely alleviated. Moreover, we do not anticipate substantial changes in psychosocial resources and emotional well-being because these domains are influenced by numerous factors that do not necessarily change as a consequence of institutionalization.

To evaluate the impact of placement, we compared pre- and postadmission data for those caregivers who admitted their relatives to nursing homes prior to

Time 4. The interview that took place immediately prior to placement is used to estimate preadmission or "baseline" care-related stress in the home setting, while the first institutional care interview is used to measure postadmission or "follow-up" care-related stress. Thus, baseline information about in-home care was obtained from Times 1, 2, or 3 for caregivers who placed their relatives between Times 1 and 2, Times 2 and 3, or Times 3 and 4, respectively. Corresponding follow-up data were obtained from placement interviews at Times 2, 3, or 4. These three sets of cases are stacked on top of one another to create a synthetic institutional care cohort sample of 185 caregivers with longitudinal data containing baseline (Time 1, 2, or 3) and follow-up (Times 2, 3, or 4) information (i.e., both pre- and postadmission data) (see Figure 9.1).

To differentiate changes associated with placement from the passage of time, data from the cohort is contrasted with data from a similar cohort of caregivers who did not place their relatives prior to Time 4. These caregivers obviously do not have pre- and postadmission data, so their baseline and follow-up data are obtained from two in-home care interviews: Baseline data are from the penultimate in-home care interview and follow-up data are from the final in-home care interview. The total sample size for the in-home care cohort is 243, which includes 86 wives, 64 husbands, 71 daughters caring for mothers, and 22 other caregivers.[3]

The following analyses pool the two synthetic cohorts, institutional and in-home care, generating a combined analytic sample of 428 caregivers with baseline and follow-up data. A dichotomous dummy variable differentiates the two cohorts and estimates the impact of institutionalization on various outcomes. Follow-up data were regressed upon baseline data and the dichotomous indicator of placement status. The impact of institutional placement, therefore, is evaluated as differences in follow-up scores between the in-home and institutional care cohorts, controlling for their baseline scores.

In addition to our expectation that placement would affect exposure to certain stressors, we also anticipated differences between kin groups (i.e., between wives, husbands, and daughters). Given the greater emotional and functional interdependence of spouses, we expected that institutionalization would be much more disruptive for them than for adult children (Cohler, Groves, Borden, & Lazarus, 1989; Rosenthal & Dawson, 1992). To assess this hypothesis, we included kin relationship as an independent variable. However, our analyses did not reveal differences in adjustment between spouses and adult children, between husbands and wives, or even between male and female caregivers. We return to these unexpected findings in our discussion at the conclusion of this chapter.

Effects of Placement on Subjective Primary Stressors

Baseline and follow-up levels of three subjective primary stressors are displayed in Figure 9.2.[4] Compared to the in-home care cohort, caregivers who institutionalized their relatives experienced statistically significant decreases over time in role overload and role captivity. In other words, obtaining institutional relief from constant demands leads caregivers to feel less confined and trapped

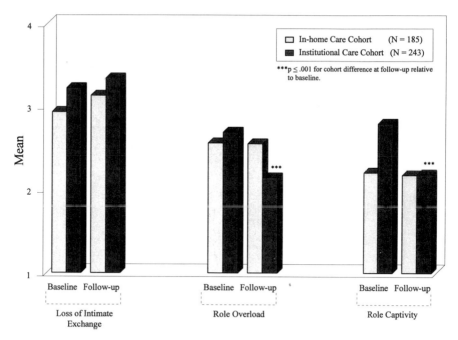

Figure 9.2   Mean subjective primary stressors at baseline and follow-up for in-home and institutional care cohorts.

by their care-related obligations than they felt previously. Placement, however, does not affect loss of intimate exchange with the patient. Instead, caregivers in both the continuing care and placement cohorts increasingly feel this loss over time.

Recall that role captivity is a powerful predictor of placement (see chapter 8, especially Table 8.2). While providing care in the home, the people who subsequently placed their relatives had higher levels of role captivity than those who continued in-home care, as shown in Figure 9.2. Following institutionalization, this sense of being confined is considerably lessened, declining to the same follow-up level as found in the continuing-care group. Thus, caregivers turn to institutionalization when feeling trapped by their care-related obligations and gain some measure of relief in this state of role captivity following institutionalization.

I'm extremely happy. I spent five years caring for my father, did my best. Now it's someone else's turn.

Role overload, in contrast, did not emerge as a significant independent contributor to the risk of institutionalization (see chapter 8, especially Table 8.2).

Hence, it is not surprising to see little difference in the baseline value of role overload between those who continued to provide care and those who institutionalized. Although role overload remains at about the same average level over time for those who continued to provide care, there is a sharp decline in overload among those who institutionalized their relatives. Therefore, although overload may not precipitate nursing home admission, it is, nonetheless, lessened by this transition.

Loss of intimate exchange neither prompts institutionalization nor is alleviated by it. Instead, caregivers tend to feel increasingly estranged from their relatives as time marches on and cognitive functioning declines, irrespective of whether their relatives live at home or in long-term care facilities.

Effects of Placement on Secondary Stressors

Because institutionalization so pervasively alters the primary stressors of caregiving, we anticipated a parallel change in secondary stressors; that is, in the amount of strain caregivers experience in their other social roles. This analysis examined three key domains of functioning: family conflict,[5] financial strain,[6] and work conflict (among employed caregivers). For the first two areas, we expected that placement would increase the amount of strain. There often are disagreements within families over whether nursing home placement is necessary or desirable, and over the financing of such care. Financial strain should increase because of the high costs of nursing home placement, especially because most caregivers in this study pay for care privately. Work strain, however, should decrease following placement, as the caregiver no longer has as many competing demands.

As in the preceding analysis, we compared levels of secondary role strains over time between the placement and continuing-care cohorts. Contrary to expectations, institutionalization does not have significant effects on changes in financial, family, or work strain. Clearly, whatever shifts occur in the caregiver's life as a result of placement do not appreciably alter the level of strain encountered in these three areas. Rather, the level of strain remains comparable to that encountered by caregivers who continue to assist their relatives at home.

In retrospect, our original hypotheses appear somewhat naive because they neglect the complex contingencies entailed in the basic stress-proliferation model. Among those who continued to provide in-home care, role captivity increases both family and work conflict (see Figure 6.1). A decrease in role captivity, such as that which accompanies institutionalization (see Figure 9.2), therefore, should alleviate these two role strains. Instead, we failed to find these effects. Apparently, whatever benefits may be derived from reducing role captivity by admitting one's relative are offset by cross-pressures that arise as a result of placement itself.

We similarly found little evidence that institutionalization affects the secondary intrapsychic strains associated with caregiving. We examined two positive assessments of the caregiving role, competency and personal gains, and one negative dimension, loss of self (i.e., the sense of losing one's identity as a result of being in the caregiver role). These three strains all pertain to the self-evaluations caregivers make of themselves with regard to their roles as caregivers. Because ties to the impaired family member and the tasks of caregiving change radically upon placement, we expected these personal assessments to change as well. Instead, we found that for all three intrapsychic strains, caregivers who institutionalized their relatives are congruous to those who continued to provide in-home care. As we saw earlier in this chapter, caregivers' dedication to their relatives generally transcends placement; their self-appraised functioning as a caregiver appears to do so as well.

These negative results are similar to those just reported for role strains. Again, it may be that the internal workings of the stress process counterbalance the impact of this major transitional event. As seen previously, loss of self is influenced by role overload and role captivity (see Figure 6.1). To the extent that placement alleviates these subjective stressors, and it generally does, loss of self should also abate. Presumably, caregivers are free to resume their precaregiving lives, reestablishing elements of personal identity that may have atrophied over the prolonged course of care. Any benefits of this type, however, clearly are offset by the very act of placement and its consequences. Hence, caregivers continue to endure these internal pressures irrespective of whether they provide care in the home or place their relatives in nursing homes.

One secondary intrapsychic strain, guilt, is intensified appreciably by institutionalization. It reflects the belief that one has not done all that he or she should have done for one's parent or spouse.

Specifically, caregivers were asked five questions: "How much do you: feel that you are not doing all that you should for your (relative), feel bad about something you said or did when your (relative) was well, regret that you didn't get a chance to make your peace with your (relative) before (his/her) illness, [and] think about the mistakes you've made in dealing with your (relative's) illness? and How guilty do you feel?" The response categories ranged from *not at all* (1) to *very much* (4). This five-item composite index has moderate reliability ($\alpha = .68$).

> Sometimes I feel guilty I let him go, but it is for the best.

As might be expected, caregivers who placed their relatives tended to experience elevated guilt, as shown in Figure 9.3. Those who continued to provide care, by contrast, remained at the same average level of guilt over time. Thus, institutionalizing their relatives appears to evoke sentiments of guilt among caregivers.

Effects of Placement on Social Psychological Resources

When we introduced the concept of social psychological resources in chapter 7, we identified three potential ways in which a stressor, such as institutional

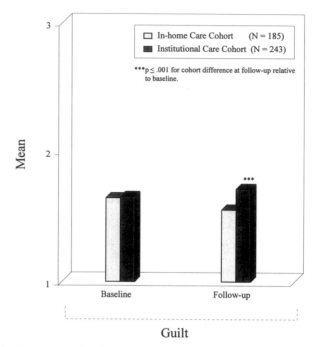

Figure 9.3   Mean guilt at baseline and follow-up for in-home and institutional care cohorts.

placement, might be associated with subsequent resources. To recapitulate, stressors may mobilize resources, deplete resources, or leave them unchanged (Ensel & Lin, 1991; Wheaton, 1985). We considered each of these possibilities for two resources, socioemotional support and mastery.[7] The same method of analysis is used to assess the impact of institutionalization: The resource at follow-up is regressed upon the baseline level of the resource and the dummy variable indicating whether the caregiver had institutionalized his or her relative.

For both mastery and socioemotional support, there are no statistically significant differences between the placement and continuing-care groups at either follow-up or baseline. The comparability between these groups at baseline is consistent with the earlier analysis of factors prompting institutionalization, which did not find a notable contribution associated with levels of mastery or support (see chapter 8). Thus self-efficacy and support neither prompt the transition to institutional care, nor become altered by this transition.

Effects of Placement on Psychological Distress

Finally, we consider the impact of institutionalization on caregivers' emotional well-being as expressed in symptoms of depression, anxiety, and anger. As with the other outcomes, we find here, too, that institutionalization has a specialized, rather than a generalized, effect on these dimensions of psychological

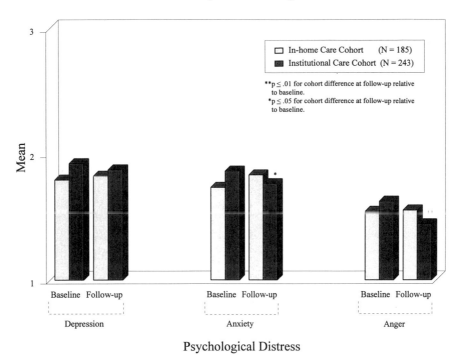

Figure 9.4   Mean psychological distress at baseline and follow-up for in-home and institutional care cohorts.

distress, as may be seen in Figure 9.4. There were significant reductions in anxiety and anger over time among the placement group. For the in-home group, anger did not change appreciably over time, but anxiety increased slightly. In contrast, with regard to depression, caregivers in both groups maintained about the same level of symptoms over time. At baseline, anxiety and anger were slightly higher in the placement than continuing-care cohort at baseline, but following placement, these types of distress declined in the placement cohort to below the follow-up level of the continuing-care cohort.

The selective effect of institutional placement on dimensions of psychological well-being is noteworthy because many studies of caregiving focus exclusively on depression. Our findings suggest that emotional well-being should be evaluated comprehensively to detect the continuities and discontinuities of transitions in the caregiving career.

A Synthesis of the Impact of Institutionalization

Admission of one's parent or spouse to a nursing home does not exert a monolithic effect on care-related stressors, psychosocial resources, or emotional well-being. For most outcomes, caregivers who institutionalize their relatives resemble closely those who continue to provide in-home care. In those instances where these groups differ, however, the advantage generally favors those who have placed their relatives. Specifically, institutionalization brings a measure of relief from role overload and role captivity, and lessens emotions of anger and anxiety. In only one instance does the advantage favor caregivers who continue to provide in-home care: Those who institutionalize appear to experience increased sentiments of guilt. Thus, there is some truth to the belief that, on average, institutionalization benefits caregivers, but to a larger extent, the burdens of caregiving are impervious to this transition.

• This synthesis of our findings pertains to the average impact of institutionalization relative to the average impact of continuing in-home care. Among those who institutionalize their relatives, though, there is considerable variability in the nature of adaptation. That is, although the overall impact of institutionalization is positive for role overload, role captivity, anxiety, and anger, some individuals do not experience this type of relief and others find these conditions exacerbated after placement. We turn now to the issue of individual differences in adaptation to institutionalization.

Caregivers' Adaptation to Placement

Compared to caregivers who continued to provide care in the home, those who placed their impaired relatives were relieved of some, but not all stressors related to their role. Although some caregivers benefited from relocating their relatives to nursing homes, many continued to endure a great deal of tension and emotional distress. The following section considers why some caregivers make the transition to institutional care relatively free of anguish, whereas others experience prolonged and even increased burdens.[8]

What Constitutes Successful Adaptation?

Depending upon their circumstances prior to placement, successful adaptation has different meanings for caregivers. To illustrate this point, a severely depressed caregiver will have a relatively successful adjustment if his or her mood improves noticeably following placement, even if he or she continues at above-normal levels of symptomatology. Similarly, a caregiver who was asymptomatic prior to placement also will experience successful adjustment if he or she remains asymptomatic. Adaptation is a relative concept that depends upon where one starts and where one ends. In essence, the meaning of individual-level adaptation postadmission is gauged with respect to preadmission circumstances.

In order to account for both regression to the mean,[9] and floor and ceiling effects,[10] we developed a procedure to assess caregiver adjustment postplacement by setting specific criteria a priori based on standardized scores regarding changes in outcomes (Whitlatch, Zarit, & von Eye, 1991). These criteria are shown in Table 9.1. To examine adaptation, we divided caregivers into quartiles,

Table 9.1 Criteria for Successful and Unsuccessful Adaptation
to Institutionalization

Successful outcomes	1. Initial baseline score is high and follow-up score is low reflecting improvement.
	2. Initial baseline score is low and follow-up score is low reflecting no change.
Unsuccessful outcomes	1. Initial baseline score is low and follow-up score is high reflecting worsening.
	2. Initial baseline score is high and follow-up score is high reflecting no change.

or four equal-sized groups (high, medium-high, medium-low, and low), based on their initial levels of each dimension of adaptation (e.g., family conflict). For each quartile, a specific criterion was set for an amount of change from pre- to postadmission that constitutes good adaptation. Caregivers with high initial scores (e.g., high levels of family conflict) had to show relatively large improvements to be rated as successfully adjusted (e.g., a substantial decline in family conflict). Caregivers with low initial scores were rated successful if their scores remained stable or increased minimally over time.

For example, caregivers with the most severe, high symptomatology must improve to at least the medium-high level of symptomatology. Caregivers with few symptoms can worsen a bit and still be considered successfully adjusted. By allowing this small increase in scores, we take into account expected regression to the mean. Finally, persons with medium-low symptomatology need only to improve slightly to be considered successfully adapted.

Using this technique, we are able to identify how many caregivers achieved clinically meaningful changes in regard to their emotional well-being, exposure to stressors, and social psychological resources. This approach assumes that the adaptation of caregivers to the transition of institutional placement is multifaceted. Thus we focus on six domains of the stress process model that span multiple levels of caregiver functioning. These domains include work strain, family conflict, financial strain, mastery, socioemotional support, and psychological well-being.

For four of the six outcomes, fewer than half of the caregivers achieved a positive outcome; that is, the majority did not successfully adapt according to the criteria specified in Table 9.1. Specifically, most caregivers did not positively adjust in the areas of work strain (59.6%), socioemotional support (54.4%), mastery (69.5%), and nonspecific psychological distress (52.5%).[11] In contrast, most caregivers successfully adapted postplacement in regards to family conflict (75.0%) and financial strain (69.8%). Thus, many caregivers experienced successful adjustment in some domains of functioning, while they simultaneously experienced poor outcomes in other domains. Again, we see that the effects of placement are specialized, rather than universal.

What Predicts Successful Adaptation?

In addition to describing the average level of adaptation, we are interested also in identifying factors that contribute to individual differences in adaptation. Five potential explanatory domains were examined: sociodemographic characteristics, objective and subjective primary stressors, nursing-home-related stressors, and secondary intrapsychic strains. The sociodemographic characteristics consist of age, income, education, kin relationship, gender, and whether the caregiver and patient lived together prior to institutionalization.

We examined objective primary and subjective stressors because the patient's behavior and the caregiver's subjective responses to it both may influence post-placement adaptation. Objective primary stressors included the impaired relative's problematic behaviors, activities of daily living (ADL) dependencies and level of cognitive impairment. The subjective stressors involved were role overload, role captivity, and loss of intimate exchange with the patient. In addition, we expanded the basic stress-proliferation model to include postadmission sources of stress. These measures assess problems experienced by caregivers in finding appropriate facilities, as well as the problems encountered once their relatives were placed (see chapter 7). The secondary intrapsychic strains consisted of guilt, loss of self, lack of caregiver competency, and absence of caregiving gains. We expected that caregivers with relatively low levels of primary and secondary stress would weather the transition to institutional care better in terms of role strains and psychosocial resources. In turn, we anticipated this successful adaptation would be associated with improvements in emotional well-being.

These elements of the stress process were examined in logistic regression analysis to explain successful adaptation. Logistic regression was used because the dependent variable is dichotomous: successful (coded 1) versus unsuccessful (coded 0) adaptation to placement. The independent variables were operationalized as baseline values and as change between baseline and follow-up (i.e., between the last preadmission interview and the first postadmission interview). Regression coefficients are presented in the tables as partial odds ratios: the multiplicative impact of a unit change in the independent variable on the odds of successful versus unsuccessful adaptation, other factors being held constant. Rather than entering all variables simultaneously into the logistic analysis, variables were analyzed in sets according to the major domains of the stress process model of family caregiving. Variables contributing significantly to the explanation of the outcome were retained when the next set of variables was added to the model. Consistent with the approach used in earlier analyses, when change variables were found to be statistically significant, the baseline variable was also included in the model regardless of its level of significance.

Effects on Secondary Stressors

We first turn to Table 9.2, which shows the models of successful adaptation related to the secondary role strains of work, family, and financial strain. The

Table 9.2   Relative Risk of Successful Adjustment 1 Year
Postplacement for Secondary Role Strains

Stressors and characteristics	Role strain		
	Work conflict	Family conflict	Financial strain
Role Captivity: Change postadmission–preadmission	.32	—	.60
Loss of intimate Exchange: Change postadmission–preadmission	—	—	1.60
Caregiver competence: Preadmission	—	2.49	—
Caregiving gain: Preadmission	—	.57	.36
Loss of self: Preadmission	—	—	.45
Loss of self: Change postadmission–preadmission	—	—	.40
Guilt: Preadmission	—	—	2.01
Problems encountered during placement	1.58	—	—
Satisfaction with facility	10.01	2.86	—
Months since admission	1.28	—	—
Spousal caregiver (/adult child)	—	2.84	—
Caregiver education (in years)	—	.80	—

chances of good adaptation with regard to work strain increase as the duration of institutional care increases.[12] As indicated by the partial odds ratio, a 1-month increase in the time since admission improves the odds of successful adaptation by 1.28 times. Only one care-related stressor, role captivity, independently contributes to successful adaptation at work: Caregivers whose sense of being trapped by their caregiver role declines after placement are likely to also experience reduced conflict between the demands of caregiving and those of work. Two facility-related stressors are related to successful adaptation at work as well: Caregivers who experience problems while searching for facilities and those who are satisfied with the facility they have chosen tend to better balance the conflicting demands of work and caregiving. The odds of adjusting successfully are affected most by satisfaction with the care facility and declining levels of role captivity.

The direction of the effect for problems in searching for a care facility is counterintuitive: Generally, we expect stressors to be detrimental to subsequent adaptation. This coefficient is easier to interpret within the context of the large effect for satisfaction. Caregivers who encountered substantial problems in searching for nursing homes, but who also are very satisfied with the facilities they select, have the best chances of good adaptation at work. Conversely, those who encounter few problems beforehand, but are dissatisfied afterwards, are most likely to have poor outcomes.

As we saw earlier in this chapter, caregivers who were employed both immediately prior and subsequent to placement tended not to have adjusted especially well at work in the immediate aftermath of the transition to institutional care. Adaptation improves, however, as time progresses. Earlier in this chapter it was also discussed that role captivity is typically alleviated by institutional placement. Here, we see that these declines in role captivity are associated with better adaptation at the juncture between caregiving and work.

Turning to family conflict in Table 9.2, caregivers who had successfully adapted (i.e., felt less family conflict postadmission than preadmission or remained low in family conflict) had lower levels of education and were more likely to be spousal caregivers than those with less positive adaptation. Satisfaction with the nursing home, caregiver competency, and caregiving gains also are related to family adjustment. Caregivers who hold positive evaluations of the care facility and of themselves as caregivers tend to have good postadmission adaptation. In contrast, caregivers who feel personally enriched by caregiving during the in-home care phase tend to have poor adjustment within the family during the institutional care phase of role enactment.

Two features of these results are especially noteworthy, one demographic and the other pertaining to the self-perceptions of caregivers during the in-home phase of caregiving. Husbands and wives are substantially more likely than adult children to have positive outcomes of institutionalization in regard to their relationships with other family members. This finding suggests that families respond to the institutionalization of an impaired spouse differently than they respond to the institutionalization of a parent. Perhaps others in the family are more judgmental and critical of sons and daughters who decide they cannot continue to provide care than they are of husbands and wives, who are themselves elderly and may also be in frail health.

The two perceptions of oneself as a caregiver exert opposite effects upon familial adjustment following placement. Caregivers who feel especially competent as caregivers tend to adjust better than those who have doubts about their role performance during the in-home phase of the caregiving career. Contrastingly, caregivers who derive a sense of enrichment from in-home caregiving tend to have more difficulty with others in the family after they have yielded in-home caregiving to institutional care. This pattern suggests that distinct elements of the caregiver's self-concept have specialized effects on family relations following institutionalization. Specifically, believing that one has done a good job as a caregiver promotes postadmission family adjustment, whereas investing one's self in the performance of the caregiving role appears detrimental.

In looking now at financial strain in Table 9.2, we see that the odds of good adaptation depend both upon the conditions prior to admission, as well as the changes that accompany this transition. Declining levels of role captivity and increasing loss of intimacy over the course of the transition to institutional care increase the likelihood of good financial adaptation. Caregivers who adapted well financially also had higher levels of guilt preadmission, retained their sense of personal identity, and did not feel they had benefited personally during the provision of in-home care. As previously mentioned, most caregivers had successfully adjusted to their altered financial situations by the time of their first postadmission interview, inviting speculation that postadmission financial strain is constrained by the fact that those who are most able financially to afford nursing home care are most likely to do so (see chapter 8).

Effects on Psychosocial Resources

We also examined predictors of successful adaptation with regard to the psychosocial resources of socioemotional support and mastery, as shown in Table 9.3. For socioemotional support, successful adaptation is linked to higher caregiver education and female caregivers tend to have the best outcomes. In addition, changes in caregiver role captivity and guilt following placement are associated with caregiver adaptation in socioemotional support, albeit in the opposite direction. Caregivers who experience a heightened burden of guilt fare better than those who increasingly feel trapped. Earlier in this chapter, we saw that role

Table 9.3 Relative Risk of Successful Adjustment 1 Year Postplacement for Psychosocial Resources

Stressors and characteristics	Psychosocial resource	
	Socioemotional support	Mastery
ADL dependencies: Preadmission	—	1.49
ADL dependencies: Change postadmission–preadmission	—	1.46
Role captivity: Change postadmission–preadmission	.62	—
Loss of intimate exchange: Preadmission	—	.65
Loss of intimate exchange: Change postadmission–preadmission	—	.59
Caregiver competence: Preadmission	—	2.13
Caregiver competence: Change postadmission–preadmission	—	2.43
Guilt: Change postadmission–preadmission	1.73	—
Problems encountered during placement	—	.73
Spousal caregiver (/adult child)	—	.45
Male caregiver	.30	—
Caregiver education (in years)	1.15	—

captivity generally declines after institutionalization, while feelings of guilt increase. Thus it appears that caregivers who have normative emotional reactions to institutionalization tend to have a better sense of social integration following placement than those whose subjective experiences run counter to that which is typical.

Turning to mastery, it is apparent in Table 9.3 that sons and daughters typically feel more efficacious following placement, whereas husbands and wives feel less so. We also see that postadmission mastery is influenced importantly by the conditions encountered during in-home care and changes in these conditions over the transition to institutional care. Caregivers who provide substantial hands-on assistance in the home and in the nursing home tend to make the best adjustment to placement in terms of their own sense of mastery. Apparently, having some control over the care one's relative receives fosters a generalized belief in one's control. Similarly, caregivers who feel competent in their roles as caregivers, including those who increasingly feel competent after institutionalization, tend to feel more efficacious following this transition.

In contrast, feeling a loss of intimacy and familiarity with the patient tends to be detrimental to postadmission mastery. Caregivers who feel this way both prior and subsequent to placement typically have negative outcomes in terms of mastery, as do those who feel this way only after they have admitted their relatives to nursing homes. Also, caregivers who have encountered difficulties in locating suitable care facilities often have less positive postadmission adaptation in terms of mastery than those who navigated this transition without encountering many problems.

These results suggest that the erosion of the persona of the care recipient tends to lessen the extent to which caregivers feel in control of important elements of their lives. For some, the inevitable process of loss over which one has no control appears to undermine feelings of mastery. However, caregivers who have control of at least some aspects of care and who feel good about how they provide this care tend to adapt well to institutionalization, at least in terms of self-efficacy.

Effects on Emotional Well-Being

The final outcome of institutionalization pertains to the emotional well-being of caregivers assessed in terms of symptoms of nonspecific psychological distress. Table 9.4 illustrates that the odds of attaining positive mental health outcomes depends upon the passage of time, exposure to primary stressors, caregiver competency, and successful adaptation in terms of mastery.

As reported earlier in this chapter, many caregivers weather the initial transition to institutional care quite well, but about one in two continue to exhibit problematic levels of psychological distress. In general, even for these caregivers, the odds of attaining good mental health outcomes increase as the actual event of admission recedes in time. In other words, the longer it has been since the dementia patient was placed in a nursing home, the more likely the caregiver is to be in a satisfactory emotional state.

Table 9.4 Relative Risk of Successful Adjustment 1 Year Postplacement
for Emotional Well-Being

Stressors and characteristics	Emotional well-being
Role overload: Preadmission	.47
Role overload: Change postadmission–preadmission	.45
Role captivity: Preadmission	.52
Role captivity: Change postadmission–preadmission	.57
Caregiver competence: Change postadmission–preadmission	2.84
Months since admission:	1.18
Mastery: Successful postadmission preadmission	.44

However, caregivers who institutionalize their relatives are not likely to improve in terms of their emotional well-being if role overload and role captivity remain elevated from the pre- to the postadmission period or when these primary stressors are exacerbated over this interval. As discussed previously in this chapter, role overload and role captivity are diminished, on average, when dementia patients are institutionalized. Caregivers who do not experience this reduction, and especially those who experience an increase instead, are particularly likely to have poor mental health outcomes. Therefore, those who do not accrue the usual benefits of reductions in primary stressors as a consequence of institutionalization are more prone to have poor mental health outcomes. Fortunately, this experience with role overload and role captivity appears to be atypical.

The findings pertaining to the impact of caregiver self-perceptions on psychological adaptation are complex. As one might expect, caregivers who increasingly feel good about how they perform the role of caregiver as they go from providing in-home care to providing institutional care tend to have positive mental health adaptations. In contrast, caregivers who have positive adaptations in terms of mastery during in-home care typically have negative mental health responses to institutionalization, the opposite of what one might expect. Increments in mastery generally tend to improve emotional well-being (see chapter 7). When mastery increases as a result of institutionalization, however, caregivers, rather than benefiting, tend to become somewhat more distressed. It may be that caregivers with high mastery feel ineffective and frustrated in dealing with the institutional setting because they have limited control over how care is provided. On the other hand, those caregivers with low mastery may feel ineffective in the home care environment, but feel relief once someone else is in charge of their relative's care.

These results point to the powerful influence of subjective primary stressors on caregivers' mental health responses to institutionalization. Most caregivers feel less overloaded and captive after institutionalization. In turn, these caregivers also become relatively less psychologically distressed. Surprisingly, experiences in searching for a facility, the patient's level of cognitive impairment, the amount of time caregivers spend visiting their relatives, and their level of satisfaction with the care facility have no impact upon their initial emotional adjustment. Secondary strains also lack a discernible impact upon psychological adjustment during the first year of institutional care.

A Synthesis of Factors Affecting Adaptation to Placement

Overall, we see that not all caregivers who place their impaired relatives adjust successfully across multiple domains of functioning, such as within work, financial, and family roles, or with regard to social and psychological outcomes. This finding has important implications for family members who are trying to assist the primary caregiver in adapting to institutionalization and for professionals who work with families in institutional settings. First, placement is often advocated by other family members and professionals to alleviate the stresses, strains, and emotional sequelae of caregiving. Although some caregivers experience relief after they admit their relatives, most caregivers continue to be vulnerable to specific types of difficulties. Moreover, many caregivers who do well with regard to one area of functioning, do not necessarily fare well with regard to other domains of functioning. Because placement alters, rather than eliminates, the stresses of caregiving, it should not be viewed as a universal panacea.

Second, specific aspects of the care-related stress process that occur during in-home care affect adjustment to institutionalization. For instance, the subjective primary stressors existing during in-home care are especially important predictors of successful adjustment after placement (see chapter 6). Similarly, the findings of chapters 6 and 8 revealed that some of the same stressors that predict psychological distress for in-home caregivers also predict who will place their family members. The findings of the present chapter extend these findings by linking these specific stressors to successful postplacement adjustment. Thus, it appears that caregivers make a decision to institutionalize because they encounter certain care-related stressors, and these stressors tend to be alleviated by institutionalization and to contribute to subsequent positive emotional adaptation after placement.

Some factors emerge as contributors to adjustment in multiple areas. Role captivity appears to exert diffuse, inhibitory effects upon adaptational outcomes. It is generally reduced by institutionalization, but when this relief is not obtained, the consequences are widespread, affecting work, finances, socioemotional support, and emotional well-being. Caregiver competence also exerts pervasive effects upon postadmission adaptation, increasing the likelihood of positive outcomes with regard to the family, mastery, and emotional well-being. Evaluations of oneself as a caregiver are not influenced substantially by the act of institutionalization, as we saw earlier in this chapter, but nonetheless are influential in determining adaptation after institutionalization. Time since admission affects only two outcomes, but in each instance, the effect is beneficial: The passage of time improves adaptation at work and emotional well-being.

These analyses produced a number of surprises. First, facility-related stressors did not extensively predict adjustment to institutionalization. This finding may be due to the generally high level of satisfaction caregivers expressed with regard to the facilities insofar as restricted variance makes associations difficult to observe. Second, in predicting successful adjustment, we found few effects of kin relationships, that is, spouse versus adult children. This finding is contrary to Rosenthal and Dawson's (1991) notion of "quasi-widowhood," which implies that adaptation to placement will be more difficult for spouses than for other caregivers. Our findings indicate that the transition is generally difficult for caregivers irrespective of their kin relationship to the patient. Although spouses undoubtedly experience many of the ambiguities described by Rosenthal and Dawson (1991), other caregivers apparently experience conflicts with similar consequences. Third, we found caregivers with higher levels of mastery after placement to be somewhat more psychologically distressed. It is possible that a high sense of mastery may be most beneficial when the caregiver is in complete charge and less helpful when others are in charge of the patient care.

These analyses have focused on the period of time immediately following placement, yet institutional care for dementia patients often lasts for several years. Our longitudinal design, which followed caregivers for three years, makes it possible to examine adaptation to placement over a longer period of time, to which we now turn.

Long-Term Institutionalized Caregiving

Thus far, we have seen that caregivers remain involved in the lives of their relatives up to 1 year after their admission to nursing homes. But do caregivers sustain their involvement after this initial period? Or does involvement gradually diminish over time as their relatives become more disabled and as the caregiver develops new routines and activities?

To examine long-term adjustment to placement, we identified those caregivers whose relatives had been institutionalized during the first year of the study and had resided continuously in nursing homes through Time 4, as illustrated in Figure 9.5. This highly select group is necessarily small in size ($n = 65$; see Figure 3.1). Other caregivers who institutionalized early in the study are not considered in this long-term follow-up because their family members died or the caregivers were lost-at-follow-up. Of the long-term institutional caregivers, 17 were wives, 10 were husbands, 27 were daughters caring for mothers, and 11 were other caregivers. To examine the dynamics entailed in long-term institutional care, we first look at the enactment of the institutionalized care role and then consider factors contributing to long-term emotional adaptation.

Change over Time in Elements of the Stress Process

Caregivers generally continued to be involved regularly in the lives of their relatives even after they had been institutionalized for up to 3 years. Nearly half of the caregivers helped their relatives to eat (40.6%), or to get around the facility

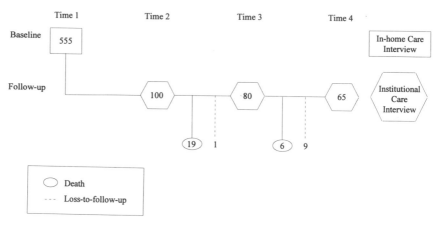

Figure 9.5 Creation of the long-term postadmission cohort.

(46.9%) or the facility's grounds (50.0%). In contrast, very few (less than 5%) provided help with changing diapers, going to the bathroom, bathing, dressing, or getting in and out of bed. The configuration of types of care provided after a lengthy period of institutionalization closely resembles that described earlier in this chapter for the 1-year interval.

> Life can never be normal as long as I go every Sunday and see a parent like that. It is not a normal life.

Although caregivers continued to visit their institutionalized relatives, they did so somewhat less frequently than during the patient's early institutional stay. One in four caregivers reported not visiting at all, although another one in four reported visiting once or twice per week. On average, caregivers to long-term nursing home residents reported visiting 2 to 3 days per week and spending up to 30 hr a week with their relatives. On average, caregivers visited 4.2 hr per week, or about 1 hr a week less than they visited immediately after placement. On weekends, caregivers visited an average of 2.0 hr, a drop of about a half hour from earlier on. Clearly, even though some caregivers have become less involved with their institutionalized relatives over the long haul, many maintained high levels of contact and involvement.

Constance

As we've already seen, Constance experiences considerable remorse over placing her mother in a nursing home, which violated a pledge she had made with herself. Her persistent discomfort with this situation is apparent in her description of visits with mother.

She's as independent and feisty as ever, and confused. I can't explain to her where she is and why. Reasoning is beyond what she's capable of. She wakes up in a strange place every morning. Every time I go there it brings back the feeling that I want to take her home. It doesn't stop hurting.

I put my face close to hers and say hi. She doesn't hear, but she smiles back. I think she recognizes me. It depends on her agitation. She'll tell me "take me home." If I come in the afternoon I go in the room with her and face her to look out the window. I have a deck of cards that I put in front of her and sometimes we'll play solitaire and she can do pretty well putting the cards in the right place. I'll hand her a magazine and turn the pages for her. I try to do something other than leave her sitting in the hall.

Sometimes she punches people who pass her in the hall. They like it when she responds like that. They're amazing people who work there. We joke about mother punching at them.

As was evident in their earlier responses, caregivers typically were satisfied with the nursing home over the long-term. Even after a longer period, a substantial majority of caregivers reported *never* being concerned with the type and amount of medication given to their relatives (80.6%), unexpected charges (71.9%), feeling that staff do not like to answer questions (72.3%), or finding people in charge to answer questions (62.3%). The biggest concern continued to be frequent staff changes. In combination, 52.4% reported having no more than one problem with the facility, 21.6% had two to three problems, and the remaining 26.2% reported four or more problems with the facility. Thus, most caregivers have few problems concerning the care facility, but a substantial subgroup experience multiple problems long after the actual admission of their relatives.

Caregivers at the long-term follow-up were also generally satisfied with the care their relatives received. For example, over half reported they were *very satisfied* with the facility's visiting hours (87.7%), smell (75.0%), cleanliness (73.8%), safety (67.7%), food (67.7%), recreational activities (58.6%), the number of staff (56.2%), the pleasantness of their relative's room (52.3%), the quality of care provided by the facility's nurses (50.8%) and physicians (44.6%), the protection of their relative's property (49.2%), and the contact they have with their relative's doctor (46.7%). On average, 57.1% of caregivers felt *very satisfied* with the care facility, 34.6% felt *fairly satisfied,* and 8.3% felt *not at all satisfied* or *a little satisfied* with the facility. Thus, the majority of caregivers who have had a family member in a nursing home for a lengthy period of time are quite satisfied with the care provided, the atmosphere, and the facility's staff, although some are quite dissatisfied even after several years of nursing home care.

Caregivers continue to manifest marked signs of good and poor adaptation in various domains of functioning. Perhaps most importantly, symptoms of nonspecific psychological distress decrease over time. Although the amount of improvement observed at the first postplacement interview was relatively small, decreases in symptoms had become substantial by the long-term follow-up (71.0%). Emotional well-being is not the sole criterion of success in adaptation. However, we limit our analysis to this single outcome because the small sample size makes extensive analysis of multiple outcomes highly speculative.

Predictors of Successful Emotional Adaptation

The factors that contribute to successful psychological adaptation for caregivers whose spouses or parents reside in nursing homes for several years are identified in Table 9.5. Adaptation is influenced both by demographic factors and by the conditions of caregiving within the home and within the institution. Older caregivers adapt less well emotionally as the institutional phase of their caregiving careers follows a protracted course. Contrastingly, income is associated with better psychological adaptation over time.

Caregivers who provide substantial hands-on assistance with ADLs to an institutionalized relative long after their admission risk poor emotional outcomes. Two patterns of continued help emerge as risks for poor adjustment: high levels of assistance that are maintained far into the course of institutional care and assistance that actually increases after institutionalization.

The erosion of the caregiver's own sense of identity also poses a threat to successful psychological adaptation in the long-term. Loss of self, as illustrated in Table 9.5, contributes to poor psychological outcomes when it emerges during in-home care and continues throughout institutional care, or when it emerges after institutionalization. In contrast, caregivers who maintain their sense of self over the transition to institutional care and its lengthy aftermath are likely to have improved emotional well-being over time, as are caregivers whose sense of self is restored following institutionalization.

These findings indicate that psychological adaptation to institutional care over the long-term is influenced by factors that differ from those that matter over the short-term (compare with Table 9.4). Over the short-term, time itself was impor-

Table 9.5 Relative Risk of Successful Adjustment 3 Years Postplacement for Emotional Well-Being

Stressors and characteristics	Emotional well-being
ADL dependencies: Preadmission	.61
ADL dependences: Change postadmission–preadmission	.50
Loss of self: Preadmission	.08
Loss of self: Change postadmission–preadmission	.30
Work strain: Successful postadmission–preadmission	.02
Caregiver age (in years)	.88
Income (thousands of dollars)	1.04

tant for improved emotional well-being, an influence that apparently dissipates as time progresses. Earlier adaptation is most strongly affected by continued and escalating exposure to subjective primary stressors, which usually are alleviated by institutionalization; when they are not, they are emotionally distressing in the immediate aftermath of institutionalization. In contrast, an objective primary stressor emerges as most salient to long-term adaptation: Caregivers who provide extensive hands-on assistance to their relatives years after their admission to nursing homes generally risk poor emotional adaptation. We saw earlier that difficult conditions experienced within in-home care can erode the caregiver's identity. Here, we see that if this occurs and identity is not reestablished after institutionalization, poor emotional outcomes are likely. In contrast, caregivers who are able to repair their damaged sense of self can anticipate better emotional outcomes over the long-term.

In sum, subjective primary stressors contribute to both placement and psychological adaptation to placement during the first year. These stressors, however, do not independently influence adaptation once the dementia patient has been institutionalized for a long time. Instead, the level of hands-on care that one continues to provide emerges as especially salient. Psychological adjustment to institutionalization, both short- and long-term, is not influenced to an appreciable degree by facility-related stressors. That is, the care setting seems to matter far less than the care-related stressors encountered while one's relative lives in that setting. It should be emphasized, nonetheless, that the institutional care sample in this study is rather homogeneous in having generally high levels of satisfaction and low levels of difficulty with the care facility. Thus, the setting may appear to be unimportant because problematic settings are uncommon in this sample. This issue deserves further investigation over a broader array of nursing home environments.

Summary

This chapter has described the postadmission phase of the caregiving career, identifying the principal ways in which caregivers enact an institutional caregiver role, examining the overall impact of placement on caregivers as a group, and differentiating caregivers who make effective adjustments to institutionalization from those who adapt poorly. The findings reveal the following:

• Most caregivers visit their institutionalized relatives regularly and continue to provide them with substantial assistance with ADLs.
• Although a small group of caregivers find their relatives' facilities less than satisfactory, caregivers more typically experience few problems and are satisfied with most aspects of the facility, including its visiting hours, cleanliness, safety, smell, and food.
• Where there are differences between those who place their relatives in long-term care institutions and those who continue to provide home care, the advantage generally favors those who place.

• Multiple domains of the stress process differentiate caregivers who make effective adjustments to placement from those who adapt poorly. These dimensions include work strain, family conflict, financial strain, mastery, socioemotional support, and psychological distress.

• Subjective primary stressors are especially important predictors of successful psychological adaptation.

• Few demographic characteristics or facility-related stressors are related to successful outcomes postplacement.

• The passage of time is generally beneficial for caregivers: As the duration of institutional care increases, caregivers are more likely to adjust well at work and in their emotional well-being.

• Caregivers who provide substantial hands-on assistance long after placement risk poor emotional outcomes.

Discussion

In this chapter, we have followed primary caregivers through the transition from home care to nursing home care. Despite the commonplace expectation of immediate relief from care-related burdens, many caregivers experience considerable stress and emotional distress long after placement. Although placement relieves stressors associated with daily care routines, it also brings with it new adaptational challenges.

Considerable individual differences in adaptation occur following placement. Some people experience substantial and immediate high levels of exposure to both primary and secondary stressors, and suffer from elevated symptoms of psychological distress. The primary demands of caregiving account for only a small proportion of this variability in response to institutional placement. Adaptation, instead, emerges from multiple processes that include primary stressors, secondary strains, and social psychological resources.

Reflecting the dynamic processes of changing characteristics of the caregiving career, the factors that influence adaptation during in-home caregiving differ from those that account for adaptation during placement and, as we will see in chapter 11, differ as well from those that affect adaptation in the subsequent course of the caregiving career. Subjective primary stressors take a more prominent role during the early phases of this transition, whereas objective primary stressors and intrapsychic strains appear to be more important to adaptation later on. These findings suggest that professionals who assist caregivers need to consider how adaptation changes over the course of the caregiving career, and to plan interventions and treatments based on an understanding of the emergence of various conflicts over time.

Finally, we have seen clear evidence of the human toll extracted from caregiving to someone suffering from dementia. Nursing home placement does not eliminate commitment, caring, involvement, or the pain associated with seeing a loved one go through a long period of decline. For a small, but noteworthy, group, intense feelings of emotional distress persist for several years following placement. Nursing home care, which places its primary emphasis on the patient, perhaps needs to be reconceptualized to incorporate the family caregiver as well. Families, as we have seen, provide regular help, and possibly could be enlisted to do so in even more constructive and mutually satisfying ways. At the same time, however, they also need help with the difficulties associated with having a relative live in a nursing home.

Notes

[1]These caregivers are not included in the analyses for this chapter because we lack detailed information about the institutional care phase of their caregiving.

[2]These activities include "eating, changing diapers or pads, going to the bathroom, bathing/showering/washing hair, dressing/undressing, brushing hair/teeth, getting in/out of bed, getting around inside the facility, getting around the outside grounds, getting going in an activity, [and] taking (his/her) medication."

[3]To make the in-home and institutional cohorts equivalent, we included in the comparison group caregivers who completed two or more in-home care interviews, but subsequently became bereaved or were lost-at-follow-up.

[4]Our emphasis is on subjective rather than objective primary stressors because institutionalization de facto lessens caregivers' involvement in personal care and behavioral management of the patient.

[5]This analysis pertains to the family's treatment of the patient and the caregiver, as these are the sole dimensions that are relevant after institutionalization.

[6]This strain is assessed as having insufficient money to meet monthly expenses.

[7]The measures of instrumental social support used in this investigation, which emphasize help with patient care, are not germane to institutional care.

[8]This analysis also is limited to those caregivers who participated in at least one institutional care interview.

[9]One technical problem with extreme scores is regression to the mean. For someone who initially scores at the extreme high or low end of a scale, measurement error can only result in movement toward the mean because that is the only direction in which change may occur.

[10]A second technical problem with extreme scores pertains to ceiling and floor effects. Caregivers who are asymptomatic at baseline are at the floor and cannot demonstrate positive change; those at the high extreme, or ceiling, cannot increase further.

[11]For these analyses, psychological distress was assessed using the composite symptom measure constructed from the individual indicators of depression, anger, and anxiety, which we refer to as nonspecific psychological distress. Although earlier in this chapter we reported a selective effect of placement on dimensions of psychological well-being, successful adaptation across these three indicators was fairly uniform among caregivers.

[12]This analysis is limited to caregivers who were employed before and after the admission of their relatives ($n = 57$).

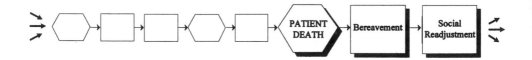

The Timing
and Settings
of Patient Death

Given the age and disability of the dementia patients in our study, the caregivers face the virtual certainty of spousal or parental bereavement. The sole exception is the premature death of the caregiver, an occurrence that is neither common nor rare, especially among spousal caregivers who are themselves of advanced age. Reactions to the death of the dementia patient present themselves in two ways: in the pain following the loss of a loved one and in the welcomed realization that their loved one has been released from the destructive course of dementia. Death of the care recipient, then, often evokes ambivalent sentiments.

Previous research suggests that dementia itself hastens death. Persons suffering from Alzheimer's disease (AD) confront a substantial elevation in mortality relative to those experiencing "normal" aging, other psychiatric disorders, and possibly other forms of dementia (Belloni-Sonzogni, Tissot, Tettamanti, Frattura, & Spagnoli, 1989; Diesfeldt, van Houte, & Moerkens, 1986; Martin, Miller, Kapoor, Arena, & Boller, 1987; Mölsä, Marttila, & Rinne, 1986; van Dijk, Dippel, & Habbema, 1991; van Dijk, van de Sande, Dippel, & Habbema, 1992; Varsamis, Zuchowski, & Maini, 1972; Vitaliano, Peck, Johnson, Prinz, & Eisdorfer, 1981). There is some evidence that reduced life expectancy occurs only for early-onset dementia (Diesfeldt et al., 1986), but other researchers do not find onset differences in survival (Mölsä et al., 1986). The increase in mortality emerges approximately 3 years after the onset of the dementia (Schoenberg, Okazaki, & Kokmen, 1981). Van Dijk and associates (1992) concluded that dementia is an independent mortality risk.

In some instances, death is attributable to the underlying disease process of dementia that interferes with brain function; in others, it results from risks associated with decreased cognition, memory, and performance (Harkness, Bentley, & Roghmann, 1990; Mölsä et al., 1986; Thomas, Bennett, Laughon, Greenough, & Bartlett, 1990; van Dijk et al., 1991, 1992). For example, dementia patients are at greater than average risk of dying following surgery because of delays in diagnosis and inability to withstand complications (Bernstein & Offenbartl, 1991). In situations such as these, dementia interferes with a person's ability to recognize that he or she is unwell and to communicate this information to others. Moreover, impairment of cognitive processes disables the capacity to participate in one's own treatment (e.g., to comply with therapies or to signal distress).

Recent research indicates quite clearly that care recipients who are institutionalized have substantially higher mortality rates than persons who continue to be cared for at home. Elevated mortality among nursing home residents has been described for the general population of older persons (Shapiro & Tate, 1988; Wolinsky, Callahan, Fitzgerald, & Johnson, 1992) and for dementia patients in particular (Aneshensel et al. 1993; van Dijk et al., 1992). Mortality rates are highest immediately following entry into a nursing home (Shah, Banks, & Merskey, 1969; Shapiro & Tate, 1988; van Dijk et al., 1992).

These patterns raise a troubling question: Does admission to a long-term care facility elevate the risk of death, or is high mortality merely an artifact of the disproportionate placement of persons about to die? These alternatives reflect *social causation* and *social selection* hypotheses, respectively, the two major competing explanations for postadmission elevations in mortality. The social causation hypothesis treats excess mortality among the institutionalized elderly as a direct consequence of institutional placement: Death is triggered by the disruptive event of admission or by the conditions of life subsequently encountered within the institution. The social selection hypothesis portrays this excess mortality following institutionalization as illusory: Death was imminent prior to institutionalization and would have occurred even if these unhealthy patients had not been presented for admission. This chapter evaluates these alternatives for the dementia patients included in this investigation. First, however, we describe the risk of dying these patients confront over the course of their illness.

Patterns of Mortality among Care Recipients

As mentioned earlier, a substantial number of care recipients died over the 3 years of this study. When considering the 555 dementia patients receiving in-home care at the start of the study, 206, or about one-third, died prior to the fourth interview, as illustrated in Figure 10.1. Slightly more than half of these

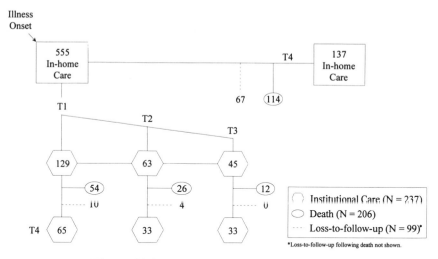

Figure 10.1   Patient deaths over time and by location.

deaths (55.3%) occurred at home; the remaining 92 deaths occurred sometime after caregivers placed their impaired relatives in long-term care institutions. At Time 4, a total of 268 care recipients were alive: about half (51.1%) were living at home and the remainder ($n = 131$) were living in institutions.[1]

At first glance, these data appear to contradict the notion that mortality is elevated among the institutionalized, given that more than half of the deaths occurred during in-home care. Such a conclusion would be mistaken, however, because it does not take into consideration the number of patients at risk for death at each location. That is, the mortality *rate* consists of a numerator and a denominator, but this viewpoint counts only the former and not the latter. Patients are at risk of dying at home *only* until they are institutionalized; patients become at risk of dying within an institution *only* after they are admitted, and all nursing home residents will eventually die in these circumstances.[2] For instance, all of the patients who died within a nursing home could have died earlier while they were at home, but they did not; they survived long enough to be institutionalized. To address this complication, it is necessary to take into consideration duration of exposure to the risk of death at both phases of caregiving, in-home and institutional.

Illness Duration and Death

As illustrated in Figure 10.1, deaths occurred throughout the interval separating the Time 1 and Time 4 interviews. It is important to note that the timing of death with respect to the timing of our data collection is not especially meaningful because care recipients had been ill for varying periods of time prior to the baseline interview. Thus, the duration of exposure to the risk of mortality following illness onset differs across patients. In essence, these interviews occurred at arbitrary points in the course of the dementia. Consequently, it is most instructive to examine mortality as a function of illness duration. In order to do so, we need to take into consideration illness duration for those care recipients who were alive at Time 4 because this group includes the longest survivors of dementia. Disregarding the length of illness for these persons would bias downward estimates of the average. This situation is another instance of the censored observation problem discussed earlier with regard to the risk of institutionalization (see chapter 8), necessitating the use of a hazard model.[3]

Figure 10.2 presents the survival distribution for the interval from illness onset until patient death. Time starts to accrue when caregivers first noticed something was wrong with their relatives (i.e., time since symptom recognition reported at the baseline interview). This value is then incremented by the time from the baseline interview until either the death of the care recipient or the case is censored (i.e., until the time of the last observation at which the patient is known to have still been alive).

This analysis pertains to illness duration as distinct from disease duration. The actual onset of the underlying disease that produces dementia usually precedes the recognition that something is wrong and the identification of the problem as an illness, as discussed in chapter 4. Consequently, disease duration typically is longer than illness duration. Also, the initial duration estimates given by caregivers are retrospective and should be viewed as estimations, thus, the time from illness onset to death inevitably is approximate.[4]

I don't feel guilty about her dying. That's the best solution.

As may be seen in Figure 10.2, most of the dementia patients included in this study survived the early years of their illness.[5] At the end of 5 years, 88.5% were still living, either at home or in an institution. This interval during which the chances of death are static, is followed by a period of continuous and uniform decline. Approximately one in four dementia patients died by 8 years after symptom recognition. One in two died 11 years after others recognized that something was wrong with their cognitive functioning; this time span is the median illness duration. Among the care recipients in this investigation then, illness typically follows a lengthy course.[6] This pattern is consistent with the known course of dementia (Zarit et al., 1986).

Peak Periods of Risk

In Figure 10.3 we present hazard rates for death: the risk of death at a specific point in time given that the patient was alive until that time, which is similar to a conditional probability. These hazard rates assess variation in risk as a function of illness duration *among those who survive the preceding phases of the illness.* The *cumulative* risk of dying obviously increases steadily with time.

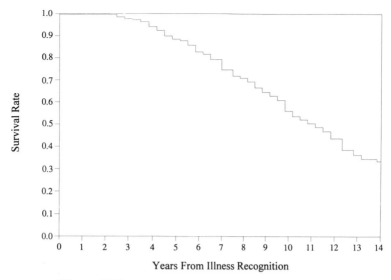

Figure 10.2   Survival until death of the dementia patient.

The risk of death is low at the beginning of dementia, but thereafter intensifies at a rather steady rate. The low initial risk corresponds to the plateau in the survival distribution seen above. After approximately 2 years, the hazard rate rises and continues to augment throughout the course of the dementia. That is, the likelihood of dying becomes greater as illness duration increases. For example,

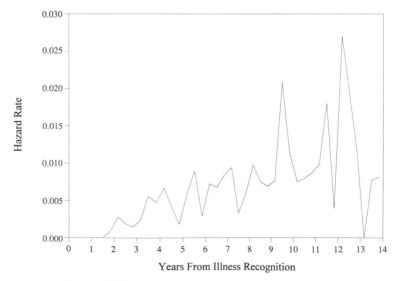

Figure 10.3   Hazard rates for death of the dementia patient.

the risk of dying during the fourth year is substantially lower than the risk of dying during the tenth year. Thus, the longer one lives with dementia, the more likely one is to die in the near future.

Rosemary

Dementia typically follows a protracted course, but death is its eventual outcome. This final period is described poignantly by Rosemary, whose husband died at home after a lengthy stay in a nursing home:

The last month he went down very fast. He didn't want to go out for rides anymore. That was not like him anymore. When he refused to respond to doing things I knew that he was going. The district nurse sent him to the hospital one day. I was very mad. I wanted him home. With the help of the doctor I got him discharged from the hospital.

I played his favorite music for him and I tried to have a warm atmosphere here. I don't know if he knew it at that time. He wasn't responding. I hope he heard the music and knew that we were around. My granddaughter came again and the last thing anyone heard Peter say, as far as I know, was on his last day at the nursing home when she'd just come and he said to her "you have such a nice . . . ", never finished it, and that was the last thing he said.

As time progresses, dementia patients are more and more likely to die. As seen previously, they also have a greater chance of being institutionalized (see chapter 8). These two outcomes, death and institutionalization, present similar cumulative pictures, but differ notably in the pattern of contemporaneous risk. For both outcomes, the risk initially is low. As time progresses, the risk of admission to a nursing home increases and then remains stable, whereas the risk of death continues to spiral upwards (compare Figure 8.2 with Figure 10.3). Dementia patients, therefore, face a uniform risk of nursing home admission over time, but an increasing risk of death.

Health Status and Mortality

Before considering the influence of institutionalization, it is important to take into account other factors that contribute to mortality, especially the impact of health status and age. The question is not whether these factors are relevant to mortality (illness and advancing age clearly elevate the risk of death), but whether these factors are the *sole* influences on mortality.

The dependent variable is the time separating illness onset and death or, alternately stated, the risk of death at any given time since illness onset. Hazard models are used to account for censored observations and for variation in the time each patient has been at risk of dying. Three indicators of the underlying dementia are included as explanatory factors: presence of a specific diagnosis of

AD, early age of onset (before age 75), and severity of cognitive impairment. Two indicators of poor physical health are included: perceived physical health status and recent hospitalization. Patient age and gender also are considered to account for aging effects and male–female differences in life expectancy.[7] With the exceptions of age at diagnosis and gender, these variables are treated as time-varying covariates.[8]

As may be seen in Table 10.1, the risk of dying depends importantly upon most of these health-related factors. The three dementia-related variables each contribute independently to mortality, but two of these relationships are counter-intuitive. Specifically, the risk of death at any given point since illness onset, given that one has not already died, is lower for care recipients who have received a specific diagnosis of AD ($p \leq .07$) and for those with early onset. Previous research had led us to expect that mortality would be elevated among those with AD and among those with early onset.

It should be noted that AD diagnosis approaches statistical significance only at the multivariate level of analysis and this occurs only when age and gender are included in the analytic model. The probability of having a specific diagnosis of AD declines with age in this sample, and men and women are about equally likely to have received this diagnosis. The emergence of the diagnosis variable in multivariate analysis, therefore, appears to be linked to age differences in diagnosis. Specifically, those with a diagnosis of AD tend to be younger and, hence, less likely to die than those with other diagnoses or no diagnosis. In this instance, then, diagnosis functions as a proxy for patient age.

> It's a long downhill slide. I can see how someone would aid a victim in ending their life. I wouldn't help him, but I wouldn't stand in his way.

Table 10.1   Relative Risk of Death by Patient Health Status

Patient health status	Relative risk	
	Full model	Trimmed model
Alzheimer's disease diagnosis (/no)[a]	.73	—
Early age of onset (/75+)	.39***	—
Cognitive impairment (0–4)[a]	1.98***	1.87***
Patient physical health status (poor [1] to excellent [4])[a]	.84*	.85*
Recent hospitalization (/no)[a]	1.82***	1.88***
Patient age (in years)[a]	1.01	1.05***
Male	1.72***	1.68***

[a]Time-varying covariate.
*$p \leq .05$.   **$p < .01$.   ***$p \leq .001$.

The early-onset effect may be understood best by recalling that the analysis considers mortality as a function of time since illness onset. Those with early onset are necessarily younger than those with late onset according to this system of measuring time and, therefore, are less likely to die at any specific time following symptom recognition. The dependency between age at the time of onset and time since symptom recognition is so pronounced that it overrides the effect of patient age, which is statistically significant only at the bivariate level of analysis. Thus, even though persons with early onset may die at younger ages than those with late onset, at any given time after the start of dementia, older patients are still more likely to die.

In contrast, the third indicator of dementia is related to mortality in the expected manner: The risk of mortality increases as cognitive impairment increases. The influence of cognitive impairment on mortality is in addition to the contributions of other health-related variables, meaning that the severity of impairment independently elevates the risk of death.

It is apparent in Table 10.1 that besides cognitive impairment, poor physical health elevates mortality. Specifically, care recipients who had been hospitalized in the past year had twice the risk of dying as those who had not been hospitalized. The caregiver's overall rating of the patient's physical health status, aside from his or her memory problems, also is strongly related to the subsequent risk of death. Patients who were rated as being in *good* physical health were 1.2 times more likely to die than those whose physical health was rated as *excellent*. Dementia patients considered to be in *poor* physical health were twice as likely to die as those whose physical health was considered to be *excellent*.

Finally, when age, physical health status, and severity of cognitive impairment are taken into consideration, male patients are substantially more likely to die than female patients.

This analysis was repeated deleting diagnosis and onset. These variables were omitted because they are dependent upon patient age and function as proxies for it. The trimmed model also is shown in Table 10.1. The main difference from the previous model is the emergence of age as a statistically significant contributor to mortality: Older patients are more likely to die. Males and patients with severe cognitive impairment, poor physical health, and recent hospitalizations also have a heightened chance of dying compared to their female counterparts and those with mild cognitive impairment, good physical health, and no hospitalizations.

The Impact of Institutionalization

Based on the findings outlined above, the social selection hypothesis appears to possess strong face validity insofar as physical health status is unquestionably predictive of mortality. Other research supports social selection as well, demonstrating that postadmission survival among dementia patients is inversely related to conditions that presumably pose a threat to their physical health: severity of dementia, severity of behavioral impairments, dependency, inactivity, physical disability, age, and possibly, age of onset and comorbidity (Diesfeldt et al., 1986; van Dijk et al., 1991, 1992; Walsh, Welch, & Larson, 1990). In general, patient mortality also is related to cognitive impairment, severe mental abnormality, urinary incontinence, need for intense nursing, functional impairment, physical dependence, and poor physical mobility (Brauer, Mackeprang, & Bentzon, 1978; Goldfarb, 1969; Kelman & Thomas, 1990; Shapiro & Tate, 1985). Indeed, the data presented above leave no doubt about the relationship between physical well-being and mortality for the dementia patients involved in this inquiry.

As previously discussed in chapter 8, the relationship between health status and institutionalization, however, is equivocal. Some studies report that elderly persons admitted to long-term care facilities are indeed in worse health than those who remain at home, others, including this inquiry, find health differences to be of secondary importance to sociodemographic factors and social isolation (e.g., Aneshensel et al., 1993; Branch & Jette, 1982; Morris, Sherwood, & Gutkin, 1988; Shapiro & Tate, 1985; Wolinsky et al., 1992). If those in poor health are not more likely to be institutionalized, then poor health cannot explain the association between institutionalization and mortality.

Moreover, even if we assume a health differential exists, it does not necessarily account for excess mortality among the institutionalized. That is, social causation effects may occur even in the presence of a selection effect. Wolinsky and associates (1992) recently considered this issue by examining deaths over a 4-year period for a nationally representative sample of older adults. They found 2.7 times higher mortality among persons admitted to nursing homes than among persons who remained in the community, even when other determinants of mortality and institutionalization, including physical health status, were statistically controlled. In an earlier analysis, a similar increase in mortality among the institutionalized dementia patients in this study was found, *net* of their health status (Aneshensel et al., 1993).

In this earlier work, mortality was considered a function of the duration of caregiving because the primary focus was on caregiver attributes. Here, we shift focus and examine life expectancy from illness onset (i.e., time from symptom recognition until death). The analytic question is whether institutionalization is related to the risk of dying when the health status of the patient is taken into consideration. This analysis entails adding institutionalization as a time-varying covariate to the previous model containing indicators of health status (see Table 10.1). Quite simply, we asked, Does institutionalization add to the risk of death already present in the form of poor health? The results of this analysis are presented in Table 10.2.

Caregivers who institutionalize their relatives are substantially more likely to become bereaved than those whose relatives continue to reside within the community. The zero-order odds of patient death approximately double following admission to a nursing home (risk ratio = 2.11). This elevation in risk is virtually unchanged when physical health status is statistically controlled, as shown in

Table 10.2   Relative Risk of Death by Patient
Health Status and Institutionalization

Patient health and institutional status	Relative risk
Cognitive impairment (0–4)[a]	1.82***
Patient physical health status (poor [1] to excellent [4])[a]	.83**
Recent hospitalization (/no)[a]	1.85***
Patient age (in years)[a]	1.05***
Male	1.61**
Institutionalized (/no)	2.12***

[a]Time-varying covariate.
*$p \le .05$.   **$p \le .01$.   ***$p \le .001$.

Table 10.2. Thus, the overall increment in mortality cannot be attributed to poor initial physical health among those who are institutionalized even though poor physical health independently contributes to mortality. Institutionalization per se is substantially associated with the risk of dying over and above the effects of poor physical health.

Mortality after Nursing Home Admission

It is quite evident, then, that nursing home patients are more likely to die in the immediate future than similar dementia patients who remain in the home. This finding suggests that postadmission survival is problematic in and of itself, as distinct from being the inadvertent consequence of a tendency to admit patients who are about to die. To examine this issue further, we consider mortality as a function of time since admission to a nursing home.

The question that concerns us is not whether nursing home patients will die, because eventually they certainly will do so. Rather, the core issue we are addressing is the *timing* of their deaths (i.e., premature death). Thus, our analysis focuses on the duration of survival within the institution. This question requires the use of hazard models because nursing home patients have been at risk of dying for unequal times and because those who did not die, a group that disproportionately contains the most long-term survivors, are censored at Time 4.[9]

Mortality clearly varies considerably as a function of time since placement, as illustrated in Figure 10.4. These hazard rates are similar to conditional probabilities: the proportion dying within an interval among those living at the beginning of the interval (adjusted for cases censored during the interval). As may be seen in the figure, the probability of dying is highest immediately following placement and declines rapidly until approximately 6 months after which it

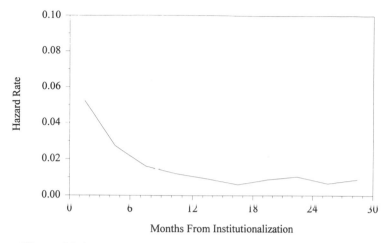

Figure 10.4   Postadmission hazard rates for death of the dementia patient.

stabilizes. The first interval, 1 to 3 months, differs significantly from all of the remaining intervals, although these later intervals are indistinguishable from one another.

The survival function, not shown here, mirrors the hazard function: An immediate, rapid decline in the proportion surviving is followed by a slow, but steady, decline throughout the remaining period of observation. Taking into account censored cases, the estimated survival rates for 1, 2, and 3 years postadmission are 67.8%, 57.8%, and 53.5%, respectively. On the other hand, a quarter (23.8%, adjusted for censoring) did not survive the first 6 months.

Frank

Frank, who has been devastated by the death of his wife, looks back with a touch of anger and irony:

One internist that I took Beth to was a great believer in euthanasia. We agreed on no heroics. He called it "studied neglect," which is a good term. That's what finally happened. She'd lost a lot of weight. Was down to 78 pounds. Contracted a urinary tract infection, then double pneumonia and went in 8 days.

By that time there was a different doctor who was on the staff of the nursing home. He pumped a lot of antibiotics into her. I was angry with him. Spent $200–$300 on drugs that he had no business to prescribe.

The most loving thought is to hope that they get out of their misery, and it lets you out of jail, too. I miss her terribly of course.

The descriptive picture is quite clear then: If one survives the first few months of institutional life, long-term survival is more likely than not, however, the odds of surviving these first few months are far from reassuring.

The Impact of Patient Health on Postadmission Mortality

These early deaths may be due to the nursing home admissions of patients in extremely fragile health, those for whom death was not unexpected. This possibility is, as previously discussed, the basis for the social selection interpretation. From this perspective, we would expect elevated mortality among dementia patients who are institutionalized for reasons of poor patient health. These patients are the *only* ones who should evidence elevated mortality if social selection accounts fully for excess mortality.

Approximately half (44.4%) of the caregivers specifically cited poor patient health as a reason for the admission of their spouses or parents to institutions. In Figure 10.5, postadmission survival is plotted for this group of patients ($n = 101$) and for those admitted for reasons other than poor patient health ($n = 130$). The latter reasons include the caregiver's belief that the dementia patient is potentially harmful to himself, herself, or others; the caregiver's assessment that he or she is no longer able to perform the tasks of caregiving; and lack of sufficient assistance from others in performing care-related tasks (see chapter 8, especially Figure 8.4). What is striking about this comparison is that a rapid decline in survival immediately following admission is seen for *both* strata.

Thus, although dementia patients admitted to long-term care facilities due to poor health are quite likely to die shortly after their admission, the pattern anticipated by the social selection hypothesis, persons admitted for reasons other

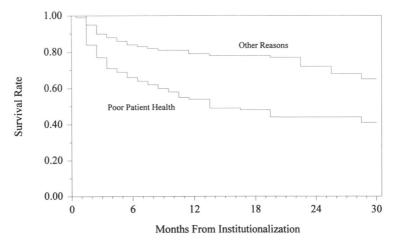

Figure 10.5   Postadmission survival by reason for admission.

than poor health also encounter a sharp initial drop in survival, a pattern *not* explained by the social selection argument. The initial rate of decline is greatest for patients admitted specifically because of poor health. The 95% confidence intervals for these survival distributions, not shown here, do not overlap.

These distinct survival functions are due entirely to differences in the mortality rate for the first 3 months of nursing home residence. For the first few months after admission, hazard rates, also not illustrated here, are substantially higher for patients admitted for health reasons rather than other reasons; these rates drop substantially over the next several months for both groups. Aside from the first 3 months, the 95% confidence intervals for the hazard rates of the two groups overlap throughout the period of observation. Thus, the reason for admission matters to the risk of death only for the first 3 months subsequent to admission; thereafter, the reason for admission is immaterial.

The most striking feature of the distribution for patients admitted specifically for reasons of poor health is the presence of long-term survivors. Roughly half of those admitted for poor health lived for at least 1 year postadmission. This figure is substantially higher for patients placed for other reasons: Approximately four out of five of these patients lived a year or longer.

The question is how I'd feel if I let her starve to death. I'm not prepared to do that.

In summary, these data demonstrate social selection processes for mortality insofar as patients admitted for poor health are most likely to die in the immediate aftermath of admission. Yet, these data also show that the admission of patients in poor health does not account fully for the elevation in mortality that occurs immediately after admission. The sharp drop in survival during this time for patients admitted for reasons other than poor health cannot be attributed to processes of social selection: These deaths are unexpected deaths.

We repeated this analysis controlling directly for preadmission patient health status to establish the robustness of these findings. The independent variables are the same set of health indicators used earlier in this chapter to predict mortality with regard to illness duration. The dependent variable, however, differs: time from nursing home admission until death. This analysis appears in Table 10.3.

Following admission to nursing homes, the patients who are most likely to die are those with severe cognitive impairments. Males do not live as long as females within nursing homes, and older patients tend to die early in their placement. Also, neither age of onset nor diagnosis is related to postadmission survival. Although poor health and hospitalization are associated with overall mortality (see Tables 10.1 and 10.2), these factors do not independently contribute to postadmission mortality. This finding is especially important because these factors are precisely the conditions that should matter to mortality from the perspective of social selection. Thus, the impact of poor physical health in the postadmission period apparently is secondary to the impact of cognitive impairment.

Table 10.3 Relative Risk of Postadmission Death
by Patient Health Status

Patient health status	Relative risk
Alzheimer's disease diagnosis (/no)[a]	1.15
Early age of onset (/75+)	.93
Cognitive impairment (0–4)[b]	2.05***
Patient physical health status (poor [1] to excellent [4])[b]	1.05
Recent hospitalization (/no)[b]	1.33
Patient age (in years)[a]	1.05*
Male	1.71*

[a]Fixed at value immediately preceding admission.
[b]Time-varying covariate.
*$p \leq .05$. **$p \leq .01$ ***$p \leq .001$.

Summary

This chapter has examined time from illness onset until patient death and the factors that are related to an elevated risk of death. The key findings include the following:

• When considering the 555 dementia patients receiving in-home care at the start of the study, 206, or about one-third, died over the next 3 years. Slightly less than half ($n = 92$) of these deaths occurred sometime after caregivers admitted their impaired relatives to long-term care institutions.

• Most of the dementia patients included in this study survived the early years of their illness: 88.5% were still living 5 years after symptom recognition.

• Although the risk of death is low at the beginning of dementia, it increases thereafter at a steady rate.

• The risk of mortality becomes greater as the severity of cognitive impairment intensifies, as physical health status worsens, and as the patient ages. In addition, males face a mortality disadvantage.

• Caregivers who institutionalize their relatives are about twice as likely to become bereaved than those whose relatives continue to live at home, even when patient health status is controlled.

• Among those who are institutionalized, the probability of dying is highest immediately following placement, and then declines rapidly and stabilizes.

• Early mortality is greatest among patients who are admitted to nursing homes because of their poor health.

• Patients admitted for reasons other than poor health also have heightened mortality rates in the first few months of institutionalized care.

Discussion

These data indicate that some of the elevation in mortality that occurs in the immediate aftermath of nursing home admission may be attributed to processes of social selection (i.e., the selective admission of patients in especially poor health). Quite possibly, these persons would have died at home had they not been institutionalized first.

However, an appreciable part of the excess mortality during this period may be attributed to social causation as well because patients who were not in especially poor health immediately prior to placement also face a high mortality risk. Their risk declines substantially after the first few months, the yardstick by which this earlier mortality may be judged as being high. By extension, not all of the early deaths among those admitted for poor health should be attributed to selection effects. Instead, only the *difference* in mortality between the two groups is clearly related to selective admissions. Thus, some of the early deaths among those who were admitted in poor health should be considered premature.

At this point, we may only speculate about the factors that might produce an excess of deaths following nursing home admission. Some of these deaths may be triggered by the disruptive event of admission, the conditions of life subsequently encountered within the institution, or both of these stressful circumstances. Admission to a nursing home epitomizes the worst features of potentially health-threatening life events: It completely disrupts ordinary patterns of daily life, requiring readjustment of virtually all behavioral patterns, including lifelong routines; it is viewed almost universally as undesirable; the patient is likely to have little or no control over placement decisions, especially when health conditions impair cognitive functioning; and it may weaken or sever social ties to family and friends that might otherwise mitigate the full force of this trauma. In addition, because of the patients' diminished resilience, the ongoing conditions of institutionalized life may put them in jeopardy; in particular, they may be exposed to undue bodily insult and infectious agents. At issue is not the specific biological mechanism that causes death, but how living conditions might shape whether such agents are encountered and if so, whether appropriate and timely treatment is received.

In conclusion, substantial mortality occurs in the immediate aftermath of institutional placement. Nonetheless, numerous persons reside within institutions for extended periods of time. This pattern suggests that if death does not occur shortly after placement, then a rather prolonged residency may well eventuate, even among dementia patients whose poor health precipitated their admission to nursing homes.

Notes

[1] The status of care recipients is unknown in those instances where the patient was alive at the time of the interview immediately prior to attrition from the study ($n = 81$).

[2] The exception is patients who return home from nursing homes. Only one patient followed this course in the present inquiry, thus, we ignore this contingency. For conditions other than dementia, the return of patients to home care substantially complicates the assessment of mortality risk.

[3] A similar censoring problem is present for those who were living immediately prior to being lost-at-follow-up.

[4] This caveat is most important to the descriptive picture of the course of dementia. It is less critical to the analysis of factors contributing to mortality because any error in these estimates occurred at Time 1, whereas all of the deaths took place subsequent to this baseline report. Thus, errors in the initial dating of symptom recognition should be random errors with regard to the subsequent death of the dementia patient.

[5] The distribution of survival times is cumulative, a running tally of those care recipients who have died. Its initial value is 1, reflecting the fact that all dementia patients were alive at the time of illness recognition. This value declines as dementia-related deaths occur and as deaths accrue from other causes. The distribution eventually will dip to 0, the point at which all of the care recipients will have died.

[6] This distribution probably underestimates deaths during the earliest years of dementia because our sampling design is more likely to result in the selection of long-term than short-term caregivers. As noted previously, when the duration of a condition is variable, the probability of selection is greatest for those with the longest duration because they are "at risk" of being sampled for a long time, whereas those with short durations are less likely to be identified "in episode." The same principle applies to disease and illness durations. Those who have been receiving care for a long time de facto did not die early in their illness. To the extent that long-term caregivers are oversampled then, the risk of death early in dementia is underestimated by these data.

[7] Although we obviously lack the laboratory-type data necessary to precisely assess the contribution of clinical factors to mortality, the available measures suffice to partition gross variation in mortality due to declining health. Moreover, these measures are typical of those usually employed in research examining mortality among the aged.

[8] The Time 1 values of these covariates were initialized and updated at each subsequent interview at which the patient was living.

[9] Nursing home patients who were lost-at-follow-up prior to death are censored at their last observation.

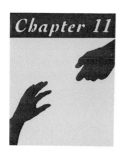

Chapter 11

Bereavement

The final stage of the caregiving career typically includes bereavement. Because AD becomes increasingly prevalent with age, most impaired relatives for whom care is provided are in the upper age ranges. As we saw in the preceding chapter, this means that the chances of having a relative die increase appreciably with each passing year. Thus, many caregivers are able to anticipate the death of their relatives in advance of the actual event. Nonetheless, when death occurs, it stands as a critical transition in the careers of caregivers.

We know that each transition and phase of the caregiving career is capable of triggering pervasive life change. Undoubtedly, the rearrangement of everyday life first occurs when symptoms of dementia are recognized and people begin to assume caregiver roles. Similarly, as we have seen (chapter 9), institutional placement often has far-reaching effects on the organization of day-to-day life. However, no transition has a greater impact on the lives of caregivers than the death of the relatives for whom they have been caring.

Despite the likelihood that caregivers will face the death of their impaired relatives, little is known about their responses to this loss or how experiences during caregiving may affect adaptation to bereavement. The few studies that have examined bereavement among caregivers have found that it parallels bereavement among noncaregivers (Bass & Bowman, 1990; Bodnar & Kiecolt-Glaser, 1994; Mullan, 1992). Among the general population, depression, sadness, and grief increase in the months right after death and then decline (see Osterweis, Solomon, & Green, 1984; M. S. Stroebe, Stroebe, & Hansson, 1993, for reviews of this literature). By the second year of bereavement, the level of depression is similar to that found among nonbereaved comparison groups (Lund, Caserta, & Dimond, 1993). However, various grief responses, such as thoughts and feelings about the deceased and yearning for them, continue well beyond the first few years (Shuchter & Zisook, 1993).

Although there is now a body of research in which this overall pattern is repeatedly found, it is important to underscore that these are average trends and that people vary greatly in their responses to the death of a loved one; some respond intensely, whereas others grieve very little (Wortman & Silver, 1989). Moreover, most studies typically examine a limited range of outcomes, primarily grief and symptoms of psychopathology, particularly depression. Thus, little is known about how other experiences might be affected by death, experiences such as feelings of role overload or mastery. Finally, and most importantly, there have been only a handful of prospective studies that have collected information on survivors prior to death (Bass & Bowman, 1990; Bodnar & Kiecolt-Glaser, 1994; Norris & Murrell, 1987; Wortman, Silver, & Kessler, 1993).

With regard to factors that contribute to variability in adaptation to bereavement, three have emerged with regularity from previous research. First, time since death is a consistent predictor of the course of bereavement: Distress increases immediately following death and then declines. Second, there is some stability in each person's adaptation; those doing well at one point in time are likely to be doing well at a later point. Third, the death of a child appears to be followed by the most difficult bereavement. Other contributors to grief are less clear-cut.

Previous bereavement research has succeeded in identifying a few characteristics that may act as risk factors or as protective factors (Sanders, 1994). For example, clinical evidence has suggested that a difficult relationship will complicate grief. Thus, we would expect that a conflictual past relationship with the dementia patient, or one tinged with guilt, would exacerbate distress when the patient dies (Bowlby, 1980; Parkes, 1987; Raphael, 1983). On the protective side, it is thought that those with strong social and psychological resources will be buffered from some of the distress that accompanies bereavement (W. Stroebe

& Stroebe, 1987). Some work has also suggested that those who have had the opportunity to prepare socially or psychologically before death will have an easier time with bereavement (Rando, 1986).

Some constructs may take on new meaning in the context of bereavement. For instance, from the perspective of in-home care, the duration of caregiving is an indicator of hardship because it assesses the length of exposure to care-related stressors (Hill, Thompson, & Gallagher, 1988). From the perspective of bereavement, however, duration may also indicate forewarning and the opportunity to prepare for the final decline and death of the patient (Roach & Kitson, 1989). The developing sense of loss of intimacy with the dementia patient is another construct whose meaning changes from the vantage point of bereavement. Although we consider it a subjective primary stressor that leads to emotional distress during caregiving, it may also reflect a realistic psychological preparation for death. Certainly, if one task of bereavement is to clearly recognize the losses sustained so that the deceased may endure in memory even as the survivor reengages with life (Marris, 1974), then those who have done this work prior to the death of their impaired relatives may be at an adaptive advantage afterwards.

> After 3 and a half years, I'm still grieving just under the surface. All I need is the thought.

In this chapter, we chart the impact of death over the short and long run along two related, but distinct lines. The first recognizes that death dramatically alters the organization of the caregiver's life. We look at the effect of death on the restructuring of daily life, especially as the absence of caregiving demands alters elements of the stress process. The second revolves around the idea that death and the losses it entails typically set in motion emotional and cognitive reactions on the part of surviving caregivers, reactions that may be characterized as expressions of grief. As we shall see, the intensity, scope, and duration of these grief reactions vary among bereaved caregivers. We consider first the restructuring effects of death and their relevance to the types of stress experienced by caregivers.

Continuities and Discontinuities in the Stress Process along the Caregiving Career

As we have seen, caregivers typically organize their daily lives around the care and welfare of their impaired relatives. Contingent upon functional dependencies, cognitive status, and the need to control and manage the behavior of the dementia patient, caregiving may produce states of role overload, feelings of role captivity, or a sense that the exchange and closeness that previously marked the marital or parent–child relationship has eroded or been entirely lost. These primary stressors, in turn, generate secondary stressors, which include strains in domains of life outside of caregiving and critical changes in the ways caregivers think of themselves. Finally, both primary and secondary stressors are reflected in the level of emotional distress exhibited by caregivers. Earlier, we saw how this stress process unfolds as caregivers continue to provide home care and as they provide supplemental care within an institutional setting.

This brief review of the components of the stress process provides a background against which the effects of death stand in sharp relief. Although the death of the care recipient brings all caregiving activities to a halt, some of the consequences of these activities linger. This is yet another instance of the continuities inherent within the caregiving career, wherein the experiences and dispositions engendered during an earlier stage influence the experiences and dispositions at a later stage. Thus, death, like other transitional events, results in both continuities and discontinuities with earlier stages. It is to the exploration of these points of convergence and divergence that we now turn, guided by a simple question: To what extent does the death of the impaired relative realign the experiences and feelings that had been created during earlier stages of the caregiving career?

Although this question is simple to pose, identifying the strategies and procedures needed to answer it is not. For one thing, experiences and feelings that had been rooted in caregiving activities and that may change following the demise of one's relative are quite varied. Among those affected are: role overload, a subjective primary stressor; secondary role strains, such as economic strains and family tensions; secondary intrapsychic strains, such as guilt and loss of self; personal and social resources in the forms of mastery and social support; and finally, symptoms of emotional distress, particularly anger and depression. Thus, the conditions that are potentially altered by death spread across the entire breadth of the stress process.

Some conditions, of course, are completely eliminated once the patient has died, such as the actual tasks of providing care. Because these conditions no longer exist following death of the dementia patient, questions about them were not included in the bereavement interviews. Questions evaluating conditions that persisted, but assumed different forms, were modified in ways consistent with this transition of the caregiver's career. For example, in the baseline, continuing in-home care, and placement interviews, we asked about familial disputes revolving around caregiving issues; however, in the bereavement interviews these questions were replaced with questions about family tensions of a more general nature.

The Immediate Impact of the Death of the Dementia Patient

The Short-Term Bereavement Cohort

To evaluate the impact of death, we compared pre- and postdeath data for those caregivers whose relatives died prior to Time 4. As we saw in previous chapters, dementia patients died throughout the course of this study. The specific interview at which we learned of a death, however, is not relevant to the assessment of its impact on the caregiver. Consequently, it was necessary to organize the data around the transitional event of death, rather than the time of data collection. This strategy is identical to that used in chapter 9 to evaluate the impact of institutional placement using a synthetic analytic cohort.

Thus, we combined all caregivers who became bereaved prior to Time 4. The data were then arrayed so that the interview conducted just prior to death is treated as the baseline (predeath) interview, irrespective of whether this interview occurred at Time 1, 2, or 3. For example, for caregivers whose relatives died between the second and third interviews, Time 2 serves as baseline. Correspondingly, the follow-up (postdeath) interview is the first interview conducted after the caregiver had become bereaved. In the example just given, follow-up is Time 3.

Figure 11.1 portrays the construction of a synthetic cohort of 206 bereaved caregivers. As indicated, these caregivers became bereaved after Time 1 ($n = 74$), Time 2 ($n = 72$), or Time 3 ($n = 60$). Baseline data are obtained from these interviews, whereas follow-up data are obtained from Time 2, 3, or 4, respectively. Thus, the caregivers comprising the bereavement analytic cohort all have baseline and follow-up data (i.e., information about both the pre- and postdeath periods).

The selection of the appropriate or best comparison group for the bereavement cohort posed a challenge. One could have simply compared bereaved caregivers with themselves; that is, as they were prior to the death of the dementia patient

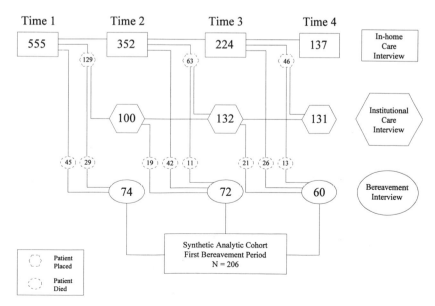

Figure 11.1   Creation of the short-term bereavement cohort.

with the way they were following this event. However, this kind of comparison leaves open the possibility that observed changes are the result of the passage of time or of withdrawal from the caregiver role, rather than the result of death per se. For this reason, it is desirable to compare change in the bereavement cohort with change observed among nonbereaved caregivers.[1]

The comparison group we used is composed of caregivers who were providing care at both Time 1 and Time 2, and who did not become bereaved before Time 4.[2] Time 1 serves as baseline for the comparison group and Time 2 provides follow-up data. This group consists of two subgroups: those who continued to provide in-home care (in-home care cohort, $n = 245$) and those whose relatives had been placed in nursing homes by follow-up (institutional care cohort, $n = 75$).

The bereavement cohort also contains caregivers who had placed their relatives in nursing homes. Of the 206 members of the bereavement cohort, almost half ($n = 92$) had institutionalized their relatives. In earlier chapters, we reported that the transitional event of institutional placement produces major changes in the lives of caregivers, leading to some relief, but generating new types of care-related stressors. We want to be certain that the changes we observe in the bereavement cohort are due to death of the dementia patient as distinct from any general relief people may experience when home care ceases. Thus, it is important to include both in-home and institutional caregivers in the bereavement group and in the comparison group.

At baseline, the comparison cohort differed from the bereavement cohort primarily in the level of impairment of the dementia patient. Compared to patients who were living at follow-up, those who died were in poorer health, were older and more severely cognitively impaired, and needed greater assistance. Caregivers also experienced a greater sense of loss of intimacy with patients who subsequently died. An additional incongruity between the bereaved and comparison cohorts is that role captivity was significantly higher among the institutional care cohort. There were no other differences between the bereaved and comparison cohorts in baseline levels of care-related stressors, psychosocial resources, or emotional distress. We control for any differences existing at baseline when we estimate the effects of bereavement on caregivers.

These effects are estimated with ordinary regression equations. The dependent variable is the condition assessed at follow-up, including stressors, resources, and outcomes like emotional distress. The key independent variable is whether the caregiver subsequently became part of the bereavement, the in-home care, or the institutional care cohort. The other independent variables assessed at baseline include background characteristics, such as kin relationship; situational factors, like the duration of care; objective primary stressors, such as cognitive impairment; subjective primary stressors, such as role overload; secondary role strains, such as family conflict; intrapsychic strains, such as guilt; the psychosocial resources of mastery and socioemotional support; and emotional well-being. We first describe the effect of bereavement controlling for these other conditions, and then consider how these conditions themselves are related to change during bereavement.

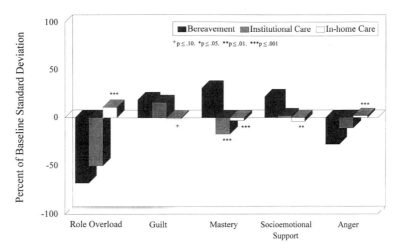

Figure 11.2   Change from baseline to follow-up for bereavement and comparison cohorts.

The Impact of the Care Recipient's Death

What generally happens to caregivers when their impaired relatives die? Most of the changes that occur are not distressing. Figure 11.2 presents the five conditions for which there were significant differences between the bereaved and comparison cohorts. In order to provide a sense of the magnitude of change, these effects are expressed as percentages of the corresponding baseline standard deviation units. A positive value indicates an increase from baseline to follow-up, whereas a negative value indicates a decrease over time.

Role overload, the first outcome on the left of the figure, decreased considerably during the first year of bereavement, an average of about 66% of the baseline standard deviation unit. This change is significantly different from the change occurring among those who continued to provide in-home care, whose average level of role overload actually increased somewhat from baseline to follow-up. Role overload decreased following institutional placement, as we saw in chapter 9, and the difference between changes in the institutional care cohort and the bereavement cohort is not statistically significant. Thus, caregivers experienced considerable relief from role overload following the death of the dementia patient, and this relief is similar in magnitude to that associated with the transitional event of nursing home placement. Because role overload is a subjective primary stressor clearly tied to the level of caregiving demands, it is understandable that it would be substantially diminished when in-home caregiving is no longer called for, either as a result of institutionalization or death.

In contrast to the change observed for role overload, guilt tends to increase among the bereavement cohort, an average of about 20% of the baseline standard deviation, as also shown in Figure 11.2. Guilt, of course, is commonly reported as a response to the death of a loved one (Bowlby, 1980). A comparable increase in guilt accompanies institutionalization, an effect described previously in chapter 9. The findings show that both transitional groups experienced increased guilt, which suggests that in both situations, caregivers look back over their family and caregiving histories and confront past resentments, inadequacies, and ambivalence. In contrast to the transition groups, the in-home care group remains fairly stable in its level of guilt.

It may be noted that neither of the other two intrapsychic strains examined, loss of self or absence of caregiving gains, nor the two secondary role strains examined, economic strain or family conflict, was affected by death of the care recipient.

In contrast, the resources bereaved caregivers are able to draw upon increase following death. Both mastery and socioemotional support, as illustrated in Figure 11.2, are enhanced relative to the in-home care cohort. For support, the institutional care cohort does not differ significantly from the bereavement cohort. Several interpretations of increased socioemotional support are possible. First, death is a normative life-course transition, and there may be more conventional or institutionalized modes of offering support in this situation than in ongoing caregiving. Also, it may be easier to support a person when a discrete event has occurred, whether death or institutionalization, than when support is needed over a protracted period of time. Moreover, it may be that this increase represents more of a perceptual than an objective change. Thus, as the demands of caregiving are diminished by institutionalization or by death, a stable level of support may be perceived as increased support. In other words, need may act as a frame of reference for judging the degree of support, with support seeming to increase as need decreases.

The change in mastery is unique in that only the bereavement cohort experiences an increase from baseline to follow-up. The bereavement cohort differs significantly from both the institutional care cohort and the in-home care cohort, both of which manifest, on average, slight decreases in mastery over time. Perhaps, once people are no longer immersed in a situation that had defied their efforts at control, their convictions about their own mastery are restored. Whatever the explanation, it is evident that they think differently of themselves once the death of the patient removes the relentless day-to-day reminders of the all-too-real limits on their efficacy.

Finally, we note in Figure 11.2 that among the symptoms of emotional distress, only anger is affected by the death, decreasing substantially from baseline to follow-up. A decrease also occurs with the transition to institutional care. This similarity suggests that diminished anger accompanies disengagement from the demands of around-the-clock, hands-on care, whether this relief is the result of institutionalization or death. Neither the bereaved nor the comparison cohorts experience a significant change in depression from baseline to follow-up, a finding to which we shall return shortly.

Generally, then, we find not only that the bereavement cohort is changing in a manner that significantly differs from the in-home care cohort, but also that the changes in the bereavement cohort do *not* differ from those taking place in the institutional care cohort. Exits from in-home care involve sharp drops in role overload, increased guilt, improved socioemotional support, and decreased anger. The exception to this coordinated pattern of changes involves mastery: The bereavement cohort improves in mastery as compared to those who are caring for someone either at home or in a facility. Thus, much of the overall change associated with death is similar to that associated with institutionalization, suggesting that these effects reflect the separation from the demands of in-home caregiving, rather than the unique cause of this separation (i.e., specific to the death of the dementia patient).

Factors Affecting the Impact of the Death of the Care Recipient

The effects portrayed in Figure 11.2 are average effects and do not convey the considerable variability that exists within each cohort. In other words, they obscure differences among those who have experienced the death of their relatives, the issue to which we now turn. More generally stated, we examine whether any characteristics intensify bereavement and conversely, whether any resources ameliorate the impact of this stressful event. In this analysis, we shall first focus on mastery and social support, resources that are thought to regulate the impact of stressors on emotional well-being (Pearlin et al., 1981; W. Stroebe & Stroebe, 1987).

Essentially, we test whether people who have high levels of mastery and social support enjoy a protective advantage over other caregivers in blunting the distressing effects of bereavement.[3] Our earlier analyses generally indicate that high levels of mastery and socioemotional support are related to low levels of emotional distress. However, these kinds of relationships describe only the main effects of resources. We are also interested in the presence of conditional or buffering effects; specifically, whether death is especially distressing to people lacking in psychosocial resources (see chapter 7). Conditional effects were assessed by adding multiplicative interaction terms to the equations predicting change in outcomes: Death × Mastery and, separately, Death × Socioemotional Support. Neither interaction term contributed significantly to the explained variance with regard to any of the outcomes. Thus, these resources do not have an especially protective effect with regard to bereavement.[4]

We also examined whether kin relationship affects the impact of death. The death of a spouse is generally assumed to be more distressing than the death of a parent because spouses' lives are most changed practically and emotionally by death. The overall impact portrayed in Figure 11.2 may obscure differential effects if, for example, spouses become more depressed, but adult children become less depressed. We tested this possibility by adding Kin Relationship × Death interaction terms to the basic regression equations, which is analogous to estimating the effect of death separately within each kin group. These terms did not add significantly to the explained variance in any of the equations except for one: Spouses became less angry than adult children following the death. We found no evidence that spouses are more distressed than adult children. This similarity across kin groups echoes our findings in earlier chapters concerning

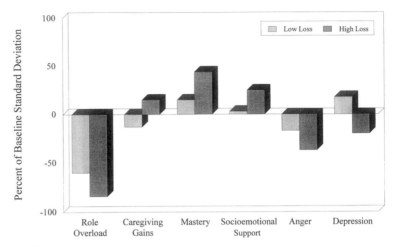

Figure 11.3 Change from baseline to follow-up for bereaved caregivers by baseline loss of intimate exchange.

stress proliferation (chapter 6), the risk of institutionalization (chapter 8), and the impact of institutionalization (chapter 9).

There is, however, one factor that protects caregivers from distress following their relative's death, and its effect is striking: the sense of having already lost the person for whom care is being provided. What is particularly noteworthy is that this sense of loss develops prior to the patient's death. Thus, a subjective stressor that surfaced earlier in the caregiving career reaches across the transitional event of death to significantly diminish its distressing consequences.

Figure 11.3 presents changes associated with death conditional upon the baseline level of loss, which is dichotomized into comparatively high and low categories.[5] Although there is variability among caregivers in the intensity with which such loss is felt, most caregivers had begun to develop this sense of loss prior to patient death, even those we have classified as low.

Those with a high sense of loss were better off in some ways than those who felt more closely connected to the dementia patient. Specifically, loss amplified the decline in role overload; elevated caregiving gains, mastery, and socioemotional support; and reduced anger and depression. Although there was a general change in these directions following the death of the dementia patient (with the exceptions of caregiving gains and depression), those who had previously experienced extensive loss of intimacy with the dementia patient tended to change appreciably more than those who had experienced less loss of intimacy. For caregiving gains and depression, both loss groups changed following death, but in opposite directions. Among the comparison cohort (not shown in this figure), prior loss is not related to changes in these outcomes. Thus, the effects of loss shown in Figure 11.3 represent true conditional effects, with prior loss altering the impact of the death of one's relative.

What determines whether caregivers develop this sense of loss over the course of caregiving? In chapter 6, we reported that loss of intimate exchange depends primarily upon the severity of the patient's cognitive impairment. As cognitive abilities wane, especially when this deterioration is rapid, caregivers tend to feel increasingly separate from the person for whom they are providing care. This sense of loss, then, appears to be a reality-based assessment of the dementia patient.

The Impact of Time

The caregivers in this study vary in how long they have been bereaved because deaths occurred throughout the interval separating the baseline and follow-up interviews. Indeed, the number of deaths is rather evenly distributed across this period of time, from a week to almost a year. The average length of time from the baseline interview to death is just over 6 months. Thus far, we have examined the overall impact of death, which averages diverse individual outcomes, combining caregivers whose relatives just died with those who lost their relatives months earlier. To get a clearer picture of the ebb and flow of reactions to death, we also examined whether time since death affects changes in elements of the stress process. This was accomplished by adding time since death to the previous regression equations, which enables us to estimate the effect of duration independent of other factors that may be incidentally associated with it. Figure 11.4 presents changes in the three variables that are most clearly affected by duration: guilt, socioemotional support, and depression.

This figure demonstrates that time is important to the impact of the death and that it exerts specialized, rather than generalized, effects. Guilt follows a simple linear course over the first year of bereavement. It is elevated immediately after

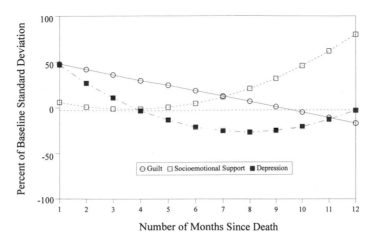

Figure 11.4   Change in outcomes by length of bereavement.

death, an increase of almost half a standard deviation above baseline (predeath) levels of guilt. It then drops at a steady rate and is slightly below baseline levels at the end of the year. Thus, the overall increase in guilt shown in Figure 11.2 may be attributed to the increase that immediately occurs around the time of the death.

Frank

It's been a while since Beth died, but Frank still grieves intensely for her:

The gap is still there. I'm just getting more proficient at handling it. I enjoy great music but too many associations with certain pieces of music. I experience my greatest loneliness out walking. I see things that nurture the memories. It's painful. One aphorism of mine is "How do you train your memory to forget?"

He is struggling to fill the gap her death has left in his life, acknowledging that he must change the way he has led his life:

I'm a loner, most of my life. But I started attending lectures and informal discussion groups on Friday morning, as part of my "rehabilitation." It's just about now I'm beginning to go out a little. I'd been turning down invitations until recently because I felt I'd be a baleful influence. Outwardly I'm a great lover of everyone. I'm an outgoing guy. My own rehabilitation may suffer by the fact that I'm a loner. I'm a mass of contradictions.

If I put my mind to it I could become more involved. This morning I thought about doing volunteer work. I'll probably try to do some traveling. I'm absolutely free right now. The problem with that is, I'd want to do it with someone. I'm becoming less of a loner. It's been thrust on me that being alone is not the best idea. Time alone or just with your wife is not always the best procedure. I mix well generally. Just haven't done it.

The time trend for socioemotional support is in the opposite direction of guilt. We saw previously (see Figure 11.2) that, on average, support increases following the death of the care recipient. Here, we see that this overall effect occurs entirely during the second half of the first year of bereavement and not in the immediate aftermath of death. This pattern is consistent with some research indicating that it is difficult to give and receive effective socioemotional support during the early months of bereavement (Stylianos & Vachon, 1993).

Like guilt, there is a pronounced increase in depression at the time of the death, as also displayed in Figure 11.4. Indeed, this elevation is similar in magnitude to that observed for guilt, about half of a baseline standard deviation. However, although guilt declines steadily over the first year of bereavement, depression follows a distinctly different course: Its *rate* of decline changes as a function of the passage of time. By the middle of this year, depression has declined to levels below baseline; the decline then levels off toward the end of the year. This pattern suggests that the temporal effect on depression is of limited duration. This temporal effect is consistent with established observations of the course of depression following the death of a loved one (Lund et al., 1993).

In summary, during the first year of bereavement, time exerts selective, rather than generalized, effects. The responses to death most affected by time are the grieflike reactions (guilt and depression) that peak immediately after the death and then decline. By contrast, responses that reflect relief, as opposed to distress (e.g., a decrease in role overload), are generally unrelated to the length of bereavement. Indeed, for most of the outcomes examined in this analysis, length of bereavement has no effect. Even in the case of reactions like depression and guilt, which show a temporal pattern, we cannot be sure that it is time itself that heals emotional distress rather than, for example, the gradual mobilization of effective support during that period.

Predeath Factors That Contribute to Postdeath Change

Thus far, we have seen that death of the care recipient affects several aspects of the stress process, specifically those identified in Figures 11.2 and 11.3: role overload, guilt, mastery, socioemotional support, anger, and depression. Moreover, we have just seen (Figure 11.4) that several of these effects vary over the course of time. Although our presentation of results to this point has focused exclusively on the impact of death, our analyses also took into consideration numerous conditions that might also affect changes in these elements of the stress process. We turn now to a consideration of how various conditions existing prior to death affect the postdeath functioning of bereaved caregivers.

We consider first the two stressors that are affected by death: the subjective primary stressor of role overload and the secondary intrapsychic strain of guilt. As shown in Table 11.1,[6] both of these stressors display a fair amount of stability over time. A substantial amount of the total variance explained by the entire set of independent variables is due to these auto-regressions (i.e., to the baseline level of the variable predicting itself at follow-up). Indeed, we should be cautious in interpreting other coefficients because the increment in explained variance (i.e., the difference between the complete regression equation and that containing only the auto-regression) is not statistically significant. This may be attributed to the large number of independent variables in the equation that do not attain statistical significance (not shown).

Two predeath factors aside from baseline role overload influence subsequent changes in role overload: caregiver health and problematic behavior. Specifically, those in better health feel less overload after death, as do those who had encountered more extensive problematic behavior on the part of the care recipient. This latter effect may be seen as another instance of relief associated with disengagement from the tasks of caregiving. The large decrease in role overload that occurs during the first year (see Figure 11.2) is not tied directly to the length of bereavement.

Table 11.1   Changes in Role Overload and Guilt as a Function
of Baseline Characteristics and Time

	Stressors at follow-up[a]				
	Role overload			Guilt	
Baseline characteristics and time	b (SE)	β		b (SE)	β
Caregiver physical health status (poor [1] to excellent [4])	−.178* (.083)	−.179		—	—
Institutionalized (/no)	—	—		−.254* (.103)	−.184
Patient physical health status (poor [1] to excellent [4])	—	—		−.104* (.054)	−.152
Problematic behavior (1–4)	−.280** (.106)	−.221		—	—
Role overload (1–4)	**.322*** (.068)**	**.399**		—	—
Guilt (1–4)	—	—		**.441*** (.091)**	**.383**
Length of bereavement (in months) Linear term	—	—		−.035* (.018)	−.162
R² Total	.318***			.319***	
R² Auto-regression	.160***			.194***	
R² Difference	.158			.125	

[a]Boldface numbers indicate auto-regression variables.
*p < .05.   **p < .01.   ***p < .001.

For guilt, the data reported in Table 11.1 demonstrate a tendency for this sentiment to be self-perpetuating and to decrease over time, as previously illustrated in Figure 11.4. Two additional factors are related to declines in guilt from the pre- to postdeath period: institutionalization and poor patient health. Institutionalization itself tends to elevate guilt, as reported in chapter 9. Here, we see that institutionalization is associated with less guilt following the death of the care recipient. This pattern suggests that guilt pertaining to placement has a limiting effect on subsequent guilt. Perhaps those who experience remorse at the time of institutionalization are protected from additional guilt at the time of death because they have already, in some sense, dealt with this issue. The patients' physical health, independent of their cognitive and functional status, affects changes in guilt following their deaths, with caregivers to someone in better health feeling less guilty.

The impact of baseline conditions on changes in resources following the death

Table 11.2 Changes in Psychosocial Resources as a Function
of Baseline Characteristics and Time

Baseline characteristics and time	Resources at follow-up[a]				
	Mastery		Socioemotional support		
	b (SE)	β	b (SE)	β	
Income (thousands of dollars)	—	—	.004* (.002)	.193	
Patient physical health status (poor ⌊1⌋ to excellent ⌊4⌋)	.065* (.031)	.139	—	—	
Problematic behavior	—	—	.153** (.052)	.219	
Loss of intimate exchange (1–4)	.107* (.044)	.171	—	—	
Mastery (1–4)	**.470*** (.074)**	**.499**	—	—	
Socioemotional support (1–4)	—	—	**.423*** (.061)**	**.470**	
Length of bereavement (in months)					
Linear term	—	—	−.038 (.034)	−.287	
Quadratic term	—	—	.005* (.002)	.496	
R² Total	.570***		.472***		
R² Auto-regression	.357***		.263***		
R² Difference	.153*		.209**		

[a]Boldface numbers indicate auto-regression variables.
*$p < .05$. **$p < .01$. ***$p < .001$.

of the care recipient is reported in Table 11.2. Again, we see that these resources display considerable stability over time. Nonetheless, these resources change following death, and these changes clearly depend upon conditions existing prior to death.

Mastery is enhanced following death among caregivers who had been caring for someone in comparatively good physical health and for someone from whom they already felt separated. Changes in mastery are not systematically tied to length of bereavement; we simply find that at some time during the first year, survivors tend to have an improved sense of mastery. With respect to changes in socioemotional support, we see that those with high incomes, as well as those who faced more problematic behavior during caregiving, feel more supported following the death. It is understandable that those with greater material resources should feel more comfortable about their social world; indeed, we observed this same phenomenon over the course of home care (see chapter 7). It is less clear why those facing greater problematic behavior should feel more supported. It may be that those encountering troublesome behaviors had reached out to others for support during caregiving and benefit from this help-seeking following death.

Table 11.3 illustrates that the final elements of the stress process that manifest an overall impact attributable to death are symptoms of emotional distress; specifically, depression and anger. Kin relationship is the sole baseline characteristic associated with changes in anger following the death of the care recipient. As

Table 11.3 Changes in Emotional Distress as a Function of Baseline Characteristics and Time

	Emotional distress at follow-up			
	Depression		Anger	
Baseline characteristics and time	b (SE)	β	b (SE)	β
Kin relationship				
Wife (/others)	—	—	−.379** (.122)	−.375
Husband (/others)	—	—	−.366** (.136)	−.309
Patient physical health status (poor [1] to excellent [4])	−.125* (.053)	−.164	—	—
Loss of intimate exchange (1–4)	−.200** (.075)	−.196	—	—
Mastery (1–4)	−.244* (.127)	−.159	—	—
Depression (1–4)	**.378*** (.104)**	**.355**	—	—
Anger (1–4)	—		**.234*** (.064)**	**.286**
Length of bereavement (in months)				
Linear term	−.172** (.061)	−.716	—	—
Quadratic term	.011* (.005)	.547	—	—
R^2 Total	.466***		.390***	
R^2 Auto-regression	.285***		.150***	
R^2 Difference	.181**		.240***	

[a]Boldface numbers indicate auto-regression variables.
*$p < .05$. **$p < .01$. ***$p < .001$.

noted earlier, despite an assumption that spouses would be worse off during bereavement, we find instead that both husbands and wives become less angry over time compared to adult children.

We have already seen that a prior loss of intimacy is related to decreased depression (Figure 11.3) and that length of bereavement has a curvilinear effect on depression (Figure 11.4). In addition, good patient physical health is related to decreased depression after death, suggesting that taking care of someone in poor health exacts a persistent toll on emotional well-being that extends beyond the boundaries of the actual provision of care. This health effect, it may be noted, is separate from the severity of the dementia.[7] Caregivers who feel efficacious during caregiving tend to have decreased levels of depression following the death of their loved one. This finding suggests that even though mastery changes in response to death, generally increasing, it also is a sign of caregivers' preexisting psychological resources, assets that help them to avoid future depression.

A Synthesis of the Immediate Effects of the Death of the Care Recipient

Our results indicate that caregivers are affected in both positive and negative ways by the death of their spouses or parents. Role overload, a subjective primary stressor, is dramatically reduced when caregiving ends. Ordinarily, other things being equal, such a dramatic drop in role overload would reverberate throughout the system of care-related stressors and lead to enhanced emotional well-being, as was the case for those who continued to provide home care (see chapter 6). Other things are not equal, however. The transition followed by the death of the care recipient entails a fundamental reorganization of the caregiver's life. These changes offset the benefit of decreased role overload and impose a high cost on the relief that may be gained from leaving the tasks of caregiving behind. Caregivers, after all, have experienced the death of a loved one and their emotional distress, not surprisingly, increases as a result. Many experience increased depression and guilt, and, as we shall see in the next section, grief reactions also occur. Nevertheless, the changes entailed in the cessation of caregiving are by no means uniformly distressful. Depression and guilt, after sharply peaking in the immediate aftermath of death, taper off steadily throughout the following several months. Both mastery and socioemotional support increase following death, while symptoms of anger decline. Certainly, by the second half of the first bereavement year, caregivers generally are less distressed than they were before the death. These effects are strengthened by a prior sense of loss, which appears to directly improve emotional well-being in the aftermath of bereavement.

Some of the changes that follow death also follow institutionalization. This similarity suggests that these two transitional events share some characteristics insofar as they entail disengagement from the around-the-clock, hands-on provision of home care. Caregivers who move to a reduced caregiving role at placement or to the cessation of caregiving at death, drop sharply in role overload, increase in guilt and socioemotional support, and decrease in symptoms of anger.

Thus, these transitional events bring some relief and some continuing difficulties. Death imposes some new burdens as well, to which we now turn.

Death and Grief

Thus far, we have looked at the death of the impaired relative as a career transition, asking how this event affects the array of stressful conditions that had surrounded caregivers' lives. However, death is more than an event that may lead to the rearrangement of activities, relationships, and feelings about oneself. It is also a stressor in and of itself. Where it involves the loss of a loved one, as is usually the case among dementia caregivers, the survivor may be left bereft, having to confront a swirling blend of unpleasant reactions. Thus, although death is a psychosocial event that marks the beginning of the role disengagement stage of the caregiving career, it is also the beginning of a parade of emotions and thoughts that may extend for an indefinite period (Shuchter & Zisook, 1993). As with virtually all other aspects of the caregiving career, we find that people differ in the intensity and scope of their grief reactions. In this section we both describe these reactions and explore some of the reasons for differences among bereaved caregivers.

We believe that some of the patterns of grief and bereavement that have been observed in general populations are relevant to those experienced by our special population of bereaved dementia caregivers. For example, we saw earlier that depressive affect declines with time among caregivers, which is the same trend detected by studies of other groups. Yet there may be features of bereavement that are unique to family caregivers for someone with dementia (Bass & Bowman, 1990; Mullan, 1992). At this time, we can only speculate as to what these differences might be. It is likely that bereavement is more difficult for caregivers than for others because, as has been shown, it besets those who are already depleted by years of caregiving. On the other hand, the lengthy forewarning caregivers typically have of their relatives' death and the psychological preparation this might afford may counter the effects of exhaustion. In the case of caregivers, too, death brings an end to the dementia patient's suffering and decline. Along with loss, death brings caregivers some relief; however, it will become amply evident in the ensuing pages that this relief does not preclude grief.

It would be well at this point to comment briefly on the two constructs central to this chapter: grief and bereavement. Although they are frequently used interchangeably, we regard them as conceptually distinct, albeit overlapping. Grief refers to the multidimensional set of cognitive and emotional responses that accompany loss and death (Mullan, Pearlin, & Skaff, 1995). As we describe below, grief is composed of multiple dimensions that are clearly delineated and measurable. In contrast, we think of bereavement as a process that includes more than grief; it entails the host of life changes that may result from death, including the many types of loss to which the caregiver must adjust (Osterweis et al.,

1984). Although traces of grief might be found long after death, bereavement is a broad process of adjustment that may continue after grief has ceased.

Our immediate task is to specify the various dimensions of grief and to describe their occurrence among bereaved caregivers. We then trace some of the conditions that contribute to the intensity of grief reactions. In dealing with these tasks, we shall employ the same analytic bereavement cohort delineated in the preceding section. That is, regardless of when the death of the impaired relative occurred between the first and fourth interviews, the interview preceding the death is considered the baseline, or predeath interview, and the interview immediately following death is considered the follow-up, or postdeath, interview.

Grief: Its Dimensions and Measurement

The losses associated with death are not uniform, grief varies in form, intensity, and duration. Most observers regard depression as the principal emotion associated with grief (Osterweis et al., 1984). It may be a low-grade dysphoria in people who continue to function well in their usual social roles or it may be more severe, psychologically immobilizing the survivor. Accompanying this sadness are more cognitive components of grief. They involve images of the deceased, thoughts and echoes from the past, and efforts to maintain ties with or to separate oneself from the deceased. These manifestations of grief can sometimes be fleeting, likely to come and go as the survivor forgets and then realizes with a jolt that a loved one is gone. In this section, we outline several key manifestations of grief along with our measures of them.[8]

I was relieved when she finally died. I was thankful.

Thoughts and memories of the deceased person commonly preoccupy the bereaved. These recollections and images may intrude into consciousness even when, or perhaps especially when, the survivor is making a concerted effort to concentrate on something else. It may be that reviewing images of the deceased person allows the bereaved to fix him or her in memory, in effect holding onto the person, even while confronting the reality of the loss. We measured what we refer to as *preoccupation* with a five-item scale ($\alpha = .83$). Bereaved caregivers were asked,

> In the *past week*, how often did you: find that many things reminded you of (him/her); remember things about (him/her) that you hadn't thought of in years; think of your times together before (his/her) illness; find yourself using (his/her) name in your conversation; [and] find that thoughts of your (relative) came into your mind, even when you were busy with other things?

The response categories were *never* (1), *once in a while* (2), *fairly often* (3), and *very often* (4).

Longing for the deceased person is a common aspect of grief. Some report

feeling the close presence of their relatives quickly alternating with the realization that the person is no longer present, which is accompanied by intense
yearning. *Longing* is a four-item scale ($\alpha = .75$) that asks caregivers,

> In the *past week*, how often did you: find it hard to accept that (he/she) is not coming
> back, find yourself doing things just because that's what (he/she) would have done, just
> feel an intense longing for (him/her), [and] feel close to (him/her) even though
> (he/she) is no longer alive?

The response categories are identical to those used for the measurement of
preoccupation.

Besides longing, those who are grieving often experience a painful sense of
loss. This is the emotional residue of memories that brings pain and emptiness,
rather than a coherent and pleasant image of a person. *Painful affect* is a six-item
scale ($\alpha = .81$). One item asked caregivers, "In the *past week*, how often did you
find it painful to recall memories of (him/her)?" Two additional items asked
caregivers how strongly they agreed or disagreed with these statements: "you
find it painful to be in places which remind you of (him/her)" and "you have
adjusted well to the loss." These questions were rated with the same response
categories used for preoccupation and longing. The final three items asked how
"accepting," "helpless," or "empty" the caregiver feels. The response categories
for these items ranged from *not at all* (1) through *very* (4). Item scores were
inverted for the two reverse- worded items (adjusted well, accepting).

Another dimension of grief concerns a lack of connection to the flow of events
in the world. As they struggle between grasping a new reality and clinging to an
old bond, the bereaved may feel disconnected internally. *Dissociation*, our label
for this aspect of grief, is measured by a five-item scale ($\alpha = .81$). Caregivers
were asked whether "time seems endless, it's hard to imagine what life will be
like without (him/her), you feel as if you've been watching everything from a
distance, [and] you have trouble concentrating on anything but (his/her) death."
Each item was rated from *strongly disagree* (1) to *strongly agree* (4). We also
asked whether they "feel numb," with response categories ranging from *not at all*
(1) through *very* (4). This unsettling mix of feelings seems to be the internal
counterpart of the external discontinuity brought on by death.

The bereaved may also experience sensory illusions, seeing, hearing, or sensi-
ng things that are not there, which sometimes cause them to worry about the state
of their own mental health. These fleeting moments, however, are often understood for what they are, misinterpretations of sound and sight. The illusions may
be part of the normal perceptual process that one employs to fill in the blanks in
the world, sustaining the continuity that had been there until the death of one's
spouse or parent. On the other hand, as attachment theorists suggest, they may be
part of a normal search in which the survivor is trying to find the deceased by
picking up some sign of him or her (Parkes, 1987). Illusions were assessed with a
four-item scale ($\alpha = .79$) that asked the caregiver,

> In the *past week*, how often did you feel as though you could walk into a room and
> (he/she) would be there, hear something you thought was (his/her) voice, react to
> things as if (he/she) was still around, [and] look for (him/her) in familiar places?

The response categories ranged from *never* (1) to *very often* (4).

The caregivers' own assessments of their states of grief are no doubt based on cultural norms and reference groups, as well as the actual intensity of their emotions and reactions to loss. With a single question, we asked people to rate their current level of grieving as *deeply grieving, grieving, grieving just a little,* or that *the grieving is mostly over.* About 40% were *grieving* or *deeply grieving* (23.3% and 17.0%, respectively). Another 26.2% were *grieving just a little* and 33.5% reported that *the grieving is mostly over.*

There is substantial cross-validation of the self-reports of grieving and the various grief reactions outlined above. The more self-assessed grief people report, the more likely they are to be preoccupied with the deceased person, long for them, feel dissociated from the normal course of events, feel pain over the death, and encounter perceptual illusions. The association between self-assessed grief, on the one hand, and these grief reactions, on the other hand, is quite strong (average $r = .55$).

How common is each of these grief reactions during the year following the death of the care recipient? Figure 11.5 presents the average frequency of grief reactions along each of the five dimensions just described: preoccupation, longing, painful affect, dissociation, and illusions. Grief reactions, as illustrated here, occur frequently, but are not ever present states. A value of 2.5 represents the midpoint for the response categories, the point halfway between *once in a while* (2) and *fairly often* (3). The average for preoccupation is somewhat above the midpoint of the scale, but the remaining grief reactions are below it. One grief reaction is substantially below the midpoint: Illusions fall midway between the response categories representing the lowest frequencies.

Thus, some of these grief reactions are more common than others. Feeling preoccupied with thoughts and memories of the deceased relative is the most common grief reaction, followed by longing for that person. Painful affect and

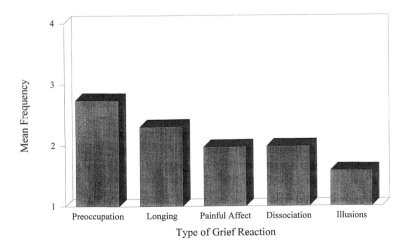

Figure 11.5 Frequency of grief reactions during the first year of bereavement.

dissociation are next and are about equally frequent reactions. Perceptual illusions occur least frequently.

It should not be inferred from these data that all memories, thoughts, and yearnings for the deceased are inherently distressful; we assume that some may be quite rewarding and soothing. Yet, memories that pinch the heart, that create a sense of deprivation, or that leave one feeling dissociated from the ordinary flow of events are unpleasant experiences. This point is substantiated by the magnitude of the correlation each measure has with depression. Preoccupation, longing, and illusions are moderately correlated with depression (average $r = .41$), whereas painful affect and dissociation are more highly related, sharing about 35% of their variance with depression (average $r = .58$).

The grief reactions we measured are conceptually related and behave similarly, so it is possible to simplify the analyses that follow without loss of information. We do this by combining preoccupation with longing, because these two measures are highly correlated ($r = .69$); the composite index is referred to as *yearning*. For the same reason, painful affect is combined with dissociation ($r = .73$); we refer to this combined index as *despondency*. Illusions remains a separate dimension.

Figure 11.6 shows that each of these dimensions of grief is most intense immediately following death of the dementia patient and steadily declines over the course of the ensuing year. Yearning is a relatively persistent grief experience. Although it declines with time, even those who have been bereaved for almost a year are likely to be preoccupied with and long for the deceased more than *once in a while,* given that the average value at 12 months is greater than 2 for this measure. Moreover, the average level of yearning at 12 months is higher than the initial levels of despondency and illusions, and illusions decline the most rapidly of all three reactions.

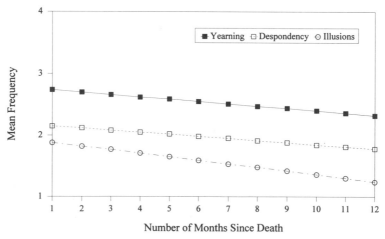

Figure 11.6   Frequency of grief reactions by length of bereavement.

Factors Affecting Grief Reactions

As a group, these caregivers are neither overwhelmed by the death of their spouses or parents, nor unaffected by it. They vary in the nature and intensity of their responses, with some grieving deeply and pervasively, and others grieving hardly at all or only in discrete realms of functioning. It is to this variability in grief that we now turn our attention, seeking to explain why some individuals more than others are affected by the deaths of their impaired relatives.

We do this by using the prospective data to predict subsequent levels of grief, ensuring that relationships do not merely reflect contemporaneous associated consequences of bereavement. The characteristics we use consist of demographic factors related to the caregiving context, objective primary stressors, subjective primary stressors, secondary role strains, secondary intrapsychic strains, psychosocial resources, prior levels of symptomatology, and the length of time since death occurred. Whereas earlier in this chapter we observed how death affected the ensuing manifestations of some of these elements of the stress process, we now examine how these elements of the stress process affect subsequent manifestations of grief reactions. Among the list of characteristics that we use to predict grief, several have a special status in bereavement research as they have been identified either as potentially important risk or protective factors. Here, we examine whether levels and forms of grief are affected by these factors: kin relationship, duration of caregiving, and loss of intimate exchange with the dementia patient. Table 11.4 presents the statistically significant predictors of grief reactions that emerged from the regression analysis. These manifestations of grief—yearning, despondency, illusions—are correlated with each other, sharing, on average, about 34% of their variance. Nonetheless, this analysis reveals that these are separate experiences with distinct antecedents.

Two baseline characteristics are related to the degree of yearning experienced at follow-up. Employment is related to a lower level of this reaction, probably because it entails involvement in a major social role structurally and psychologically unconnected with caregiving and death. The demands associated with working may interfere with being preoccupied with the past and the loss of one's relative, or may provide substitutes for longing for a lost loved one. In contrast, experiencing a high degree of role overload prior to death tends to increase yearning following death. It may be that those who were less drained by caregiving had sufficient energy before the death to prepare for separation and, therefore, experienced less preoccupation and longing later. The other predictor of yearning is the length of time one has been bereaved. Consistent with our expectations, yearning is highest immediately after death and then declines linearly over the course of the first year of bereavement (see also Figure 11.6).

Despondency is the most fully explained of all the grief reactions, with almost 50% of its variance being explained versus roughly 30 to 40% for the other reactions. This is probably because it is a measure directly involving distress, as are many of our baseline predictors. Several care-related stressors are positively and independently related to this dimension of grief: role overload, loss of self, and guilt. Caregivers were most likely to feel painful affect or dissociation when

Table 11.4 Grief and Grief Reactions as a Function of Baseline Characteristics and Time

Baseline characteristics and time	Grief reactions							
	Yearning		Despondency		Illusions		Self-assessed grief	
	b (SE)	β	b (SE)	β	b (SE)	β	b (SE)	β
Caregiver physical health (poor [1] to excellent [4])	—	—	—	—	.182* (.074)	.200	.299** (.117)	.201
Employed (/no)	-.315** (.127)	-.202	—	—	—	—	—	—
Institutionalized (/no)	—	—	—	—	—	—	-.349* (.163)	-.152
Difficult relationship (1–4)	—	—	-.128* (.060)	-.147	—	—	-.251* (.121)	-.156
Loss of intimate exchange (1–4)	—	—	-.120* (.059)	-.148	—	—	—	—

	b (SE)	β	b (SE)	β	b (SE)	β	b (SE)	β
Role overload (1–4)	.123* (.063)	.159	.099* (.048)	.151	—	—	.243** (.096)	.201
Loss of self (1–4)	—	—	.170*** (.060)	.218	—	—	—	—
Guilt (1–4)	—	—	.153* (.072)	.147	—	—	—	—
Mastery (1–4)	—	—	−.294** (.101)	−.236	—	—	−.424* (.205)	−.185
Depression (1–4)	—	—	—	—	.227* (.105)	.233	.334* (.167)	.210
Length of bereavement (in months)								
Linear term	−.038* (.019)	−.163	−.034* (.014)	−.175	−.053** (.013)	−.261	−.203* (.099)	−.559
Quadratic term	—	—	—	—	—	—	.015* (.008)	.521
R^2 Total	.340***		.474***		.317***		.371***	

$*p < .05.$ $**p < .01.$ $***p < .001.$

they felt overwhelmed by caregiving during the predeath period, their sense of identity was eroded by caregiving, and their memories are imbued with guilt. At the same time, three conditions appear to protect people from despondent reactions. Among these factors is a strong sense of mastery, which inhibits subsequent pain and dissociation. Consistent with our earlier findings, having developed a sense of loss of the person prior to death also protects against later despondency. Finally, in contradiction to the theories that a difficult past relationship with a deceased relative complicates later bereavement, those reporting difficult pasts in our study actually felt less despondent.[9] Death that follows a problematic history or an exacting period of decline may be perceived as a relief. During the first year of bereavement, despondency declines linearly at about the same rate as yearning.

Table 11.4 also shows the baseline factors affecting sensory illusions following death. Caregivers who were depressed prior to bereavement subsequently experienced more of these misperceptions, which are also common among those who were in better physical health. The number of sensory illusions declines steadily over the first year of bereavement.

Finally, the self-assessments caregivers make of the state of their grief is influenced by previous caregiving experiences and by characteristics of the caregiver; more than one-third of its variance is explained by these variables. Numerous specific variables attain statistical significance, most of which also are important to one or more of the specific dimensions of grief. For example, good caregiver health is related to more intense grief and to illusions. The effect of depression, similarly, is shared between sensory illusions and self-assessed grief: Those who are depressed prior to bereavement, grieve more intensely following it.

Self-perceptions of grief and despondency share three antecedents. First, those who had a difficult relationship with the care recipient prior to the onset of the dementia experienced less grief following the death of this person. Second, role overload during caregiving is related to increased grief, an effect that is shared with both despondency and yearning. Third, mastery appears to contain grief.

In contrast to the effects that are shared with specific grief reactions, one factor emerges as a separate contributor to the caregivers' self-perceptions of grief. Those who had institutionalized their relative were grieving less at follow-up than those who had continued to provide in-home care. As we suggested earlier in this chapter, the emotional reactions caregivers have to institutionalization may, in some ways, serve as a form of grief or preparation for the final separation of death.

Length of bereavement is related to grieving in a curvilinear manner, in roughly a U-shaped curve. The most recently bereaved grieve the most intensely, those bereaved 5 to 7 months earlier grieve the least, and those bereaved just less than 1 year begin to grieve more intensely once again. It may be that grieving drops quickly in response to the cessation of the demands associated with caregiving, but that people reengage in the grief process after a break from it. The upturn may also coincide with something of an anniversary reaction occasionally reported in the literature (Osterweis et al., 1984).

The Long-Term Impact of the Death of the Dementia Patient

During the first year of bereavement, then, caregivers generally are less distressed than during the earlier stage of home care. Most notably, once caregiving demands cease, there is a dramatic decrease in role overload. However, other ongoing stressors and intrapsychic strains change very little during the first year of bereavement. We now consider how elements of the stress process play out over a longer period of time and how grief reactions change as time passes.

The Long-Term Bereavement Cohort

To obtain a lengthy trajectory, we examined the subset of 74 caregivers who became bereaved early in our study (i.e., between Time 1 and Time 2). As illustrated in Figure 11.7, we followed these individuals for three bereavement interviews (i.e., two interviews more than in the previous analysis). This procedure extends follow-up to a maximum of 3 years following the death of the care recipient. Recall that the mean time between death and the first bereavement interview was about 6 months. Follow-up took place at yearly intervals, resulting in bereavement reinterviews that occurred, on average, at about 18 months and 30 months after the death. Although most of the bereaved caregivers were successfully reinterviewed at each subsequent occasion, a few were lost-at-follow-up, which reduced the sample size to 63. This strategy allows us to chart long-term trajectories, but at a price: There are far fewer caregivers available for this analysis than for previous ones. Although the small sample size limits the kinds of analyses that may be conducted, it nonetheless provides a glimpse of the long-term postdeath phase of the caregiving career.

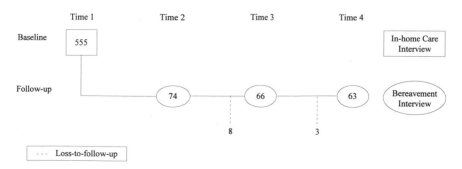

Figure 11.7 Creation of the long-term bereavement cohort.

Stability and Change over the Long-Term

We observe three patterns of stability and change in elements of the stress process over the 3-year span from Time 1 to Time 4 (i.e., from the predeath interview to the third bereavement interview). The first pattern is one of general stability: Loss of self, lack of caregiving gains, financial worries, and family tensions are not affected by the death of the care recipient either immediately or in the ensuing 3 years. Of course, this group profile does not necessarily mean that individuals within the group are not changing, only that these changes are not tied systematically to death or to the duration of bereavement. Indeed, as we saw previously, some people show improvement in these domains, whereas others encounter increased difficulties, a pattern that continues over the long-term. For the bereaved cohort as a group, neither death nor the passage of time since death is consequential to these stressors.

> It's time to move on to something else.

The other two time trajectories entail change, either in the immediate aftermath of the care recipient's death or sometime thereafter. Both patterns are evident for stressors and for resources, as shown in Figure 11.8. In one pattern, the death of the dementia patient has an immediate impact that does not change appreciably as time progresses. One stressor and one resource follow this pattern: guilt, an intrapsychic strain, and mastery, a personal asset. As we described earlier, for the total bereavement cohort, mastery and guilt both increase follow-

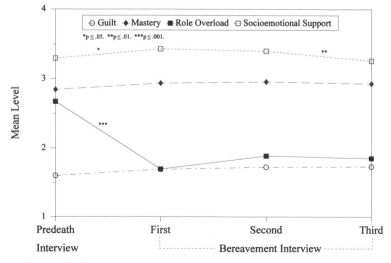

Figure 11.8 Long-term bereavement trajectories of stressors and resources.

ing the transitional event of death.[10] The long-term data add to this picture the permanence of these initial changes over an extended arc of role disengagement.

The final pattern, followed by role overload and socioemotional support, is the most complicated one, entailing changes in the second or third years following the death of the impaired person. Here we see change occurring *after* the initial period of bereavement. Role overload significantly increases between the first and second years of bereavement, but the magnitude of this change is quite small compared to the decline in role overload that occurs from the predeath to the immediate postdeath periods. This pattern may reflect a rebound effect as people reengage in other activities and social roles. Changes in socioemotional support follow a slight curvilinear path, increasing in the first bereavement interval, remaining flat during the second, and decreasing thereafter. This course may reflect the changing configurations in social relationships that occur as people reintegrate themselves following the death of a loved one; the support offered and received during the earlier bereavement period may not be sustained over time.

The same two patterns of change are found with regard to two forms of psychological distress, as depicted in Figure 11.9. Depression, as we saw earlier in this chapter, does not change, on average, in the first bereavement year, partly as a consequence of the curvilinear trend that occurs within this short interval. During the second bereavement year, however, depression declines and then remains at about that same level, on average, during the last year of follow-up. In contrast, anger declines substantially in the immediate aftermath of the death of the care recipient, but remains steady thereafter. Thus both of these states of distress decline following death, but the decline in anger evolves over a shorter

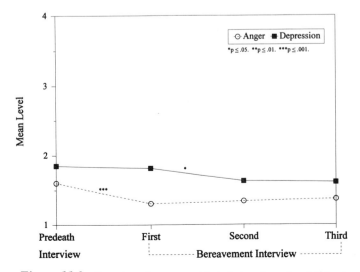

Figure 11.9   Long-term bereavement trajectories of emotional distress.

period of time than the decline in depression. In each instance, the decline appears to be permanent insofar as the reduction in symptoms of distress from the role enactment stage to the role disengagement stage is maintained over time, irrespective of whether this change occurs immediately or after a lag in time.

Thus, 3 years after the death of the impaired relative, people are functioning as well as or better than they had been functioning during caregiving. Although guilt remains slightly elevated and socioemotional support, after rising, seems to decrease once again to caregiving levels, survivors generally feel less over-whelmed by the demands of their lives; they have a greater sense of being in control, and they have fewer symptoms of anger and depression.

There is some danger that these average patterns overemphasize the uniformity of individuals' experiences during bereavement (cf. Wortman & Silver, 1989). Thus it is important to underscore the complex and varied nature of the responses of individuals. For example, although role overload, on average, increases from the first to the third bereavement year, many individuals remain stable (20.6%) or decrease (28.6%) in this stressor during this time. Similarly, 15.9% remain stable and another 30.2% increase in their level of depression even though the average level of depression decreases as bereavement extends over time. Moreover, changes in these elements of the stress process are barely or not at all related to one another (e.g., for changes in role overload and depression, $r = .19, p \leq .15$; changes in socioemotional support and depression, $r = -.01$, N.S.).

The Extended Course of Grief

Changes in levels of grief over the three bereavement interviews reinforce the general patterns described above, but complicate it slightly. Figure 11.10 displays the average level of the grief reactions, yearning, despondency, and illusions, over the three bereavement interviews. Three aspects of these plots are worth noting. First, along all three dimensions, grief reactions continue to decline as time progresses. Second, these declines are greatest early on, and become quite slight thereafter. Third, having noted these declines, it is also important to point out that these distributions do not dip to the lowest possible level (1), although by the end of the third year, few people report perceptual illusions. Thus people remain caught up in memories and images of their relatives, and, for some, these are painful experiences.

The general decline in grief reactions is accompanied by lessened self-assessed grief at each succeeding bereavement interview. Recall that 40.3% reported that they were grieving or deeply grieving at the first bereavement interview, which occurred about 6 months after the death of the care recipient. At the subsequent interview, an average of a year and a half after death, 20.6% reported grieving or deeply grieving. By the third bereavement interview, two and a half years after the death, only 11.1% felt that they were grieving or deeply grieving and 33.3% felt that they were grieving only a little. Indeed, by this time, well over half felt that their grieving was mostly over.

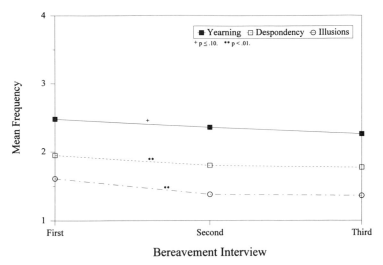

Figure 11.10 Long-term grief reactions.

These average patterns, of course, mask considerable individual variability. First, an individual does not necessarily change in a uniform manner across the various dimensions of grief reactions. Although grief reactions change in similar ways, this alignment is not as strong as one might imagine. For example, over the 3-year bereavement follow-up, change in yearning is only modestly correlated ($r = .23, p \leq .07$) with change in despondency. Change in illusory experiences, however, is correlated more strongly with yearning ($r = .55, p \leq .001$) and with despondency ($r = .38, p \leq .001$). Nevertheless, even the strongest correlation, between change in illusions and yearning, indicates that these experiences may change relatively independently of each other at the individual level.

Although the small sample size precludes multivariate attempts to disentangle the sources of such variability, it is useful to consider the continued relationship between changes in elements of the stress process described previously and changes in grief. Briefly, change in depression is the only one of the stress process elements that is consistently correlated with changes in grief reactions, and these correlations are in the moderate range for changes in yearning ($r = .37$, $p \leq .01$), despondency ($r = .41, p \leq .001$) and illusions ($r = .25, p \leq .05$). Thus, long-term changes in grief reactions are rather separate from elements of the care-related stress process, a pattern observed previously for the short-term follow-up. Although we can only speculate about the sources of this independence, we suspect that as the death becomes a temporally distant event, and as family members reorganize their daily routines and activities, other factors begin to regulate the stress process, beyond their grief and their ties to the memories of their impaired spouse or parent.

Summary

The death of the dementia patient represents a crucial transitional event in the caregiving career, signaling the beginning of the role disengagement stage. Over the course of this stage, we observe both reactions shared in common by many caregivers and considerable variation at the individual level. Disengagement from the caregiver role clearly does not mark the end of psychological involvement with the deceased person.

• Common grief reactions during the first year of bereavement include preoccupation with thoughts and memories of the person; feelings of closeness and longing for him or her; painful affect associated with some memories; feelings of dissociation from daily life; and perceptual illusions.
• Guilt and depression increase around the time of the death, but diminish toward the end of the first year.
• Following the death of the dementia patient, feelings of role overload decline as do symptoms of anger.
• The psychosocial resources of socioemotional support and mastery increase during the first year.
• Some of the changes during role disengagement appear to be tied to relief from around-the-clock care insofar as they also occur among those who have institutionalized their relatives: relief from role overload, increased guilt, improved socioemotional support, and decreased symptoms of anger.
• Changes in mastery, however, appear to be specific to death.
• Experiencing loss of intimacy with the care recipient prior to the patient's death mitigates the distressing consequences of death during the first bereavement year.
• Although mastery and socioemotional support are generally related to less emotional distress, neither of these psychosocial resources buffers the impact of the death.
• Spouses are no more distressed or grief stricken than adult children who lose their parents, which is consistent with our earlier analyses of stress proliferation and institutionalization, but contrary to our initial expectations.
• After an initial period of bereavement and recovery, most elements of the stress process remain, on average, relatively stable, although change also occurs late in the role disengagement stage for role overload, socioemotional support, and depression.
• The bereaved differ from one another in the amount of grief they experience, the ways they grieve, and the factors contributing to their grief.
• Predeath characteristics that increase some aspects of grief include role overload, depression, guilt, loss of self, and, surprisingly, caregivers' good physical health. Conversely, a prior sense of mastery, an already developed sense of the loss of the care recipient, and a difficult past relationship with the patient protect against grief.
• Thoughts and feelings about the deceased person persist years after their

death, whereas the more painful aspects of grieving are less common and tend to be more closely linked to depression.

• Although grief reactions are still present up to 3 years after the death, on average, survivors do as well during bereavement as they had been doing during caregiving.

Discussion

One striking finding concerning the role disengagement stage pertains to the caregiver's preexisting sense of loss of the impaired person and of the relationship with that person. This sense of loss develops as caregivers confront the destructive transformation brought about by a progressive dementia. These sentiments are a recognition of the cognitive losses that have already occurred, not an anticipation of death. Although this recognition may lead to heightened distress during role enactment, it serves as a psychological preparation for the physical death of one's parent or spouse. These "mental" losses are probably unique to progressive dementias in which caregivers have a long time to recognize the irreversible decline of their relatives, and to realize its interpersonal and emotional consequences.

Earlier, we treated this sense of loss as a subjective primary stressor that develops alongside role overload and is influenced by many of the same conditions that affect role overload. Yet, in the context of bereavement, loss and overload function differently and within distinct time frames. For example, the two stressors are only modestly correlated at baseline ($r = .24$, $p \leq .001$), and unlike role overload, loss is not strongly related to depression prior to the death of the care recipient. Moreover, during active caregiving, loss appears to be a negative experience when judged in terms of its effects on depression. During bereavement, however, when people are dealing concretely with loss, the importance of earlier, similar experience appears beneficial.

It is also important to note that psychosocial resources, mastery, and socioemotional support change in response to the death of the impaired family member. We often treat these resources as stable assets that people may draw upon when difficult situations emerge. The fact that mastery and support change in response to bereavement challenges our conventional understanding of these concepts and the ways we study them. This added complexity, nonetheless, also leads us to more realistic models of how situations and transitions affect the careers of caregivers.

I was isolated from society. I had to work myself back into it. I had forgotten my social mannerisms.

The variability in reactions among bereaved caregivers merits special emphasis. We believe this variability results, at least in part, from the fact that survivors experience different kinds of losses upon the deaths of their impaired relatives.

At this transition, caregivers confront the final loss of the spouse or parent. Although the experience of loss may emerge for the first time at death, we have seen that it is quite likely to have arisen beforehand. With death, too, comes the loss of the caregiver role, a role that had structured daily life and may have provided a rewarding sense of purpose. Death may also bring the loss of those elements of self that came from close identification with one's spouse or parent.

One nonfinding should be noted. The bereavement reactions of the adult children in our study do not differ from those of the spouses. Also, there was no evidence of any conditional effects involving the relationship of the caregiver to the dementia patient. Why do adult children react similarly to spouses?

We propose four general explanations for the lack of differences between these two groups of caregivers. First, children who become caregivers may be different from children who do not take on such tasks. They are a self-selected group and perhaps are already deeply involved in the lives of their parents. Thus, the impact of the loss of a parent for them is greater than what we would expect for most adult children. Second, providing such intimate care for so long may bring about an emotional bond, or reactivate an old one, so that caregivers grieve more intensely than do other adult children. Third, it is possible that caregiving children do not differ from other adult children, but that caregiving spouses react less strongly to widowhood than do other spouses. They may grieve less than do other bereaved spouses because the sense of loss developed over the long illness may mitigate their grief.

Fourth, it may be that the question is irrelevant: Why should one expect large differences in the grief reactions of spouses and adult children? Cohler (1983) has argued that we tend to underestimate the bonds between adult children and parents because our culture values autonomy. One indication of this may be the scarcity of empirical research on the responses of adult children to parental death, despite the ubiquitousness of this loss (Moss & Moss, 1989). If, as some have argued, we have overemphasized and exaggerated bereavement reactions among widows, perhaps we have underemphasized and minimized the impact of parental death among adult children.

Rosemary

Dementia often robs its victims of their personalities long before death takes their bodies. Under such circumstances, death may be welcomed, as we saw in the previous chapter, but any release or relief provided by death is not without pain. Rosemary is surprised at the course her grief has taken:

Peter had been gone mentally for so long that I thought I'd not find his passing to be a big thing, but it was! I was very much surprised. I'd had him physically there. He was a big person. Having him physically disappear was an experience I didn't expect.

I thought that now that he was gone I could forget the Alzheimer's and think of him as he was. But it's not worked that way. The recent events are so powerful that they took over. When he was still alive and physically present I could think back to what he had been. After he went I could no longer do that. He became a mythic figure rather than a real figure and this disturbed me very much.

The last few months I'm just getting over it and being able to get by the Alzheimer's. I went to see a number of old friends. A month with these old contacts broke this spell. I was very pleased with that. The memories were in our minds that Peter shared life with us. This began to break the spell of the myth and bring Peter back to me.

I'm beginning to break through and get back to the past. I grieve more and more. Almost a physical sense of loss and holes in my life and wanting to turn to him and not being able to. Almost a physical sense of something wrong.

The whole experience of Peter's passing has been very different than I thought. I thought that I'd grieve a lot at first and that it would tail off. I thought I'd remember Peter as he was as a real person. At first I wasn't mourning so much as being confused and then the shock of having the Alzheimer's take over in my memory rather than the real Peter. As I've worked myself out of this I find myself grieving more and more, as I work out of this. It's a very strange feeling.

Rosemary and her family have found their own way to remember Peter:

We scattered Peter's ashes on the mountain top, as he wished, with all the family there. I was very dubious about the ashes scattering thing — it's not the thing that people do. I'd never heard of a family ash-scattering ceremony. There was no telling how family members would react. I didn't know how I'd react. It might have been awful. In fact it was very lovely and satisfying. We took a picnic and had a nice family gathering at sunset.

My sons wanted some place that marked Peter's being there. I vetoed it. I didn't want a plot in a cemetery. They wanted some spot that said "Peter." Finally we found a perfect solution. We decided to build a mountain cairn of stones. We all found stones and I collected a lot of stones and fossils, and I put on some that Peter had enjoyed a lot. Now anyone who wishes could add a stone. I think Steven's daughter will bring one home from my husband's family home in Atlanta. She's planning on bringing a stone from there for the cairn. Everyone is happy with the cairn.

Rosemary now wants her own ashes handled the same way.

. . . in the same place, I realize now. At the top of the mountain where our cabin lies there's a road to the top, so that everyone could get up there. Of course we're all mountain climbers.

Notes

[1]Compared to other studies, our study design offers several advantages in looking at the effects of bereavement. Our design is truly prospective, permitting a true assessment of change among bereavement caregivers. In addition, because our comparison group is composed of people from the same study, the caregivers are sampled in the same way and asked identical questions about their functioning. Thus, we know a great deal about them and can control in our analyses for any preexisting differences between the bereavement and control cohorts.

[2]This group maximizes sample size because it includes caregivers who subsequently were lost-to-follow-up. The disadvantage of this strategy is that none of these caregivers were providing institutional care at baseline and, therefore, could not have experienced the care of a relative in a nursing home for very long. An alternative was to use data from the third interview as baseline data and the fourth interview as follow-up data respectively. This comparison group would have been smaller and somewhat different from the original sample, because it omits those who dropped out of the study after the second or third round of interviews. It does, however, contain caregivers who have been caring for relatives in nursing homes for longer periods of time and, in this respect, may be more like some of the bereavement cohort. We conducted sensitivity analyses across alternative comparison groups and the findings reported here are robust.

[3]In the following analyses, there was no difference between the in-home care and institutional care cohorts. Therefore, we treat them as a single comparison group.

[4]We also tested a second kind of conditional effect, involving prior experiences that might make caregivers *more* vulnerable to the death. We tested four such effects: prior levels of depression, role overload, past relationship difficulties, and guilt. None of these separately or together added significantly to the explained variance.

[5]These categories are defined as being one standard deviation above or below the mean (3.08 + .86).

[6]Only statistically significant coefficients are tabled because these regression equations contain a large number of statistically nonsignificant coefficients.

[7]The level of cognitive impairment is controlled statistically in this analysis, but is not shown in Table 11.3 because it is not related to postbereavement changes in depression.

[8]Our measures of grief were derived from pilot interviews with bereaved caregivers who were not part of this sample. The questions we asked were guided by the bereavement literature (Bowlby, 1980; Marris, 1974; Parkes, 1987; Raphael, 1983; Zisook & Shuchter, 1986). Although not everyone experiences all of these reactions, nor each with the same intensity, some probably are experienced by most people following the death of a close relative.

[9]Past difficulty in the relationship was assessed using a two-item scale that asked about conflict and lack of closeness in the relationship prior to the illness ($\alpha = .54$).

[10]These changes do not always reach statistical significance with the smaller, long-term bereavement sample size ($n = 63$).

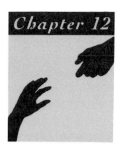

Chapter 12

Clinical Interventions and Caregiving Careers

Caregiving to those suffering from dementia is without question one of the most difficult challenges to emerge during the adult life course, especially when the caregiver is at an advanced age. After having plotted the course and consequences of care-related stressors, we must now look to the question of how these hardships and their repercussions may be alleviated. Our analyses have focused upon abstract concepts and their interrelationships for caregivers as a group, emphasizing themes and topics that typically surface in the experiences of the average caregiver. In the quantitative treatment of these topics, it is easy to lose sight of the individual, the person who occupies the role of caregiver. The informed clinician, however, can and should attend to the whole person, taking into consideration both the elements shared in common with other caregivers and those that uniquely characterize individual caregivers. Toward this end, we now examine the implications of our findings for clinical practice and intervention.

Intervention Strategies across the Caregiving Career

Our approach to clinical interventions builds upon the two core themes developed throughout this book: the caregiving career and the stress process. The concept of career embodies a basic principle of intervention: The form, content, and timing of intervention should depend to a considerable extent on where caregivers are in their careers, and involve an understanding of what has passed before and what is likely to lie ahead. That is, the problems encountered today should be viewed against the backdrop of yesterday and with an eye towards tomorrow.

As the caregiving career progresses, the types of hardships encountered mutate, spawning unforseen adaptational challenges. This conclusion rests upon the nature of dementia: Its degenerative course means that the demands impinging upon the caregiver are transformed over time, altering the constellations of primary and secondary stressors, psychosocial resources, and outcomes. Clinical interventions must evolve in unison with this process.

Thus, the types of interventions required to ease the shifting points of tension necessarily vary as caregiving continues over time, a premise illustrated in Figure 12.1. As shown, three intervention strategies are especially important during the role acquisition stage of the caregiving career. Because most novices at caregiving are not well informed about dementia or caregiving, education is of paramount importance in enabling them to perform their roles and to perform them well. The period of role acquisition can be immediately difficult as a result of the massive changes in daily life occasioned by the start of care. It also is a crucial time with regards to the future. Interventions at this time should be preventive in function, focusing on the avoidance of problems that commonly emerge later in the course of dementia. The implementation of preventive intervention rests, obviously, on planning for the future, both the immediate contingencies that are likely to arise and those that will emerge only at later points in the dementia.

The role enactment stage typically is of lengthy duration and often encompasses the admission of the dementia patient to a nursing home. Stress management is a key element of intervention during this time for two reasons. First, as we have demonstrated, caregiving can be enormously stressful, especially over the protracted course of most dementia care. Second, the transition to institutional placement in caregivers' lives is often very difficult. As we have seen, institutionalization itself is stressful and although it alleviates some tensions, it also generates new ones. Because caregivers face a prolonged period of exposure to chronic stress, they may deplete or exhaust their social, personal, and economic resources. Interventions over the course of caregiving, therefore, should emphasize the reinforcement of these resources.

Role disengagement is initiated by the death of the care recipient. It is appar-

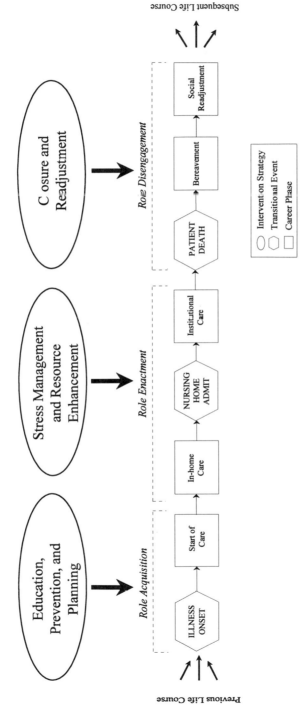

Figure 12.1 Intervention strategies across the caregiving career.

ent in Figure 12.1 that two basic adaptational challenges are posed by death: (1) bereavement, dealing with the loss of one's relative; and (2) social readjustment, coming to terms with the end of caregiving and with the start of the postcaregiving portion of one's life. Interventions during this stage, therefore, should have a dual focus of bereavement counseling and establishing the foundation for the future.

Clinical Intervention and the Stress Process

The clinical implications of our findings also flow from the second theoretical perspective guiding this research, the stress process model; in particular, from its approach to differences in adaptation to the demands and stressors of caregiving. Our research demonstrates that people exposed to similar stressors, in this instance, the severity of the symptoms of dementia and the need for care these symptoms create, have highly dissimilar modes of adaptation. Some people manage reasonably well over time; others are overwhelmed from the beginning and remain so; and still others fluctuate, sometimes appearing in control of the situation and sometimes having marked difficulties. Our results show that variation in the outcomes of caregiving depend, at least in part, upon the extent to which stress proliferation is constrained by psychosocial resources.

Variability in adaptation is a key to understanding how clinical interventions can aid caregivers. Objective primary stressors, the actual demands imposed by caregiving, account for a surprisingly small portion of caregiver well-being and most of this effect is indirect, transmitted via secondary stressors. Dementia creates the circumstances in which care-related stressors may develop, but whether or not a caregiver actually experiences these stressors is the result of other factors, including the caregiver's social, personal, and economic resources.

Understanding variation in response is especially important in the instance of dementia. The progression of Alzheimer's disease (AD) and similar disorders is unrelenting. Currently available treatments do not consistently provide symptomatic relief or appreciably alter the long-term course of the disease. As a result, it might erroneously be assumed that little may be done to help caregiving families because the source of their stress, the patient's illness, is unremitting. If adaptation were determined solely, or even primarily, by the course and symptoms of the disease, this conclusion might be warranted.

We have seen, however, that disease-related burdens do not necessarily portend escalating stressors. Instead, as dementia progresses, the care situation may deteriorate, remain the same, or improve. These outcomes depend, at least in part, upon the resources available to the caregiver, especially socioemotional support and mastery. By extension, clinical interventions to enhance these resources should serve to stem the expansion of care-related difficulties and their emotional sequelae.

Figure 12.2 illustrates some of the techniques that may be used to this end and the locations in the stress process where these methods are especially relevant.

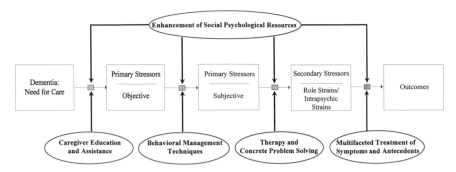

Figure 12.2 Clinical interventions and stress proliferation.

As mentioned previously, most caregivers are not well informed about dementia when a spouse or parent is diagnosed, making education a necessity. Also, the dependencies prompting the need for care can easily and rapidly overwhelm the novice caregiver who requires, in addition to instruction on how to manage the patient and the dementia, some tangible relief from the full burden of hands-on, around-the-clock care.

The objective conditions produce subjective states requiring a second juncture of very different clinical interventions. Our findings demonstrate that providing substantial assistance to someone who resists aid and acts in a disruptive manner may result in states of role overload, role captivity, and loss of intimacy with the patient. This transformation may be contained by the use of behavioral management techniques to break the cycle of stimulus and response that reinforces difficult patient behavior.

In the same manner, the primary stressors of caregiving may create secondary role strains, such as family conflict and secondary intrapsychic strains, such as doubts about one's competence as a caregiver. Intervention in this process is likely to take two forms, therapeutic processing of emotional issues (e.g., family counseling) and concrete problem solving (e.g., financial planning). Finally, intervention may help prevent the accumulation of primary and secondary stressors from producing emotional distress. A multifaceted approach is required at this time to (1) relieve states of distress and (2) address the conditions generating distress.

Thus, clinical interventions may target modifiable features of the caregiving situation, thereby reducing stress proliferation and increasing the likelihood of stress containment. The specific types of interventions that are undertaken will depend upon two sets of circumstances: the specific issue that is problematic (e.g., exposure to a particular stressor) and the stage of the caregiving career in which exposure occurs (e.g., whether a caregiver is confronting problems during in-home care or during institutional care). Our application of the career concept thus serves as a heuristic device to assist clinicians in organizing their understandings of the conditions encountered by caregivers and the evolution of these conditions over time. This long-term view of caregiving should make it possible to plan and implement preventive interventions.

Our study may be viewed as the observation of naturalistic interventions. In contrast to planned interventions that entail deliberate attempts to manipulate features of situations, we have observed the spontaneous functions of resources in containing stressors and how their absence contributes to stress proliferation. In naturalistic interventions, access to resources might be limited as a result of social and economic circumstances, differences to which clinicians need to be sensitive. The clinical interventions we suggest below target varying junctures in the caregiving career and, building upon the small but growing literature on planned interventions with family caregivers, focus on issues of stress containment.

We address clinical interventions in the broadest sense, both in terms of the professionals who may become involved and the types of interventions that may be implemented. Clinicians who work with family caregivers and dementia patients have diverse professional backgrounds, including not only psychologists, social workers, nurses, physicians, and other health personnel, but also legal and financial agents. In some cases, caregivers may similarly benefit from assistance provided as part of ongoing professional relationships, such as between nurse and caregiver, that is not directly intended as a service to caregivers.

We want to emphasize at the outset that caregivers generally do not have access to enough of any of the types of help they need. Certainly, we have found that caregivers use meager amounts of formal health and social services. Given the serious, intractable, and complex problems caregivers face, we do not hesitate in advocating more intensive and focused help.

Basic Premises

Our examination of clinical implications begins with five fundamental premises that emerge from the main findings of this research. First, the stress process is characterized by multiple dimensions that interact with one another in often complex and subtle ways. It follows, therefore, that clinical interventions should begin with a multidimensional assessment that encompasses the diverse ways in which care-related stressors may adversely affect a caregiver's life. This type of assessment should identify the unique constellation of issues found within a particular family. It is not sufficient to know that a patient has AD or that a caregiver feels stressed, nor is it sufficient to know that caregivers generally experience select sets of issues at particular times in their careers. Rather, the clinician needs to assess how caregiving has affected each individual at specific points in his or her caregiving career.

The second premise follows logically: Goals and procedures for treatment should be based on the particular configuration of conditions that exist for each individual caregiver at a specific time in his or her caregiving career. Although self-evident, this principle unfortunately represents an ideal not often realized in practice. For example, many clinical interventions focus on the emotional well-being of caregivers, especially depression. At any given time, however, most caregivers do not have pronounced symptoms of depression. As a consequence, interventions to alleviate depression have limited potential efficacy and may leave more pressing problems untouched. In essence, we are merely suggesting that caregivers do not all face the same issues or experience the same concerns and dynamics. Therefore, goals for treatment should emerge from caregivers themselves. By starting with an overview of the stress process, the clinician can identify the constellation of problems and goals that uniquely characterize the life of a specific caregiver and family.

Third, broad and comprehensive interventions are needed. Our results document that the stressors associated with caring for dementia patients often permeate other areas of life. As a consequence, clinical interventions cannot focus exclusively on a narrowly defined set of difficulties that entail the direct provision of care (i.e., those problems that we identify as objective primary stressors). Instead, interventions need a dual focus: the immediate problems associated directly with the tasks of caregiving and the consequences these problems have on the caregiver's life (i.e., the creation of secondary sources of stress). As we have seen, the main concerns facing caregivers change over time, meaning that clinical interventions should target both the most pressing current problems and those that are emergent.

Fourth, because the reasons for clinical interventions vary from caregiver to caregiver, it follows that methods of determining whether treatment has been effective must also differ. It makes no sense to use an evaluation that measures the utility of a treatment for relieving depression if depression is not problematic. Clinical research with family caregivers, however, has often employed this approach (Haley, Brown, & Levine, 1987; Zarit, 1989). As a result, studies have frequently not shown clear advantages of one type of treatment over another (Zarit & Teri, 1991). Because we cannot assume all caregivers have the same problems or concerns, we should use multiple criteria to evaluate interventions.

Finally, although a thorny issue, it must be recognized that the interests of the caregiver and the patient sometimes diverge. These disparate interests are most apparent with regard to institutionalization. We have shown that nursing home placement relieves some elements of distress for caregivers, but increases the short-run risk of mortality for patients. Patients, however, cannot be effective advocates for themselves. To dismiss the perspectives and needs of patients as irrelevant because the patients are brain injured is inappropriate and unethical. Caregivers themselves often are searching for strategies to reconcile their needs with those of the patient. There is no simple answer or straightforward clinical approach that solves this conundrum. Rather, the clinician needs to consider both perspectives and formulate strategies that, whenever possible, help both the caregiver and the patient. When these interests cannot be reconciled, clinicians must, at the very least, be aware of the implications of their decisions and of their own biases regarding whose interests should prevail.

The Need for Early Intervention: Role Acquisition

Although intervention during role acquisition could prevent some of the common problems that usually emerge later in the course of caregiving, we know little about the process of assuming the role of caregiver because most research studies begin after the role has been assumed. However, based on observations and retrospective accounts, it is evident that early assistance would have been welcomed and useful. Intervention during role acquisition can facilitate caregiving by providing immediate relief and preventing future problems.

A critical turning point in role acquisition is diagnosis of the patient's dementia, a juncture that provides an opportune time and setting for early intervention. A formal diagnosis forces caregivers to recognize that the problems they have observed are not transitory: The impairments will intensify along with dependencies and the need for care. Unfortunately, this opportunity is more often missed than exploited. Despite some exceptions, the initial medical examination mainly focuses on the medical aspects of dementia. Physicians do not routinely address in any detail the family's emotional needs or practical issues of care, nor give referrals to appropriate services. These circumstances delay families from making plans and taking necessary actions.

> When he was first diagnosed I used the slightest excuse to get away.

Core Issues That May Be Addressed during Role Acquisition

Understanding the Disease, Its Possible Causes, and Options for Its Treatment

Families often have a multitude of questions about the disease itself, many of which are not resolved during the diagnostic evaluation. They often need to take some time to think about the situation and gather information before they are able to articulate their concerns. For example, caregivers may want to know what causes dementia and if they or other members of the family now face an elevated risk of developing dementia. Anticipatory stress over what lies ahead often surfaces at this time and typically is complicated by the dementia patient's own awareness of his or her decreasing abilities. Although not denying the inevitable progression of the disease, the clinician needs to focus on identifying practical and realistic steps that may be taken to enhance the functioning of the patient and to facilitate the family's adaptations to the changes that already are underway.

Rosemary

Social embarrassment is a luxury caregivers can no longer afford, as evidenced by the advice Rosemary has for other caregivers:

Another thing I'd tell people is to accept the fact that the patient won't be able to live up to even minimum standards of etiquette behavior. You can waste a lot of good living time and emotion thinking that they have to meet the standards they would have earlier. Let it go. That's the way it is. Let a lot of things go. I never knew what would happen but I finally decided that wasn't a reason to not do things. I realized he wouldn't always look the way I'd like, but I let it go. He was happier and I was happier if the ordinary standards of life just didn't apply.

Identifying Potential Financial and Legal Issues

It is imperative that families review their financial and legal situations as soon as possible after a dementing illness is diagnosed. Among the steps that should be considered are obtaining durable power of attorney for both management of assets and health care, completing advanced directives for health care that address the conditions under which the patient would prefer treatment not be given, writing or modifying wills, and making financial arrangements that protect the interests of the patient and the patient's spouse. By acting while the patient is able to give consent, families can eliminate at least some problems that would otherwise arise later. When families wait for too much time to pass and the patient is no longer competent to consent to legal proceedings, the alternatives can be very time-consuming and costly, and the decisions may not be in accord with the patient's wishes.

Locating Help for the Patient and Family

Familiarizing the family with options available for aiding them with patient care may be very useful at this time and prevent later difficulties. For example, the patient may benefit from early interventions, such as therapeutic activity programs, exercise plans, or support groups (Yale, 1991). By establishing some routines early, such as attending day care, patients may have fewer problems accepting similar services necessary during later stages of the disease. Likewise, caregivers may be more likely to use services when the illness is advanced if they begin to seek help early on.

Easing Social Interactions

One of the most difficult problems faced by caregivers is explaining the disease to family and friends. We have seen that family conflict can emerge over issues concerning the severity of the patient's condition, the methods for managing his or her behavior, and the sharing of care-related tasks and responsibilities. Many of these conflicts arise because other family members are not well informed about dementia or the steps the caregiver has already taken. In addition, caregivers sometimes feel stigma associated with dementia, and withdraw from social contacts or keep the patient isolated. Other people may not understand the problems caused by dementia or know how to act around the patient. Family and friends may avoid the caregiver and the patient, increasing the caregiver's sense of stigma and fueling a cycle whereby the caregiver and patient become increasingly cut off from their normal social life. Interventions aimed at helping caregivers discuss the disease with family and friends may be helpful.

Solving Problems Specific to Role Acquisition

Problems specific to assuming the caregiving role also need to be addressed. Some people are reluctant to take on this responsibility, or there may be disagreement within the family over who should provide care and who is excused. A major dilemma that often arises concerns whether or not to move the dementia patient to the caregiver's geographical location or into his or her household. On the positive side, relocating patients reduces some concerns about patient supervision and simplifies dealings with doctors and other service providers. On the negative side, the family may find that care is more demanding and intrusive than they had expected, especially if there was an expectation that the impaired elder would become relatively independent in a new community, for instance, joining activities and making new friends. These acts are very difficult, if not impossible, for dementia patients. Also, some families come to realize that they have made a much bigger commitment than they can manage. A useful strategy in this early stage is to help caregivers explore their capacity to commit to the caregiving role, including their own preferences and needs. Providing families with information about the disease and available resources is especially important in enabling them to make realistic decisions about care and to prepare them better for what lies ahead.

In summary, caregivers confront two sets of challenges during role acquisition: adaptation to current circumstances, including confirmation that dementia is present; and preparation for what lies ahead as a result of this illness. Given that families are unlikely to have a thorough understanding of the disease and its consequences, key objectives of intervention at this time for the patient and the family members should be education about the disease, its treatment, and options for accommodating its progression. Interventions should also address the potential impact of the dementia on the family as a whole and upon its individual members, especially those who are most caught up in the provision of care. Although dementia inevitably runs its degenerative course, the path of caregiving need not deteriorate as well. Thus, early interventions should be preventive in orientation, aimed at helping caregivers curtail the proliferation of care-related stressors and avert future crises.

Interventions for the Long Haul: Role Enactment

There are multiple points in the stress process at which clinical interventions could reduce tensions and increase resources as caregivers go about the tasks of providing long-term care (see Figure 12.2). Because dementia care typically continues for lengthy intervals, clinicians need to consider both the present and the future. Addressing concurrent problems can bring immediate relief, as well as curtail some problems from exacerbating as the disease progresses. Long-term objectives should focus on maintaining and enhancing the psychosocial resources that are so crucial to the containment of care-related stressors, especially social support and mastery. Structural barriers to these resources, such as economic limitations, also need to be addressed. In this section, we identify clinical issues that arise during the phases and transition of the role-enactment stage: matters surrounding the provision of care in the home, hospitalization as a crisis, the decision to place the dementia patient in a nursing home, and the caregiver's continuing involvement in patient care following placement.

A first step in effective intervention during this stage is to determine what caregivers know about dementia and about the care options and services available to them. As we mentioned earlier, clinicians cannot assume that caregivers possess basic information of this sort. Yet, caregivers need a solid comprehension of why their relatives behave in unsettling and disturbing manners before they can effectively evaluate the ways in which they might manage their situations more effectively (Zarit, Orr, & Zarit, 1985). A crucial issue for families, for instance, is to understand that dementia patients have limited abilities to change or regulate their actions. Caregivers must initiate change, rather than passively hope their relatives will learn to remember or behave better.

Strategies for Alleviating Primary Stressors

Although the underlying dementia and its associated functional impairments cannot be halted or reversed, the primary stressors of caregiving may be remedied, at least in part. Because behavior problems are major determinants of poor caregiver outcomes, reducing the frequency of these problems should ease some of the tensions entailed in providing in-home care. The potential for better management of these problems, however, is frequently overlooked. Families and clinicians alike may feel impotent in the face of this degenerative and irreversible disease. Yet, although dementia makes certain kinds of behaviors likely, such as wandering, some behaviors may be more or less regulated according to the nature of the patient's environments, routines, and interactions with others, all factors that may be altered.

Numerous environmental interventions have been proposed to make the home environment safer and less confusing for the dementia patient (e.g., Gallagher-Thompson, 1994; Heagerty & Eskanazi, 1994). For example, to control wandering, special locks may be placed on doors, or buzzers or bells may alert the caregiver to a door being opened. Similarly, dangerous items, such as power tools, may be removed or disabled to reduce the potential for injury.

Furthermore, behavioral management techniques employed by counselors or taught to families have considerable potential to reduce problematic behaviors (Gallagher-Thompson, 1994; Zarit & Teri, 1991). This strategy involves first identifying the pattern of events and circumstances that occur around problematic behaviors and second, changing or disrupting this pattern. By modifying the events leading up to or reinforcing troublesome or disruptive behaviors, the rates at which these behaviors occur may be lowered, at least in some instances. For example, agitated behavior may follow lengthy periods of inactivity. Increasing activity levels before patients become agitated may reduce the frequency of these outbursts. Also, disturbances of this type often garner immediate attention, thereby inadvertently rewarding the patient, a cycle that could be broken by altering caregiver reactions.

A related strategy is teaching caregivers effective modes of communication with patients. Because cognitive impairment severely impedes the individual's ability to converse coherently, previous patterns of interpersonal interaction are disrupted. For example, dementia patients often make statements that contradict reality. These occurrences may be relatively inconsequential, such as insisting that it is an incorrect day or year, but others may be extremely troubling to caregivers, like insisting upon visiting a parent who is deceased, but whom the patient believes to be alive, or wanting to be taken home when one already is there. Caregivers often respond to such predicaments by trying to correct reality. This approach usually is not productive because the ability to process correcting information has been impaired by the dementia. To continue the example of wanting to see a deceased parent, caregivers sometimes remind the patient that the parent is dead and may show the patient an obituary or other evidence. These approaches usually leave both the caregiver and the patient upset. An alternative is to acknowledge that although the patient's ability to organize facts and memories is damaged, these communications, nonetheless, connote important emotional states. Reactions which attend to these feelings, such as offering reassurances and comfort, or reminiscing about the past, may be helpful.

Another potential intervention is to medicate the dementia patient, which is sometimes effective in alleviating agitation and depression. However, these medications do not consistently have positive effects and sometimes can, paradoxically, increase behavioral problems. Thus, families may expect immediate relief from the administration of medications, only to be deeply disappointed if these agents do not remedy behavioral problems or if they create new ones.

Although there is still much more to be learned about the effective management of behavior problems among dementia patients, the pivotal role these problems play in the proliferation of care-related stress makes it incumbent upon the clinician to take appropriate steps toward their reduction and management. Unlike many other mental health issues, solutions in this case involve encouraging caregivers to intervene actively while the patient is relatively passive. Families are sometimes unwilling to take this initiative or may believe that it is the patient's responsibility to act in a more appropriate manner. Thus, the clinician must address both the practical issues of behavioral management and the caregiver's attitudes about implementing such strategies.

Families can support the primary caregiver in behavioral management by learning about the techniques that help to reduce disruptive or troublesome behavior and by working with the caregiver to implement these strategies. All too often, however, families vacillate between not wanting to acknowledge the seriousness of the behavioral problems and giving advice to the caregiver without fully understanding the situation. These reactions undermine the effectiveness of behavioral management techniques.

One other strategy for diminishing the primary stressors of caregiving, which is discussed in detail below, is to reduce the caregiver's exposure to these stressors by employing respite care.

Strategies for Alleviating Secondary Stressors

The possibilities for intervention extend well beyond the concrete demands and tasks entailed in providing care, encompassing as well the intrusion of caregiving into other spheres of adult life. Interventions that contain the proliferation of secondary sources of stress, therefore, represent potentially very powerful methods of improving the overall well-being of caregivers. Strategies for reducing secondary sources of role strain depend, obviously, upon the variety of other social roles configured in the caregiver's life (e.g., whether he or she is the parent of small children, employed outside of the home, embedded in a cohesive social network, and so forth). It is thus necessary first to identify how caregiving affects other aspects of the caregiver's life. This step entails determining not only whether the caregiver is an incumbent of a specific social role, but also the impact caregiving has had upon the quality of experiences within that role. For example, caregivers who are employed outside of the home risk conflict between the demands of caregiving and those of working. However, the fact that a caregiver works does not necessarily mean that he or she is beset by role conflict. Indeed, we have seen that work provides appreciable benefits to some caregivers.

The strains between work and caregiving may be addressed, at least in part, by identifying appropriate respite services, such as adult day care and in-home respite, that will provide care for the dementia patient during the caregiver's working hours (Scharlach & Boyd, 1989). Respite care programs have been expanding rapidly, although the availability and quality of these services varies considerably from one community to another. Despite these problems, working caregivers who are able to obtain respite find it extremely beneficial (Berry, Zarit, & Rabatin, 1991; Scharlach & Boyd, 1989).

Secondary intrapsychic strains constitute a crucial focal point for clinical intervention. Our findings reveal that caregiving presents some potent threats to self-concept. Because the amount of care required is considerable and continuous, the commitment caregivers make often seems completely absorbing, leading to what we have called loss of self, a wearing away of identity that has depressive consequences. Furthermore, caring for someone with severe cognitive impairment may not produce the same rewards found in other types of caregiving. Patients usually do not acknowledge or thank caregivers for their help and may, indeed, resent and resist being assisted. In fact, the disintegration of the persona of the care recipient is a key contributor to the caregiver's loss of identity. Also, families may be quick to criticize, rather than to praise, the primary caregiver, for no matter what the caregiver does, the deterioration of the care recipient cannot be halted or reversed. As a result, caregivers have few benchmarks against which to evaluate their own competency or feel good about their efforts.

In such situations, counseling may assist caregivers in identifying reasonable standards and setting limits for the care they provide. This intervention entails recognition of their own limitations and acknowledgment that they cannot do everything. Caregivers often need help in realizing that it is in their best interest to take breaks from caregiving. Clinicians may also assist caregivers in identifying and prioritizing goals, and making self-appraisals of their performance that are based upon these goals. These steps move caregivers away from unrealistic goals and expectations that they could never achieve.

Clinical interventions that address self-doubt, negative evaluations of self, and a sense of worthlessness may be useful. In particular, they may help the caregiver recognize that the course of dementia often resists the most motivated and skilled efforts and this resistance lies in the nature of the disease, not in the failures of the caregiver. In instances where the relative's illness has exacerbated an already fragile self-esteem, long-term counseling may be appropriate.

Obstacles to Intervention

A variety of health and social services can shoulder some of the burden of care that would otherwise fall entirely upon the family, but these services often are underutilized as a result of practical and attitudinal barriers. For example, respite programs, including adult day care, in-home respite care, and overnight or short-stay nursing home care, provide temporary relief (Friss, 1990; Heagerty & Eskanazi, 1994). However, many families are reluctant to take advantage of these services (Caserta, Lund, Wright, & Redburn, 1987; Lawton, Brody & Saperstein, 1989). In some instances, services are not used because families believe they should provide all the help required or think the patient will not accept outside help. Moreover, these services are not always able to accommodate dementia patients or the hours of service may not be compatible with the caregiver's work schedule. Uncertain quality, too, may discourage utilization. In this regard, some families report that respite services are not reliable or that staff are not trained in the care of individuals with dementia (MaloneBeach, Zarit, & Spore, 1992). In some cases, families fear losing control of the care situation, for example, when they have little or no say in who the agency will send to their home or the days and times they will receive assistance. Depressed caregivers are less likely to use services, suggesting that the caregiver's own level of distress may be still another barrier to receiving appropriate help (Mullan, 1993).

Financial strain is a barrier in and of itself to intervention. There are several sources for this strain. In some instances, the patient's illness results in a loss of income, and some caregivers leave the workforce or reduce their working hours to accommodate caregiving. The use of health and social services may deplete economic resources as well. Cost may be another barrier to these services because they usually are not covered by Medicare or other insurance. Caregivers often lack information about the alternatives available to them for financing care. An important component of such interventions, then, is to help caregivers identify mechanisms by which they may obtain subsidies or other monies to pay for services.

Clinical interventions to increase service use may be complicated and difficult. One issue concerns differentiating between realistic barriers, such as a truly incompetent and unreliable service provider versus reluctance on the part of the family to employ any kind of help. A second problem is determining the focus of intervention. In some cases, the clinician may consult with an agency to work out arrangements for the dementia patient that will be suitable or acceptable to the patient and his or her family. In other instances, however, the primary interest of intervention will be the caregiver. In either case, the clinician may be of assistance to caregivers in navigating the off-putting labyrinths of community-based care systems.

A counseling intervention that examines underlying beliefs about why accepting help is wrong may sometimes be used for overcoming attitudinal barriers (Beck, Rush, Shaw, & Emery, 1979; Zarit et al., 1985). The therapist may discuss the types of services that are available in order to aid caregivers in identifying their apprehensions about obtaining help for themselves or for their relatives. Examples of the issues that arise include caregivers should be able to do everything by themselves, they are weak if they accept help, no one else can provide the same quality of care, and the patient will not accept help from anyone else. At a more abstract level, caregivers often are demanding perfection of themselves and of any helpers who might be brought into the situation when they have such expectations.

Once the specific beliefs a caregiver holds are recognized, the therapist can help him or her examine alternatives and determine more realistic ways of looking at the situation. As an example, a caregiver who believes she must do everything herself and who also wants to keep her mother at home as long as possible can be helped to identify the contradiction between these beliefs (i.e., to realize that fulfilling the latter may require compromising the former). Similarly, when examining the belief that no one else provides care as well, caregivers may recognize that service personnel do a reasonably good job and that this assistance will enable the caregiver to be more effective over a longer period of time. Caregivers also may learn to accept that it is not possible to have everything done exactly as they want. The process of examining beliefs, of course, must be carried out in a supportive and nonjudgmental way. The method developed by Beck and associates (1979) conveys support without making clients defensive by using questions to draw out the beliefs of caregivers, and examining and developing alternatives.

Easing the Crisis of Hospitalization

Hospitalization of the dementia patient constitutes a significant crisis and, as we have empirically shown, it can trigger nursing home admission. Several factors combine to make long-term placement a likely outcome of hospitalization. The patient's functioning may be markedly worse immediately prior to or during hospitalization. Dementia patients are especially sensitive to the effects of both illnesses and medications. Symptoms of dementia may worsen when the patient is ill or develop into full-blown delirium. The ability to perform activities of daily living (ADLs) may decline substantially, and cognitive and behavioral symptoms may be exacerbated. Once in the hospital, similar factors may contribute to apparent declines. Changes in routines, unfamiliar surroundings, and medications or other treatments may adversely affect functioning. Hospitals are not always able to manage dementia patients in an optimal manner. When there is insufficient staff to manage a disturbed dementia patient, many hospitals resort to restraints or tranquilizing medications, both of which can hasten decline.

Problems incurred as a result of hospitalization are at least partially reversible. Because dementia is a degenerative disease, however, families often interpret any increase in symptomatology during hospitalization as the next step in the dementia. As a result, patient deterioration may signal to the caregiver that long-term placement is necessary or unavoidable. Similarly, these declines may prompt physicians to advocate institutionalization.

A practical issue also influences nursing home admission following hospitalization. Patients who go from the hospital directly into nursing homes for medical reasons usually qualify for short-term (up to 120 days) Medicare reimbursement. Thus, it may be financially advantageous for families to place patients in nursing homes following hospitalization. For these reasons, placement of the dementia patient may be premature, but make practical sense. It is regrettable when these factors contribute to a decision that would be better made based on the true level of the patient's functioning after the medical problem is resolved. In general, more effective efforts need to be made in identifying, treating, and preventing the temporary exacerbation of dementia associated with illnesses, medications, and hospitalization. Approaches that maximize the comfort of patients may provide them with reassurance; those that minimize the use of drugs and restraints may reduce the severity of reactive symptoms. Caregiving families should be educated about problems associated with illness and hospitalization so that they are able to make informed decisions about placement. In sum, admission to a long-term care facility following a crisis hospitalization may indeed be the best choice for some families, but clinicians should be prepared to prevent placement for the wrong reasons, as well as to support those who decide to continue in-home care.

Deciding to Place a Relative

The decision to place the dementia patient in a nursing home, assisted living facility, or other supervised setting is wrenching for many families. For some caregivers, placement represents failure, a promise never to use a nursing home made to one's impaired relative and oneself that is broken when home care becomes untenable. The guilt evoked by such circumstances can be formidable. Caregivers also face practical issues regarding paying for care and finding a suitable facility.

Our research demonstrates that the stressors impinging upon caregivers, especially the sense of being held captive by caregiving, are at least as important as the behavior and functional status of the dementia patient in determining whether placement occurs. Although some have proposed that there is a certain time or stage in the course of dementia when placement is appropriate, families arrive at this transition on their own schedules. Clinical interventions should not hurry this decision based on a mistaken sense of what is best for a family, nor should clinicians delay placement when a family is ready to make this change. Instead, clinicians should make it permissible to consider placement as an option throughout the course of the disease and provide practical information about alternative settings, costs, and mechanisms for payment. Clinicians may also help caregivers consider placement against the background of different criteria, for example, as a step to be taken when certain impairments arise (e.g., incontinence). As part of this process, caregivers may need to reexamine the promises they made to the patient and themselves at an earlier time about not resorting to a nursing home. When that commitment was made, neither party envisioned the severe mental and physical disabilities characteristic of dementia, nor the burden they would eventually impose.

Placement decisions may also rekindle family conflict. It is not uncommon for families to be divided on this issue. Some relatives may strongly attack the primary caregiver regardless of whether the decision is to institutionalize or to keep the dementia patient at home. In some instances, the level of communal guilt is so intense that everyone acts defensively rather than in an understanding and supportive manner. Whatever the constellation of family forces, this transition is another point in the caregiving career when family counseling may be of substantial value.

In any discussion about placement, caregivers need to be fully informed about costs. Particularly for spouses, failure to take the proper steps when placing a husband or wife may result in a loss of assets. Finances will also dictate the choice of nursing home or other facility. Some facilities do not accept Medicaid. Patients who use up their available resources at one institution may then have to be moved to a different facility that accepts Medicaid. Families with limited financial resources need to consider these issues when selecting a nursing home.

Increasingly, families may select from a range of care settings. An important trend is the development of special units designed for the care of dementia patients (Sloane & Mathew, 1991). These facilities are usually locked or have alarms to prevent patients from wandering. Patients do not have to be monitored continually and can move about freely within the unit. Structured programs and the environmental design of the facility are frequently used to maximize the patients' remaining abilities and minimize the need for restraints.

An alternative to nursing home placement is assisted living facilities, such as board-and-care homes. These settings sometimes provide a high quality of care in a more homelike setting and at a lower cost than nursing homes. The main difference between these types of facilities is that assisted living homes are not required to have the same trained medical personnel as nursing homes (e.g., health aides versus registered nurses). Because most dementia patients do not have other serious medical problems that necessitate continuous skilled nursing care, assisted living homes that can manage dementia are a practical alternative. In Oregon, a substantial effort is being made to divert potential nursing home admissions to these facilities (see chapter 13).

A valuable step in the decision-making process is to encourage caregivers to visit facilities and obtain firsthand experience with the available alternatives.

This may challenge the popular image of nursing homes as snake pits. Indeed, given the limited resources available to them, many nursing homes do a very credible job. This is reflected in some of our data, which suggests that the anticipation of and preparation for placement are more stressful than the later conditions of actual institutional care.

Facilitating Adaptation to Nursing Home Care

Caregiving does not end at the door of a nursing home. Rather, placement changes the kinds of involvements caregivers have with their relatives. Although some stresses are relieved, especially those most directly tied to the tasks of daily care, new difficulties often emerge. Unfortunately, caregivers may receive little formal or informal support following placement as a result of the mistaken assumption that nursing home placement has relieved all stressors. Interventions following placement, however, may enable caregivers to make better adjustments, improve relationships between families and nursing home staff, and in the end, contribute to better quality of care for the dementia patients.

Problems that arise at placement include coping with the immediate psychological and emotional reaction to the transition, sorting out the amount and type of involvement to have in the nursing home, learning how to deal effectively with nursing home staff, and anticipating long-term adjustment issues. Following placement, some caregivers experience intense emotions. Guilt, depression, anger, and a sense of abandonment are common. Even if the patient no longer was able to communicate prior to placement, not having that person at home may create intense feelings of loneliness.

The caregiving role is redefined by placement. The social expectations concerning the involvement of families after this transition are indistinct; there are no set norms for how often to visit or how much help to provide in the nursing home. We have seen that families typically visit frequently and assist their relatives with ADLs on a regular basis.

Helping the patient may bring caregivers into conflict with staff. Caregivers will inevitably feel that the nursing home cannot give the same quality of care they provided at home. As a result, they may become extremely demanding or critical of nursing home staff, which, in turn, may diminish, rather than enhance, the care their relative receives. Therefore, it is crucial that caregivers and staff learn to work together effectively.

There usually is some basis for the belief that caregivers provided better care at home, so it is best for clinicians not to deny it outright, but to find ways to reframe the issue in a more productive manner. In particular, caregivers can be encouraged to think strategically about working with staff toward meeting the needs of the dementia patient. Also, it may be helpful to identify which staff should be approached about which issues: Sometimes it is best to talk with the aide on duty and at other times it is best to talk to the nurse in charge of the unit. In some instances, caregivers can ask the head of a unit who should be consulted about a particular concern.

From the perspective of the nursing home, it is useful to determine the most proficient ways of working with families and to create an environment where families are valued and welcomed. Families can be a resource, personalizing care and facilitating staff efforts. The time nursing home staff spend in orienting and training families on how to help, as well as finding ways to address the excessively critical caregivers, should pay off in terms of better programs.

Once past the immediate adjustment, caregivers need to strike a balance between a continuing sense of obligation to the patient and the need to reestablish their own lives. This step may be most difficult for spousal caregivers, whose ambiguous position, as discussed in chapter 9, has been described by Rosenthal and Dawson (1991) as "quasi-widowhood." Still married, they do not have the companionship of a spouse, yet may feel they cannot take steps towards a new life with someone else.

There is no formula for what caregivers *should* do to resolve this dilemma. Giving advice, such as telling the caregiver to get out more or visit the home less, is often not helpful. As with the decision to place, the ways caregivers decide to resolve their long-term roles are a matter of values. The starting point for aiding caregivers is understanding their values and how they perceive their situations. Clinicians should create nonjudgmental atmospheres to explore the ambiguities of these situations.

The evolution of the postplacement caregiving role varies considerably. Some caregivers may immediately initiate new activities or resume old ones. Spousal caregivers sometimes undertake new romantic relationships. Some caregivers face anger and hostility from other family members, which may make therapeutic intervention appropriate. Although a number of caregivers choose to visit the nursing home on a minimal basis or not at all, others prefer greater ongoing involvement. In these latter situations, clinicians can help establish a balanced schedule of visits that does not exhaust the caregiver, as well as encourage occasional breaks or vacations. In any case, we want to emphasize that clinical interventions should facilitate, not dictate. Caregivers find diverse ways to resolve the tensions of the postplacement period, and not all of these practices are what we would choose for ourselves.

Adjustments during Bereavement: Role Disengagement

Throughout this volume, we have emphasized the continuity of the caregiving career, even as major events or changes occur. Continuity is evident even after the death of the dementia patient, with the events of caregiving having an enduring impact on the process of readjustment. As with other transitions, caregivers need continuing support throughout bereavement.

An extensive body of literature has developed on the effects of bereavement in later life (Gallagher, Breckenridge, Thompson, & Peterson, 1983). Historically, widowhood was seen as a problematic social status, with widows having high rates of depression and widowers being at high risk of mortality. Recent studies suggest that bereavement is associated with a short-term increase in emotional distress, but only a relatively small minority of people are at risk for longer lasting problems in adjustment (Gallagher et al., 1983). Most studies focus on the death of a spouse and thus, little is known about the loss of a parent during adulthood.

A majority of bereavement studies also use samples where the duration of disability prior to the patient's death was relatively brief. There is minimal research examining bereavement following a long period of decline and disability, as occurs with dementia. This latter type of decline results in very different conditions prior to death: intense involvement by the caregiver, exposure to multiple stressors, and for many, separation for an extended period of time. Although we cannot compare the relative risk of bereavement after lengthy or brief periods of morbidity, our findings show how prior experiences contribute to the course of bereavement and recovery. Notably, caregivers who were worn out by the care process experienced more grief and preoccupation with their losses, and those with more personal resources, especially a strong sense of mastery, experienced less grief.

A particularly important issue to clinical interventions at this time is the connection between a caregiver's prior loss of feelings of connection or intimacy with the care recipient, and subsequent better adjustment to his or her death. In a sense, this caregiver has already mourned the person he or she once knew. Under these circumstances, death may be viewed as the release from a terrible illness, greeted with a certain amount of relief.

Does this finding suggest that we should encourage caregivers to disengage from the patient earlier in the disease process? Such a conclusion would be a gross misinterpretation and overgeneralization of our findings. Recall that loss of intimacy is depressing, especially to the extent that it contributes to a loss of personal identity. This linkage suggests that it is more appropriate to focus on maintaining the integrity of the caregiver's self-concept over the course of dementia care.

An additional issue that arises following lengthy caregiving is the sense of having missed experiences and opportunities because of the patient's illness or because of care responsibilities. Spousal caregivers may not have done the things they had hoped to do during retirement, such as travel, and may regret both the loss of time and the loss of their companion. Daughters and other family caregivers may regret lost involvements with their own nuclear families and occupational lives.

I regret not getting to know my grandchildren.

In the end, some caregivers may need assistance in developing new activities and new focuses in their lives. For others, the loss may raise issues of identity and self-esteem. No longer a caregiver, nor a spouse or child, these individuals may question their social identities. These processes of discovering new activities and re-creating identities may go hand-in-hand. Tentative explorations of new involvements may be useful in fostering this transformation. We should also not overlook the fact that some caregivers will now be facing practical problems they are not prepared for, such as managing an inheritance or living alone.

Finally, we should not assume that the loss of one's spouse or parent can or should be completely overcome. The death of a significant other leaves a permanent void. Activities that recall the person, or in some way honor the person's memory, may be helpful in acknowledging the meaning the relationship continues to have for surviving relatives. It may be pacifying to find ways of remembering the person as he or she once was, before the onslaught of this terrible disease. Although dwelling only on the past is problematic, a balance between memories, acceptance, and adjustment is undoubtedly helpful in recovery.

Types of Clinical Approaches

We have addressed the implications of our research in broad terms to illuminate problems that caregivers bring to a variety of clinical and service settings. Counseling approaches, including family sessions, have been emphasized as a treatment strategy. This intervention, however, is certainly not needed by all caregivers, nor is it necessary throughout the caregiving career. Many times, a helpful discussion with a nonjudgmental professional, whether a physician, nurse, activities director, or another caregiver may give caregivers the boost they need to cope more effectively with their current situations. When caregivers need more than informal assistance can provide, counseling by a professional knowledgeable in issues of caregiving is warranted. Although the amount of research is still limited, the available studies suggest that short-term counseling is a very proficient way of lowering stress on family caregivers (Gallagher-Thompson, 1994; Zarit & Teri, 1991).

Frank

Frank, who describes himself as a loner, reports that a support group for caregivers helped him survive difficult moments during Beth's illness.

Marvelous! I was in a depression and I'd say that two of the women in particular, the leader and her assistant, and the group itself were enormously helpful. That group saved my life. I don't have suicidal tendencies but it does go through your head as you see life disintegrating.

Although few caregivers in our study sought professional counseling, a somewhat larger group attended support group meetings. Since the late 1970s when the first AD support groups were established, these groups have become a seemingly ubiquitous phenomenon and form AD and Related Disorders Associations' (ADRDA) centerpiece of community activities. Groups are very popular among caregivers and may be especially helpful in disseminating information about the disease and about resources. Groups may also guide caregivers in putting their emotional reactions into perspective by demonstrating that the situation is stressful for caregivers.

Research on support groups, however, has had disappointing results (Haley et al., 1987; Whitlatch et al., 1991). Generally, counseling is more effective in the short run than support groups in lowering feelings of strain and distress. The available studies, though, have focused only on short-term outcomes. The benefits of groups may become more apparent over longer periods of time. Studies have also not tended to measure outcomes in terms of the processes groups are most likely to affect, such as the caregiver's understanding of the disease or knowledge of and use of resources. Given their enduring popularity, support groups should not be dismissed without more extensive research. When a caregiver is emotionally distressed, however, referral to professional therapy, rather than a support group, is the better course of action.

Concluding Comments

Research necessarily presents a picture of caregiving in a piecemeal way. Theories and research strategies are useful for highlighting key processes and examining their relationships to one another. The clinician has the opportunity to integrate and extend these findings, bringing us full circle to the caregiver as a whole person coping with a unique situation. We began our study impressed with the difficulties and often heroic struggles of families of dementia patients. Nearing the end, we strongly believe that more concerted clinical interventions are needed to improve the circumstances of both patient and caregiver.

Clinical endeavors may be informed in two primary ways by our research. First, our work has provided a conceptual framework for understanding caregiving and care-related stress. Basic concepts, such as individual differences in response to similar situations, can guide how clinicians think about, plan, and assess interventions for family caregivers. Second, our research suggests specific ways in which interventions may help. In the broadest sense, primary goals for intervention are reducing stress proliferation and increasing stress containment. Determining optimal methods of attaining these goals is a complex task given the unremitting demands on caregivers and the wide range of individual differences in how caregivers respond to these demands. Nonetheless, a critical next step in the caregiving field is to identify those interventions that most effectively achieve these goals. Creative partnerships among families, clinicians, and researchers can yield valuable information about new directions for intervention.

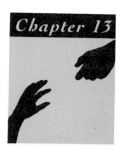

Implications for Public Policy and Society

Our investigation of the caregiving career has focused for the most part on individual caregivers as members of various social groups defined by characteristics such as gender, kinship, and socioeconomic status (SES). We move now to a different level of analysis, the implications of caregiving for public policy and society in general. Family caregiving is problematic not only for the families with the misfortune of having a disabled elder, but for society as a whole. Moreover, it is a difficulty that can only grow in magnitude and complexity in the coming years and decades. Informal caregivers stand at the juncture between the impaired person and the formal service system. The manner in which public policy shapes formal services, especially its impact on the interface between the formal and informal care systems, greatly affects the care families can provide. Given the demographic trends we described in chapter 1, it is clearly time to establish policies that assure a workable system of long-term care for individuals, families, and society, rather than waiting until current shortcomings escalate to a crisis level.

Much of the debate on public policy and aging has been dominated by economists. It is understandable that their proposed solutions often appear preoccupied with economic considerations, such as the reallocation of financial resources from one program to another. Our investigation of the social, psychological, and behavioral aspects of caregiving over the long-term provides an alternative vantage point. It has identified problems and needs that emerge, grow, change, and recede over time. We believe that the policy debate needs to start here, with a realistic appraisal of the duration of caregiving and the evolving constellation of problematic conditions it imposes upon families. With a clearer idea of what needs to be done, we can proceed to a more productive discussion of how to build political and financial support for the systematic relief of at least some of these burdens.

As discussed previously, family caregiving has become a prominent social issue because demographic trends have dramatically increased the likelihood that sustained caregiving will be needed during a person's lifetime. With the growth of the older population, larger numbers of people are living to ages when significant disabilities are likely to emerge. People also are surviving longer after the onset of disability and, hence, are living with more severe and complex disabilities than in past generations. As the need for elder care grows, the family remains the first line of defense. When a disabled elder has a spouse or children, these family members usually assist in myriad ways, often coordinating the efforts of formal service providers as well. Families are probably providing more extensive and complex care than ever before and doing so for longer periods of time.

Current public policies concerning care of the disabled elderly are inconsistent with one another and often have cross-purposes. For example, for many years the stated federal policy has been to encourage older persons to remain in their own homes. Yet, community-based services to assist disabled elders and their families are fragmented, with little or no third-party payment available through public (i.e., Medicare and Medicaid) or private insurance.

Additionally, the hidden costs of this system of family care are numerous. Our study has highlighted some of the impact on primary caregivers, including both tangible costs, such as lost wages, and adverse effects on emotional well-being. There undoubtedly are tangible and emotional tolls extracted from other family members as well, especially those persons who assist the primary caregiver. The lack of a systematic plan for the delivery and financing of long-term care services means that costs are distributed in unequal and unplanned ways with some families paying disproportionate amounts. Similar inequalities may also exist within families as some members bear more than their fair share of the financial burden.

I feel there's always something left for me to do.

The experiences of the families in our study appear fairly typical: The majority received little, if any, formal assistance over long periods of time, and those that did receive services usually paid for most or all of them out-of-pocket. Relief from care-related burdens and expenses often comes only from resorting to nursing home care because Medicaid will pay the cost of care after the older person has exhausted his or her own assets. These financial practices, therefore, counteract the explicit policy goal of maintaining the patient in the community. It is a situation where practice undermines policy.

Although the focus of our discussion concerns the United States, comparable public policy issues have been voiced in numerous other developed countries as a consequence of growing populations of disabled elderly. Despite differences across countries in the developmental state of their formal service systems, their concerns are converging. Although policy discussions in the United States appropriately emphasize the need for increasing services and benefits (McConnell & Riggs, 1994), countries with well-developed service systems contemplate how current programs may be extended to meet exploding demand. The cost of care is a major concern in either scenario. Some projections indicate that the major bottleneck in extending services will be the lack of sufficient numbers of trained formal service providers to staff community and institutional long-term care programs (Thorslund, 1991). In countries with strong social welfare programs, such as Sweden and Denmark, families can expect to take on more of the burdens of care in the coming years. The critical question globally is how to arrange supportive and equitable systems that encourage families to help, but do not impose an overwhelming responsibility on them.

The Policy Conundrum: Addressing Diverging Interests

Given the typically long duration of caregiving and the numerous demands it places on the family, the logical first programmatic step is to increase the types and amounts of available and affordable services (McConnell & Riggs, 1994). There is no question that a better-developed and coordinated system of community and institutional long-term care is needed in the United States, along with a reasonable payment method combining public and private funding. As was discussed in chapter 12, the magnitude and duration of care-related stressors means that weak or circumscribed interventions will have minimal benefits. Too little, too late is perhaps the costliest system of all.

Family caregiving presents a unique challenge to policymakers because it is a group issue in a society that emphasizes individuals in its legal and financial systems. There are few precedents for policies that must consider both the disabled elder *and* his or her family. This situation is complicated by the fact that the interests of the dementia patient and those of the family diverge at key points. Moreover, the interests of each may also differ from the interests of the society at large. We discuss these issues in more detail in the following sections.

The Individual Focus of Policy

The main exception to the United States' public policy focus on individuals rather than families concerns parents' obligations toward their minor children.

Adult-child care of parents poses a dilemma in this context. Daughters and sons are expected and encouraged by society to assume responsibility for an aged parent, but there is no legal obligation to do so. State laws that at one time required children to provide parent care have been repealed or fallen into disuse. In contrast, spouses have legal and financial obligations that pose potential economic hardships.

The primary emphasis on individual rights creates difficulties in situations like family caregiving that involve two or more adults. For example, the family requires information about the patient's medical condition and other needs in order to provide appropriate care. Yet, confidentiality in doctor–patient relationships means that the family, including a spouse, does not have a legal right to this information. In effect, physicians and other health service providers are obligated to deal directly with the dementia patient. There are remedies to this situation, such as obtaining durable power of attorney for health care or, in some situations, guardianship. In some instances, clinicians share confidential information with families without formal consent. Moreover, the right to receive and refuse treatment, including social services, rests with the individual. These examples point out that the individual, not the family, has primary rights and protection and as such, these are instances wherein important principles are inappropriately applied.

Likewise, there has been ambivalence about extending benefits and services to the family of a disabled person. For instance, Medicare pays for medical care for the dementia patient, but not for respite care or other services that might relieve caregivers. Expanded mental health coverage in Medicare can now be used by caregivers if they are over age 65 themselves and if they have received a psychiatric diagnosis. Unfortunately, Medicare reimburses family therapy at lower rates than individual psychotherapy, although the former may be especially helpful for caregivers (see chapter 12). For adult children or spousal caregivers under age 65, health insurance (if they have any) is likely to provide limited mental health coverage and no other benefits to assist in their caregiving efforts. Similarly, many home care programs and services have been reluctant to provide help directly to the caregiver rather than to the designated patient. In some states, priority has been given to serving elderly who live alone because they are the most vulnerable to becoming institutionalized. This approach tends to penalize family caregivers whose impaired relatives live with them by providing little or no help. Fortunately, this tendency may be changing, enabling families with disabled elders in the households to qualify for some services.

Probably the most important recent policy change for families has been the 1989 modification of the spousal impoverishment provision in Medicaid (McConnell & Riggs, 1994). Prior to this change, spouses were completely responsible for nursing home costs; the patient only became eligible for Medicaid reimbursement after the *couple* had spent down to the poverty level. Not surprisingly, spousal caregivers with limited financial resources feared becoming impoverished by the costs of nursing home care. Since the policy modification, the spousal caregiver can retain some assets (approximately $65,000) and a house, if the couple owns one.

Adult children do not have the same legal obligation to contribute financially to parent care. This situation may be advantageous, but also may penalize these caregivers. The advantage, obviously, is that parents can qualify for financial assistance without their caregiving daughters and sons having to spend down their own resources. On the other hand, children who incur costs in parent care are not identified as needing financial assistance because they are not legally obligated to make this contribution. Aside from a small tax credit for dependent care which reimburses a maximum of $720 a year (McConnell & Riggs, 1994), these voluntary contributions are not usually supported or reimbursed. Ambiguity about familial obligations impedes the development of programs that directly support caregivers, such as subsidies for services that assist them (e.g., housekeeping, baby-sitting, and counseling), even though these programs would enable them to be more effective caregivers and thus, indirectly benefit the person with dementia.

Diverging Interests of Patients, Families, and Society

An issue that flows directly from our findings concerns the contrasting interests of patients and families at key points in the caregiving career. Extending this perspective, the interests of society as a whole in minimizing the cost of formal services competes at times, as well, with the concerns of the dementia patient, the caregiving family, or both of these parties. A major point of divergence involves the decision to place a dementia patient in a nursing home or similar facility, or to continue to provide care at home. This issue entails balancing costs and benefits for patients, caregivers, and society.

From the family's perspective, there are some obvious risks associated with continuing in-home care. As we have seen, caregivers may experience considerable strain and disruption of work, social, and family life, in addition to incurring substantial out-of-pocket expenses for formal services. Feelings of depression, anger, and anxiety may increase to clinically significant levels. Continued exposure to such chronic stressors is, without doubt, potentially harmful.

Balancing these costs are the satisfaction of motivational imperatives and other intrinsic rewards associated with caring for an ailing spouse or parent. As we have seen, some caregivers gain a sense of competency or feel they are fulfilling an important family obligation. Others simply minimize feelings of guilt or social disapproval by providing care at home.

For patients, the scale rocks back and forth between the costs and benefits of continued home care, but typically the positives outweigh the negatives. This is partly because dementia patients usually prefer to remain at home. Given the progressive nature of dementing illnesses, individuals should function better in familiar settings than in new environments where they need to learn new spatial information and routines. On the other hand, as their disease progresses, many dementia patients no longer recognize these environments. They may, for example, insist on being taken home when they are in fact already at home.

He gets better care with me.

However, it cannot be assumed that continued home care is without risk to the patient. For example, situations of abuse and neglect have been documented (Pillemer & Suiter, 1994). Patients who are not monitored adequately may risk injury or trouble by leaving a stove on, wandering off, falling, and so forth. Families confront the dilemma of assuring the safety of a patient whose reasoning is impaired, while not taking unnecessarily restrictive steps that limit meaningful activities that the patient can still perform.

By contrast, there also are considerable risks to patients who are admitted into nursing homes. As we have documented, the primary danger is excess mortality during the first months of placement. Over the long haul, patients in nursing homes also face the possibility of overmedication, restraints, and other iatrogenic problems. The lack of meaningful and stimulating physical and mental activity in some nursing homes may take its toll as well, hastening decline in remaining functional abilities. As discussed in chapter 12, special Alzheimer's units are designed to provide appropriate stimulation while containing active and agitated patients through environmental design, programming, and staff training (Sloane & Mathew, 1991). The degree to which they minimize the risks associated with the institutional setting, however, remains to be determined. This is not to argue, of course, that home settings are uniformly stimulating: Families with few social and material resources and little energy may find it difficult to keep patients active.

The nursing home is a living cemetery.

While emphasizing points where the interests of patients and caregivers diverge, we want to call attention also to the fact that in most respects, these interests tend to converge and are consonant. Just as the majority of family caregivers assume their responsibilities willingly, nursing homes typically do a very credible job, especially given their limited resources. Indeed, in some instances and at certain periods during the progression of dementia, they provide better conditions than continued home care. In other words, this situation is not one of diametrically opposite interests, but rather one in which there are differences at critical times and in particular circumstances. The ideal that should be supported by public policy is to help both families and institutional settings function at optimal levels of quality in caring for impaired elders.

Turning to societal concerns, a primary policy objective has been to keep taxpayers' costs down, which translates into a preference for home care. Nursing home placement has been discouraged by limiting benefits under Medicare to brief stays following hospitalization. A recent, additional barrier is the require-ment of preadmission screening for Medicaid-eligible patients. These screenings are designed to identify people who could be managed at lower costs in less intensive care settings, particularly those with primarily mental health problems.

Many policy initiatives have sought to increase the availability of community services as a way of reducing nursing home placement. Some have argued that this approach is cost effective because the expense of community services would be offset by reduced nursing home expenditures. This argument is flawed, how-ever, because the rate of nursing home placement already is quite low compared to other developed countries (Doty, 1990). In effect, our system uses financial disincentives to keep placement rates low. Consequently, community services probably will not reduce already low placement rates. Indeed, any increase in Medicare or private coverage of long-term care may increase placement rates.

Current social policies in the United States, however, also encourage institu-tional placement in some ways. For example, we have reported a substantial increase in placement following hospitalization, which is not surprising given that Medicare pays for nursing home placement following hospitalization. At least some families take advantage of this opportunity to save on nursing home costs. The patchwork of community services, which is especially inadequate for dementia patients, acts as an inadvertent incentive for placement as well. For many families, home care ceases to be a viable option because they simply cannot provide enough help themselves and the kinds of community-based assis-tance needed are not available.

Certainly, the biggest incentive toward institutionalization is funding of nurs-ing homes by Medicaid. This "safety net," which is triggered when nursing home residents have exhausted their own resources, makes long nursing home stays possible. Medicaid coverage is the most consequential public policy for elder care and a major financial cost to states and the federal government. Without Medicaid, large numbers of severely disabled older persons would be without necessary care. Finally, the attitudes of many professionals encourage placement without adequate consideration of the resources needed to provide care at home effectively.

Is it likely that policies can be developed that reconcile these diverging inter-ests, practices, and policies? An example from a different area of research may provide the answer to this question. Mirowsky (1985) has studied the relationship of depression to the distribution of decision-making power in married couples. Depression follows a U-shaped curve as an individual goes from having no power, to shared power, to having complete power. That is, both husbands and wives are most likely to be depressed when they make all of the decisions or none of the decisions, and least likely to be depressed when decision making is more or less equally shared. There are separate curves for husbands and wives, how-ever, with different optimal points. Specifically, the lowest risk for husbands, on average, occurs when the husband has somewhat more power, whereas the re-verse is the case for wives. Thus, there is no particular point where depression is equally minimized for both partners.

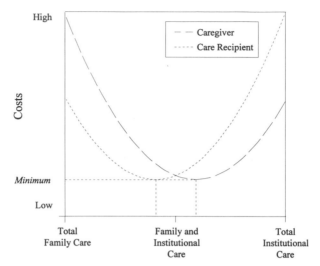

Figure 13.1   Hypothetical costs of family versus institutional care.

We cannot make a comparable empirical analysis of diverging interests between caregivers and care recipients with our data. We suspect, however, that the results of such an analysis would be similar to those observed for marital power; that is, there would be no single solution that maximizes everyone's best interest.

This possibility is illustrated in Figure 13.1[1] for a hypothetical continuum extending from total family care through a mix of family and institutional care to total institutional care. The "costs" portrayed in this illustration are composites of numerous dimensions that include the following: financial expenditures; foregone earnings; social repercussions, such as withdrawal from social activities and conflict with other family members; and damage to health and emotional well-being. The relative mix of these types of costs is likely to differ across the continuum of care, at various points in the caregiving career, and between the caregiver and care recipient.

As we have documented throughout this book, the costs to caregivers of providing all of the care required by their impaired relatives are very high. We anticipate that these costs will decline as some of this burden is shared with sources of support outside of the family, including such services as day care and respite care. We do not expect this decline to be limitless, however, as the mix of care moves increasingly in favor of institutionalized sources of care. As we saw in chapter 9, institutionalization relieves some burdens on family caregivers, but initiates others.

This point is especially evident for the most extreme case: complete nursing home care without supplemental family care of any type, including mere visits. In this instance, the average family caregiver is likely to incur certain new costs. For example, this situation might be viewed by others as abandonment, producing negative social sanctions. Alternately, caregivers may experience intense feelings of guilt, remorse, or other emotionally painful states. Thus, we hypothesize that the costs for caregivers follow a U-shaped curve, such as that shown in Figure 13.1. Although this view needs empirical verification, we believe that at some stage of the caregiving career, most families and patients benefit from a reasonable mix of family and institutional assistance.

A similar U-shaped curve is postulated for care recipients. As discussed earlier, although dementia patients typically prefer to remain in the home, this type of care is not without cost to the patient (e.g., being left unattended and insufficient stimulation). Thus, care recipients would benefit from additional care provided outside of the family, but within the community, to supplement the care caregivers are unable to give within the home. The best example of this would be day care specifically designed for dementia patients.

Although institutionalized care is seen as generally beneficial to caregivers, care recipients are hypothesized to incur greater costs as their care becomes increasingly institutionalized. We expect these costs to be highest in the instance of complete institutional care in the absence of any supplemental family care. It has been emphasized that nursing homes typically do a credible job with limited resources; however, the fact that they are "limited" means that the patients often do not receive optimal care. Family care that supplements nursing home care, which occurs somewhat to the left of total institutional care in Figure 13.1, is expected to decrease costs to the patient.

The most important feature of this illustration, however, is the presence of two separate curves, one for caregivers and one for care recipients. As may be seen, there is no single combination of family and institutional care that minimizes the costs for *both* parties. The optimal point for caregivers is to the right of the optimal point for care recipients, meaning that caregivers are best off when there is a strong contribution from outside sources of care, whereas care recipients benefit most when this balance is tipped in favor of family contributions. As caregivers move left from their minimum point, they incur excess costs; as care recipients move right from their minimum point, they incur excess costs. A few scenarios are possible: costs may be minimized for one party and greatly increased for the other, or both parties may incur costs somewhat in excess of their own personal minimum.

Constance

Constance's reflection on her decision to place her mother in a nursing home reflects the ambivalence that can arise when there is no good solution to an intractable problem:

I often wonder if we'd left her there [at home] what would have happened. Maybe it would have been better. Maybe if something had happened, it would have been over with and not gone through this long prolonged period. It's not an alternative that occurred to me at the time, but looking back . . . I wonder, what if we'd done something differently? . . . At one time I "hoped," . . . Mother gardened and she would literally go up in a tree to prune the branches. I thought she's got to go some way, some day, how neat if she fell out of the tree. That would be so typical of her and suddenly it would be over. Something along that theme, that it would suddenly be over for her instead of this long drawn-out process that I see going on.

This example is meant only to illustrate the competing interests of the caregiver and care recipient. It is theoretical, not empirical. For instance, the curves may be closer together than shown here, or farther apart. The most important point to be taken from this example is that there is no single mix of services that is best for both sides of the caregiving dyad.

In conclusion, policy discussions should acknowledge explicitly how interests diverge. Also, these discussions need to be based on honest estimates of the costs, financial and otherwise, involved in alternative strategies. Because there are no cost-free solutions, it is necessary to be realistic about the implications of various policies and to make informed choices about which risks we are willing to accept.

Public Policy and the Elusiveness of Establishing Need

The need for assistance by family caregivers to dementia patients is rather difficult to establish. It cannot be based on disease duration or stage of illness because the functioning of impaired individuals neither remains stable over time, nor necessarily increases linearly. Thus, indicators of need for help are highly variable, making it difficult to rely solely on concrete signs, however appealing these pseudomedical markers might be. Family burden, although certainly related to objective conditions, is ultimately a subjective state that cannot be equated with a single configuration of objective conditions.

As a consequence, public policies for the support of family caregiving need an unprecedented degree of flexibility. They must be based not only on the presence of a specific set of objective primary stressors, but also on the presence of secondary stressors, resources, and unique features of the situation. Additionally, policies need to target especially vulnerable groups, such as working caregivers. Support, however, should not be limited to such groups; a system that denies services to large numbers of people outside these categories would be unfortunate. Identifying some caregivers as needy and others as not would inevitably seem inequitable because there is no clear calibration of need in this instance. Some observers have argued that the best approach is to give families credits to spend as they prefer (J. J. Callahan, 1989a), a straightforward approach to variability in need. Rather than proposing a specific solution, however, we want to emphasize that caregiving requires new and flexible ways of thinking about benefits and services, precisely because individual differences in needs and resources are so great.

If I worked, I'd pay it all to a sitter.

The issue of establishing the level and context of need touches on another important matter: the specific diagnosis and health problems of the patient. Is a policy necessary specifically for dementia, or should public policies collectively address all disabled elderly? There is a tendency to think of need in terms of medical categories, a tendency nurtured by the fact that advocacy groups are typically organized around diseases and limit their efforts to their own constituencies. Alzheimer's Disease and Related Disorders Association (ADRDA), though founded only in 1979, has had a profound influence on Congress, research funding for dementia, and, to an extent, public policy (Fox, 1989). However, this impact is somewhat circumscribed, not extending, for example, to families caring for members with stroke or head trauma.

An exception to the pattern of disease-specific advocacy and programming is the Family Caregiver Alliance (formerly, Family Survival Project). A grassroots organization founded in the mid-1970s, it has successfully established 11 California Resource Centers (CRCs) throughout California. These CRCs, funded by the state's Department of Health Services, provide services to caregivers of cognitively impaired adults (e.g., head trauma, Parkinson's disease, stroke, and dementia). This organization maintains that service and policy issues are sufficiently similar to pool resources and advocacy efforts. A more detailed description of their program appears later in this chapter. The largest advocacy organization for the elderly, the American Association for Retired Persons (AARP), also takes a broad perspective on health-care issues and caregiver needs.

Is the care of dementia patients so different from other disabled elderly that separate programs and policies should be encouraged? Probably not. Some other groups, for instance, the mentally ill elderly, pose equally severe challenges to their family caregivers (Pearson, Verma, & Nellett, 1988), who presumably would benefit from a similar package of services. Although care for someone without cognitive impairment is, on average, somewhat less stressful than dementia care, some families are overwhelmed by this kind of care in the same ways as dementia caregivers are overwhelmed. It seems more sensible to build a national policy to support families, irrespective of the cause of the elderlies' disabilities. Where specialized programs are needed, such as in dementia units in nursing homes, these components may be added to a basic support system.

Directions for Public Policy and Caregiving

In the following sections, we discuss the implications of our findings for specific policy directions. We consider goals for policy, as well as some promising initiatives. We also return to the question of nursing home placement because it is so central an issue to both caregiving and policy discussions.

A Partnership of Families and Support Services

The most direct ramification of our findings for policy is the need for a comprehensive approach that supports caregivers throughout their careers as caregivers. Policy issues arise quite early in the course of dementia, certainly by the time of diagnosis when the initial accommodations families make establish the basic parameters of the course of caregiving. The stage of role acquisition also commands policy attention because of its potential for stemming the tide of stress proliferation that might otherwise intensify or accelerate. Policy needs to address, as well, the changing needs of dementia patients and their caregivers as time goes on. If, for instance, a key policy objective is the encouragement of in-home caregiving over institutionalization, then programmatic efforts need to consider such issues as early financial planning and the types of expenditures that are most salient at various points in the progression of the dementia.

Moreover, policy must take a multipronged approach for several reasons. First, the needs and resources of the impaired elderly and their caregivers are diverse; even those at the same stage of their illnesses and their caregiving careers differ considerably in their requirements for assistance and support systems. Thus, a wide range of service alternatives are necessary. Second, concerns change over time, and new challenges arise and reside in one's multiple domains of functioning. The mix of services, therefore, must be able to evolve over time in response to changes in the patient's condition and the family's ability to provide appropriate care. Third, policy initiatives also ought to consider the interconnection of the multiple parties affected by dementia. It is not sufficient to address patient needs in isolation from the primary caregiver, nor those of the primary caregiver in isolation from the patient or the rest of the family. Given the heterogeneity of needs, resources, and structural composition of families, a variety of services should be flexibly and selectively available. These services should provide treatment and stimulating activities for patients, respite and relief from caregiving for the care provider, and support and counseling to families as they build their resources for the long haul. Another component would be a viable program of insurance for nursing home care (see Wiener, Hanley, Spence, & Murray, 1989, for an incisive analysis of how to fund long-term care). Although not ignoring medical aspects of dementia and economic implications, policy must primarily address the social and behavioral consequences of dementia.

Whatever the specific form new programs and services take, a major policy goal should be to establish a partnership with families. Services should enable and enhance what caregivers already are doing by providing relief both from certain tasks and from extended periods of caregiving. If service providers approach caregivers in rigid ways, they will become a new stressor and undermine the very efforts they are attempting to make. Informal care should be viewed as a resource to be nurtured, not subverted or displaced.

> Can't talk to the staff. They speak Spanish.

Drawing upon the work of Litwak (1985), Noelker and Bass (1989) have developed a useful framework for examining the interface of informal and formal services. They empirically identify five kinds of connection between formal and informal assistance: kin independence, where the family provides all home care tasks without any formal services; formal service specialization, where agencies take on tasks not being performed by the family, but family and service agency provide some other tasks jointly; dual specialization, in which family and service agency perform different tasks; supplementation, where agencies assist with tasks that families also perform; and substitution, in which formal care totally replaces family care. A fruitful direction for research is to consider which combinations of formal and informal help are most beneficial to what kinds of families, under what circumstances, and at what stages of their careers.

A partnership of families and formal providers demands that services be organized in ways that facilitate the continued involvement of families. A primary goal for policy should be to establish a "user-friendly" system of services. By this, we mean that eligibility, subsidies, and costs for services are organized in a straightforward way that is understandable to the ordinary consumer. The categories of service also have to be reasonably flexible to address the full spectrum of care-related needs. Under the current patchwork system, families have a great deal of uncertainty about available services and their eligibility for benefits (MaloneBeach et al., 1992). Categories of service may not match needs, and unless agencies are reasonably flexible in interpreting guidelines, many families who might benefit from programs end up being excluded.

A favorite service approach of policy-oriented gerontologists has been case management. The rationale behind case management is that services are often available, but individuals or their families are unable to locate and access these services. By matching people and services, a more efficient use of current resources could be effected with little increase in cost. Unfortunately, the results of large-scale demonstrations of case management suggest that there may be few advantages over what families achieve by themselves (J. J. Callahan, 1989b; Carcagno & Kemper, 1988). In any event, case management, by itself, does not address the underlying need for more comprehensive and flexible services.

A related issue is that service programs also have to be "dementia friendly." Families often report that service workers do not have any idea about the appropriate ways to care for dementia patients (MaloneBeach et al., 1992). Although we do not believe dementia requires a completely different service system, providers must be knowledgeable about dementia and how to interact with patients and their families. The brief training that many home health aides currently receive prepares them inadequately for assisting families in the complex situations that often arises in the case of dementia.

Part of the goal of user-friendly services is to support the family's feelings of mastery over the care situation. Some current approaches undermine this sense of control. For example, when arranging for someone to come into the home to assist the dementia patient, families are often told they cannot choose the aide or the time the aide will arrive (MaloneBeach et al., 1992). Moreover, the same aide may not return for the next visit. Although these arrangements may make sense from the perspective of organizational efficiency, they are hardly appropriate for families or dementia patients, for whom developing a personal relationship with a provider is important. Furthermore, from the family's perspective, having strangers come into the home can be a source of anxiety. To feel that one has no choice about arrangements for these intrusions further undermines confidence and mastery, which generally exacerbates care-related stress and its emotional sequelae. In-home care often is viewed as a matter of matching resource to family without consideration of the personal dimensions involved.

Valerie

Valerie not only provides home care for her husband Donald, she works to support both of them. One of the strains that impinge upon her is arranging for respite care:

They can only send someone from 1–4 P.M., but I need someone from 2–5 P.M. 1 to 4 just doesn't work. Can't be home from work by 4 P.M. What will I do?

In contemplating a vacation, she is stymied by the lack of flexible alternatives for Donald in her absence.

I wouldn't put him in a hospital. It's outrageous to have him get used to something different for a short time. Need someone in the home. They're going at it from the wrong end.

A particularly daunting challenge is to support working caregivers. Adult day care may be a reasonable solution to role conflict for many working caregivers if extended hours are available. Programs like these have expanded enormously in recent years and now exist in most metropolitan areas. Transportation and cost, however, remain barriers for many families. Day-care programs may also be unable to accommodate dementia clients who exhibit high levels of behavior problems.

A central question concerning the interface of formal and informal help is whether families should be required to provide a certain amount of help and, if so, how much help should be required. Spousal caregivers typically provide extensive assistance, but in the case of adult children, there is more variability. The daughters and sons in our study all assumed major responsibilities. Most lived with the dementia patient and provided extensive assistance, even after nursing home placement. This care was all done voluntarily and without any monetary or other tangible reward. Given scarce resources, social programs tend to help first those elders who do not have good informal care. Should the family that does more receive less help or obtain help only later in the caregiving career? Such a strategy may well prove to be inadvertently counterproductive. An alternative approach is to formalize the involvement of the family, developing care plans that include contributions from both informal and formal providers. Because families are so heterogeneous, it is unlikely that a single formula or approach can encompass a sufficient range of types of informal assistance. In the end, however, it is most important that policymakers recognize and support those families who are able to make significant contributions to care, and not penalize them for their efforts by setting higher eligibility standards for services or benefits.

Promising Initiatives and Trends

There are several favorable initiatives and programs that currently serve family caregivers of dementia patients. These programs have been developed from local and sometimes state resources, and suggest possible models for more large-scale initiatives. Given their local roots, these programs also incorporate unique features of the community in which they operate, a factor that also should not be overlooked in national initiatives.

Perhaps the oldest program addressing needs of family caregivers is the previously mentioned Family Caregiver Alliance (Friss, 1990, Heagerty & Eskenazi, 1994), which has united people caring for adults with any type of brain impairment, such as AD, stroke, and head trauma. The program emerged in response to the lack of attention paid to these groups in existing policies. Although services for brain-injured children were available, no comparable programs were available for adults or their families. A distinctive feature of the program is that the family caregiver is the client. Programs and services are designed to support the family, including educational programs, respite care, and development of an information clearinghouse. Family Caregiver Alliance also has had a pioneering role in identifying legal issues affecting caregivers and lobbying for changes in Medicaid rules to prevent the impoverishment of spousal caregivers.

Legislation in California in 1984 established a statewide network of CRCs, also described earlier, based on the model of the Family Caregiver Alliance. These CRCs serve specific regions of the state, making it possible for caregivers residing anywhere in California to receive similar packages of information and support services.

Another innovative program is Legacy's Family Support Center, based in Portland, Oregon. Like Family Caregiver Alliance, this center emphasizes education, support, and respite services for caregivers (Heagerty & Eskenazi, 1994). A distinctive feature of the program is that it is located in a large medical center, which facilitates referrals from physicians. This arrangement also makes feasible collaboration with physicians in the development of educational programs and training materials. The center also is connected to the Oregon Alzheimer's Disease Center, serving as a technological resource base. This linkage of medical, research, and family caregiving services is unique. Instead of being dwarfed or intimidated by medical and research programs, Legacy's Family Support Center has exercised considerable leadership in the development of programs and advocacy. Its success suggests an approach that bridges some obvious gaps in the service system.

Local chapters of the ADRDA also have played major roles in the development of services for families (ADRDA, 1992). Using seed money from the national organization and local funds, 51 chapters have developed respite programs, including both in-home and day care. In some instances, the programs consist of subsidies for families to use existing services along with dementia-specific training for providers. In other instances, where suitable services are not available, local chapters have taken the lead in initiating programs.

The programs described thus far all have strong voluntary and community ties. Each grew out of needs not being met by formal service providers and developed in response to specific local circumstances. Part of the success of these programs is undoubtedly due to the sense of mission embodied by families and professional staff. Summarizing the characteristics of innovative programs, Heagerty and Eskenazi (1994) suggested several common elements. These programs all began on small scales with clearly defined foci; develop diversified sources of funding; possess strong advocates; respond to new trends; and most importantly, design their own innovative approaches to meet their unique goals. This blending of private and public efforts is difficult to legislate and duplicate because it largely depends on local talent and initiative.

A somewhat different model for mobilizing community-based support is a partnership between state government and existing service organizations. For example, the Department of Health in New Jersey used funds raised from taxes on local gambling casinos to develop several programs for dementia patients and their families. One such program subsidizes the use of an approved adult day-care program (Engström, Greene, & O'Connor, 1993). Subsidies are based on the income of the patient and pay up to 100% of the costs for as many as 5 days per week. They are paid directly to the day-care providers, who, in turn, lower the fees paid by families. Eligibility and enrollment are relatively simple. Patients must have a diagnosis of dementia or related disorder and meet income requirements. Unlike similar caregiver programs in other states, no separate assessment or evaluation is needed beyond that used by the day-care center.

The Timing of Placement

A comprehensive policy to support family caregivers also will need to address the issue of nursing home care, which we know to be not only expensive, but also laden with emotional and social significance. Without an equitable and affordable solution to this part of the care continuum, many families will continue to meet great hardship in the face of caring for a demented relative in need of placement and live in doubt about the future. If public funding of nursing home care is expanded, or some combination of public and private financing for institutional care is developed, eligibility and timing of placement will be key points of concern. As we emphasized earlier, the interests of caregiver, patient, and society may diverge on this issue.

From the family's perspective, placement makes sense when the strains associated with daily care outweigh their resources and resolve to continue. Many caregivers reach a point when they are no longer willing or able to meet the demands placed on them. This process depends more on caregivers' subjective responses than on objective indicators of severity of disease or care demands. Consequently, pressures to institutionalize do not increase steadily over the course of the disease, but ebb and flow as a result of the conditions of caregiving.

There are certain junctures involving the patient's condition at which placement makes convincing sense. As dementia progresses, patients become increasingly unaware and unresponsive to the environment. When they no longer recognize their home or loved ones, including the primary caregiver, placement seems
to be a reasonable alternative. Similarly, placement becomes a more attractive
option, as indicated earlier, when the family can no longer provide adequate care,
abuses the patient, or otherwise places the patient at risk. The agitated dementia
patient may also do better in a structured, protected environment, such as the one
provided by special Alzheimer's units in some nursing homes.

> The memory I live with and the reality
> I see when I go there is always a shock.

The optimal timing of placement does not necessarily correspond for patient
and caregiver. The decision to place, and the ways in which policies encourage or
discourage placement must be sensitive to the diverging needs of patients and
caregivers. Indeed, although it has not been a topic of this research, we suspect
that decisions regarding placement are often difficult precisely because caregivers struggle to balance their interests with those of their loved ones. Although
an optimal solution maximizing everyone's concerns may not be possible, we
also should not deal with the situation blindly by promoting the interests of
caregiver over patient, or vice versa. As we have stressed throughout this chapter,
policies must engender a system with sensitivity to individual preferences and
circumstances that allow families some control over this difficult decision.

Because of the high costs of nursing home care, alternative approaches are
likely to focus on containing expenses. For the past few years in Oregon, preadmission screenings have diverted many people eligible for Medicaid from nursing homes to small board-and-care homes, as described in chapter 12. Board-and-
care homes have been found to provide high quality, personalized care (Eckert,
Namazi, & Kahana, 1987). They may be better settings than nursing homes for
some dementia patients because they have a more homelike setting, and emphasize ordinary activities and routines. On the other hand, their small-scale and
small-profit margins may mean that staff become overwhelmed. Regulated far
less than nursing homes, these facilities may also have more potential for abuse.
It is important to note, therefore, that a comprehensive evaluation of the Oregon
program has yet to be conducted.

A similar approach has been developed in Sweden. "Group homes," small
facilities designed for dementia patients, are alternatives to nursing homes and
other intermediate forms of care (Malmberg & Zarit, 1993). A primary impetus
for their creation was the belief that the medical emphasis in nursing homes does
not provide sufficient social and physical stimulation for dementia patients.
Group homes consist of individual apartments for each resident, which are linked
to common areas and secured to the outside. The staff-to-patient ratio is quite
high by American standards (1:3 during the daytime), and staff undergo extensive formal training. Programs emphasize engaging in everyday activities, such

as assisting with cooking, cleaning, and laundry. A distinctive feature is that residents have considerable autonomy. Patients lease and furnish their apartments, and can go inside or outside when they like, locking the door behind them. This autonomy is integrated with security features that enable group homes to serve moderately to moderately severe dementia patients.

A somewhat different approach allows "aging in place." Life care communities are the prototype of this kind of facility. Older people move to these facilities when they have little or no impairment. The amount of help they receive is then adjusted upwards as they become more disabled. Recently, assisted living programs have been developed in some states that have similar features. These facilities are organized like retirement homes, but have the flexibility to increase the amount of assistance residents receive as needed. This type of program may be especially appropriate for patients in the earlier stages of dementia. A patient with mild dementia still has the ability to adjust to a new environment and routine. Then, as the person's impairments and dependencies increase, the program can make the necessary accommodations. This idea of aging in place would be particularly reassuring to older people who cannot rely on family for help.

Ethics and Public Policy

In the final analysis, caregiving raises questions of ethics that go beyond discussions of what services might be created or how they could be financed. We have already raised some important ethical issues, such as the diverging interests of patients and caregivers, and the question of equitable assistance when caregivers' situations are so heterogeneous. Those discussions addressed the various risks and costs involved in choices available to caregivers and patients, a point to which we now return.

Risks Associated with In-Home Care and Institutionalization

As described previously, many of the dementia patients' behaviors during in-home or institutional care are self-destructive. Some of these behaviors, however, threaten the safety of others as well. For example, if a patient leaves the stove on, it could cause a fire, or if a patient drives when he or she is no longer able to do so safely, he or she may crash into another car or pedestrian. Instead of pretending these dangers do not exist, we should make informed and conscious decisions about which ones are tolerable. When risks are identified in a home-care situation, the argument is often made that placement is necessary. This tactic, however, often substitutes one set of dangers for another. The same event families or providers fear that could harm the patient at home, such as a fall, could well occur in an institution, especially during the transition period when our data on mortality indicates that patients are at considerable risk of mortality.

The decision to place has to take into account two questions: What is the probability of danger, and is this a risk that the family is willing to incur? Given the variability in the behavior of dementia patients, the fact that one patient may leave a stove on does not mean that another will do the same. If a patient has not had a particular problem in the past, there is no reason to assume he or she necessarily will have that problem in the future. Also, as addressed earlier, there may be simple ways of reducing risk, such as attaching an automatic shut-off to a stove or taking away a patient's access to car keys.

The question of the family's willingness to incur risk is a more complex issue. Because no choice is risk free, families should make decisions based on their values, not solely on the recommendation of a physician or other provider, or societal expectations. Families may believe it is better to run the risk that something might happen when the patient is left at home alone than to institutionalize. When analyzing this risk, families should be encouraged to consider what the patients themselves would have wanted or, if possible, to involve patients in the discussion. We do not advocate neglect, but, instead, in the absence of perfect solutions, choosing an alternative that is the most comforting to all involved.

The Trade-offs Involved with Dementia Patients

Regrettably, the decisions about dementia patients sometimes involve compromises between longer life and quality of life. In order to continue in-home care, it may be necessary for the caregiver to go against the dementia patient's wishes. For example, a caregiver may need to counter a patient's resisting efforts to take his or her car away, or restrict his or her driving privileges if he or she is putting him or herself or others in jeopardy. Some states now even consider a diagnosis of dementia or related disorder a sufficient reason to take a license away, or will do so with a statement from a physician indicating the patient can no longer exercise the necessary judgment to drive safely.

The issue of trading longer life for quality of life is central to decisions about medical treatment. Treatments may be initiated that extend life, but that also contribute to the continuing downward spiral of quality in the dementia patient's life. For instance, in early and middle stages of dementia, patients may need surgery to correct problems, including some that may be life threatening. Surgery, especially when a general anesthetic is used, may result in hastening the decline in cognitive abilities. Additionally, the benefits of surgery may be limited if patients are unable to engage actively in rehabilitation efforts needed for recovery. This problem, however, has not received sufficient attention and should be investigated further. Thus, for some families, choosing between difficult alternatives will not be easy. Appropriately, they will feel placed between a rock and a hard place.

The Dilemma of Prolonged Medical Treatment

Trade-offs are not the only issues in medical treatment of dementia patients. Later in the course of the disease, families may be asked about life-sustaining measures, such as inserting feeding tubes when patients can no longer swallow on their own. The family may refuse to have this procedure initiated because, given current guidelines, it is very difficult to remove a feeding tube or similar device once it is in use. Another issue is whether to resuscitate. Advanced directives can address this issue, but must be on file with physicians or the nursing home.

What once was heroic care has now become routine care. Infectious diseases, such as pneumonia, which had previously been a major cause of death in old age, can be treated routinely with antibiotics, thereby prolonging dementia patients' lives. The continuing growth of new treatments is expanding what was once ordinary or expected care. Ethicists and health-care providers have debated the issue of prohibiting medical care after a particular age (Binstock & Post, 1991; D. Callahan, 1987; Jahnigen & Binstock, 1991). Many European countries either formally or informally restrict certain treatments at advanced ages. Extending life even through routine and widely accepted medical procedures is a complicated matter. On one side are advocates who support the sanctity of life, arguing that any compromise leads to a slippery slope where a variety of disadvantaged groups, including the elderly as a whole, may selectively be denied the full benefits of medical care. On the other side are those who argue the utilitarian viewpoint that we currently do not provide adequate medical care for children and pregnant women, and using scarce resources to improve the health of these groups is more important than prolonging the life of severely disabled older persons. Many people would make a quality-of-life judgment not to have their own lives needlessly extended with treatment should they have a debilitating disease like dementia. From this perspective, patients should be made as comfortable and pain free as possible, but active treatments should not be undertaken. Finally, there are discussions of euthanasia, such as currently practiced in the Netherlands (Humphry, 1984). Euthanasia, however, might not give dementia patients control over how they die unless advanced directives that were drawn up when they were competent are honored.

Concluding Comments

In the end, we must confront the ongoing tragedy of dementing illnesses. We have detailed the terrible toll that these diseases take on the family, but we should not forget the primary victim, the person suffering from dementia, who loses control, dignity, and his or her very sense of self. Current procedures are more the result of unplanned responses to a series of changes and developments in medicine and society, rather than a thoughtful strategy for addressing the consequences of degenerative diseases in later life. Because modern medicine can keep people alive longer, even in the face of chronic degenerative conditions like dementia, should we passively allow this to happen? If so, should we not provide adequate support to the families and to the institutions caring for these patients? We need to remember that providing medical care in these circumstances represents a choice over withholding it. We need to consider if it is a choice we want to make and accept the consequences of that decision.

In the face of the protracted and terrible dementing diseases, the real heroes are the family caregivers, whose exhaustive efforts go a long way in preserving dignity and honor. In a situation in which there is no good solution, where the disease is relentlessly debilitating and ultimately terminal, caregivers struggle to give meaning to their efforts and to the lives of their loved ones. They deserve an informed and intelligent debate on policy and ethical questions—free from the hysteria of television sound bites—that leads to a compassionate system of supports for caregivers and patients.

Notes

[1]The precise form and location of the curves are unknown, (e.g., their shapes might be flatter than shown here or the endpoints may differ in elevation).

A Review and Overview of Caregiving Careers

Cutting through many of the substantive findings that have been presented, some of which we shall highlight in this chapter, is a compelling theme: Caregiving is not merely a set of tasks; instead, it is a career that can envelope one's very being over a considerable span of time, often continuing in its effects long after the death of the care recipient. Caregiving involves not so much an array of responsibilities as a recurrent redirection and reorganization of one's life. Although threads of continuity are found throughout the course of caregiving, it is also evident that careers are dynamic. Underlying much of this change is the progressive character of the dementia, which drives the shifting needs for care and pulls both caregivers and patients through major transition points. At each turn and twist of their career trajectories, caregivers are faced with new circumstances calling forth different behaviors and modes of adaptation.

There is a pair of intriguing questions that emphasize the magnitude of the commitment made by caregivers: Why do people engage in this career in the first place and, once embarked on it, what keeps them going with such dogged determination? We did not design the inquiry to address internal motivations and, hence, answers to these questions do not flow readily from our data. Inevitably, however, one is led to ponder these matters. Had we found that people tended to treat the role with indifference, keeping it on the peripheries of their lives, or that people usually withdrew from the role quickly, explanations might be easier to find. After all, as the title of the book indicates, people typically do not expect that they will be immersed in providing assistance to their spouses or parents whose cognitive deterioration prohibits them from caring for themselves. And, as we saw, a fair number of caregivers are unwilling participants of the role; they would much prefer to be free of caregiving demands. Against the background of an essentially onerous disruption of the expected life course, it is difficult to explain the intense determination and commitment demonstrated by most care-givers at every step of their careers. From our qualitative interviews with care-givers, we are quite sure that it is not merely a sense either of obligatory debt or a desire for self-sacrifice that motivates people to become and remain caregivers. Instead, we are ready to accept that the most obvious explanation may also be the best explanation of the powerful grip of the caregiving career: It is an expression of the binding attachments that are established over decades of marriage or, in the case of adult children, from the earliest moments of life. It is an expression, too, of the normative imperatives that stake one's own well-being on that of the other family members.

A disclaimer needs to be offered, however implicitly, whenever statements are made concerning the motivations of caregivers or the structure of their careers. Virtually nothing of substance can be asserted that will be applicable to all caregivers under all conditions. Throughout this volume we have emphasized the diversity of careers: their circumstances and the directions and timing of their trajectories. This diversity is not only manifested in the inevitable uniqueness of caregiver–care recipient dyads but also in the patterns that differentiate social and experiential subgroups of caregivers. This disclaimer needs to be kept in mind as we recap some of our findings at different stages of the caregiving career.

The Caregiving Career

Role Acquisition

Entry into the role of family caregiver typically has a nebulous quality. In many families, the exchange of affection, attention, and assistance shifts from reciprocal to unilateral without immediate notice, a shift that may be recognized only in retrospect. The blurred beginnings of caregiving can be explained, in part, by the character of the very conditions creating the need for care. Thus, the underlying cognitive disorder, such as Alzheimer's disease (AD) or multi-infarct dementia (MID), typically has been present for some time before its symptoms are recognized as symptoms. Concomitantly, families may make spontaneous adaptations to deviations in their relative's memory and behavior long before realizing that these changes are out of the ordinary. As a result, many caregivers take up the tasks of caregiving before they come to see themselves as being a caregiver. In addition, as we saw in chapter 4, medical treatment often is not sought for substantial periods of time following symptom recognition.

The sequencing and timing of transitional events within the role acquisition phase is consequential because most of what we know about caregiving is information gleaned after symptom recognition and after diagnosis. Certainly this is the case with the present inquiry: all caregivers saw themselves as caregivers and most of their relatives had received a diagnosis. Other research suffers from this limitation as well because it is difficult to identify in advance who will become a caregiver.

We have demonstrated that many caregivers do not consult a physician until long after they realize that something is wrong with their relatives. Studies of diagnosed patients, therefore, should take into consideration illness duration prior to diagnosis. Similarly, studies of self-identified caregivers should take into consideration not only how long care has been provided but also illness duration. We make these self-evident points only because issues of timing, sequence, and duration often are overlooked in caregiving research.

Role Enactment

Although caregiving is often thought of as being synonymous with home care, we have seen that enactment of the caregiving role is not confined to this setting. Instead, this career stage encompasses decisions about nursing home placement as well as the provision of care within an institutional setting. Furthermore, home care, preparation for placement, and institutional care exist not as separate entities but are woven together to form a cohesive pattern of experience extending through time. The conditions encountered in providing in-home care shape, at least partially, decisions about institutional placement and adjustment to this transitional event. Consolidating these elements into one stage of the caregiving career emphasizes the continuity of experience that permeates each separate segment.

The decision to institutionalize one's parent or spouse cannot be understood in isolation from the situational context that leads caregivers to consider this option in the first place. As we saw in chapter 8, most of the caregivers who earlier were loathe to place their relatives ultimately do so, an action that goes against the grain of their earlier sentiments. The unrelenting degenerative course of dementia contributes to institutionalization, especially when it is manifest as troublesome and disruptive behavior. Characteristics of the dementia are less important to the risk of institutionalization, however, than the extent to which the dementia creates conditions of stress for the caregiver. Role captivity is particularly important in this respect: caregivers who feel trapped by their caregiving responsibilities tend to seek relief from institutionalization and, moreover, tend to feel relieved following this transition, as shown in chapter 9. In addition, the conditions encountered within the home prior to institutionalization shape the caregivers' understanding of why they have turned to institutional care, an action they attribute to demands that exceed their resources (i.e., to the stressful nature of caregiving).

Nursing home admission connects home care and institutional care. It can be seen as an act of coping with caregiving demands because this step frequently is taken to alleviate stress associated with home care. However, the implementation of the decision to place is often a source of stress itself. Thus, caregivers typically experience considerable anticipatory stress, many have difficulties in locating a suitable facility, and some are burdened by intense guilt. As we saw in chapter 8, these problems flow from the conditions of in-home caregiving existing immediately prior to admission; that is, placement difficulties are most likely to arise when there are other problems in the caregiver's life, especially when the caregiver is in poor health, when there is family conflict, and when financial resources are tenuous. Indeed, financial strain generally impedes institutionalization. The extent to which such problems emerge during placement is more directly related to dimensions of care-related stress than to the state of cognitive or functional impairment of the patient.

The encouragement given the caregiver by others to place their relatives in nursing homes typically is grounded in the belief that placement will alleviate the burdens associated with caregiving. This expectation generally is met, but only to a limited degree. In many respects, institutionalization alters the types of stressors encountered by caregivers rather than alleviating care-related stress overall. As we saw in chapter 9, caregivers usually do not depend on the institution for the entirety of care needed by their relative. On the contrary, they are likely to continue to provide substantial supplementary assistance, sometimes at the considerable expense of their own time and energies. Moreover, although the caregivers in this study generally were satisfied with the care their relatives received, some encountered substantial difficulties long after admission. In this regard, institutional care emerges as a new source of stress, replacing rather than eliminating the stressors encountered during home care.

Caregivers differ substantially from one another in how well they adapt to institutionalization; occasionally, too, caregivers who adapt well in one domain of functioning do less well in other domains. As would be expected, this variability can be attributed partially to the conditions of institutional care, especially the degree of satisfaction with the care facility and the services it provides. Adaptation also depends to some extent on the linkages between home care and institutional care. This is illustrated best by the carryover of role captivity. Elevated levels of role captivity prompt institutionalization, which generally alleviates this source of stress. When role captivity remains elevated following placement, however, adaptation is likely to be poor. Thus, the conditions of home care and their continuity influence the quality of caregiver adaptation to institutional care.

Role Disengagement

During the course of our study only a very small number of caregivers withdrew from the role, either leaving it entirely to other family members or to institutional staff. Yet, for most caregivers, the eventual demise of their spouse or parent acts inevitably as a lever for role disengagement. Despite the fact that the caregivers are likely to greet death with a sigh of relief for themselves as well as for their deceased relative, the involuntary cessation of the role does not immediately allow the caregiver to embark on a fresh start. Death is a discrete and clearly discernible event, but the disengagement that follows is a process that extends over time and only gradually winds down. For some the process may come to a comparatively quick conclusion, but for others, grief may continue for the remainder of their own lives.

Disengagement can be described at multiple interrelated levels. Thus, it can entail the confrontation and resolution of various dimensions of loss—for example, loss of an established role that filled one's life, of a shared past and a planned-for future, loss of status and material resources, and so on. Death, no matter how clearly or for how long it was forecast, is also likely to let loose currents of unpleasant grief reactions of various kinds, each of which may run its course at a different pace. Disengagement certainly entails coming to terms with grief in all its forms, whether this means learning to live with it or resolving it. In the long run, disengagement from the role may initiate a reengagement with one's self, reflected, for example, in the establishment or activation of network ties, reinvestment in occupational life, the discovery of new interests, and the elevation of self-concepts, such as mastery.

We have emphasized that the conditions experienced during each phase of the caregiving career may be influenced by those in preceding stages and are potential sources of influence on succeeding stages. This is nowhere more evident than in the case of role disengagement brought on by death. The extent to which caregivers previously felt that their relative had already been lost to them is pivotal in this regard. The early sense that the quintessential character of the dementia patient has been lost to the caregiver has a bearing on the subsequent disengagement process and adaptation to death. For example, the early acknowledgment of this loss helps to diminish the intensity and duration of grief reactions and of depression. Clearly, caregivers do not shed what they have acquired in one career stage after transition to another; and what they carry forward influences that which transpires during the new stage.

I feel like I have a life ahead of me.

What we have learned without any doubt is that the cessation of the caregiving activities is not coterminous with the cessation of the caregiving career. It continues on through what might be a lengthy period of emotional and behavioral disengagement and the reorganization of life without the presence of a caregiving role.

The Care-Related Stress Process

Whereas the construct of career is useful in understanding the continuities and discontinuities of the organization and reorganization of caregivers' lives through time, the construct of the stress process orients our attention specifically to experiences having the potential to exert deleterious effects. The two concepts are highly congenial and conceptually synergistic, of course, for the stress process is an experiential reflection of careers and their changing trajectories. What we have been able to learn about the stress process from the longitudinal study of caregivers to someone suffering from dementia has implications reaching far beyond this group. Although the particular circumstances we have examined pertain strictly to caregivers, we believe that the components of the process and their interconnections are applicable to other groups embedded in situations that give rise to chronic stressors.

At the same time, the application of the stress process framework to a population of caregivers has served as a guide to certain practical issues. As spelled out in chapters 12 and 13, the framework has helped to bring to light the panoply of hidden material and psychological costs often incurred in the course of caregiving. Some of these costs can be reduced by informed intervention on the part of professional workers, and the stress process framework serves as a useful map showing the way to potentially effective points and modes of intervention. Similarly, it provides an heuristic backdrop for making explicit the often unrecognized choices bound up in the development of public policies.

One of the key features of the stress process framework is the distinction between primary and secondary stressors, the latter viewed as problematic conditions lying outside of caregiving activities but that are, nevertheless, the consequences of caregiving. As indicated by the findings that are highlighted below, the causal links between primary and secondary stressors, reflecting stress proliferation, are critical elements of the stress process.

The Impact of Primary Stressors

The degenerative course followed by dementia functions as a catalyst, initiating and maintaining a process of stress proliferation. Cognitive abilities—such as remembering recent events and understanding simple instructions—decline with time, of course, a trajectory characteristic of dementia. The most direct and prominent casualty of this decline is the caregiver's feeling of having already lost one's husband, wife, father, or mother. Waning cognitive abilities and the accompanying erosion of the patient's persona coalesce to exert inexorable pressure on the caregiver's own sense of self, and, ultimately, on his or her emotional well-being.

The cognitive decline of the dementia patient, however, is not the sole element propelling the stress process. A distinct contribution to stress proliferation is made by the actual tasks impinging upon the caregiver, as was evident in chapter 6. The demands confronting caregivers are shaped by the underlying dementia and the dependencies it fosters. In general, the greater the dependency, the greater the assistance that is provided. This alignment is far from perfect, however: as demands escalate, some caregivers reduce their own involvement in care, some by recruiting other informal caregivers, others by turning to formal sources for supplementary assistance. Indeed, how family members respond to escalating demands often depends less upon the course of the dementia per se than upon characteristics of the care recipient, the caregiver, their shared history, and the social, economic, and cultural contexts within which they find themselves.

Assistance provided by the caregiver with activities of daily living (ADLs) proves to be consequential largely because performing these tasks engenders role overload. The sense of being overwhelmed by caregiving increases as the tasks of caregiving become more extensive and more frequent, especially among caregivers whose initial responsibilities were circumscribed. Role overload, in turn, affects emotional well-being through its links to secondary stressors, in particular damage inflicted upon the caregiver's own sense of self. Caregiving tasks sometimes interfere with outside employment as well, providing an additional link to the stress-proliferation process.

The management of troublesome, disruptive, and oppositional behavior also plays an essential role in the development of caregiving stress and its emotional sequelae. Such behavior occupies a prominent place in the caregiving experience as it evolves over time, including actions like wandering, waking the caregiver, and being uncooperative. Unlike cognitive impairment, however, problematic behavior does not necessarily increase with time, nor does the extent to which caregivers must supervise and control erratic behavior. The fact that behavioral problems are not always linked to the state of cognitive deterioration means that behavioral management exists as a separate source of caregiving stress in and of itself.

As indicated in chapter 6, the management of behavioral problems is especially noteworthy because it contributes to stress proliferation over both the short- and long-term course of in-home caregiving. Over a 1-year period, the control of behavioral problems, especially problems that escalate at a rapid rate, produces an intensification of role captivity. When unmanageable patient behavior escalates over 3 years, it generates not only role captivity, but role overload as well. And, as we have demonstrated repeatedly, these subjective stressors bear importantly upon the caregiver's emotional well-being and upon decisions regarding admission of the patient to a nursing home.

The objective primary stressors of caregiving matter to the mental health of caregivers in large part because these conditions generate subjective primary stressors and because these subjective stressors, in turn, affect emotional well-being. The demands imposed by the unrelenting course of dementia require not only behavioral responses from caregivers, but also elicit internal cognitive, attitudinal, and emotional responses. These internal reactions are products of the meaning caregivers attach to the conditions they encounter and to the circumstances in which they find themselves. In general, the greater the assistance provided, the greater the sense of being overwhelmed and engulfed by the caregiving role. However, some assiduous caregivers are not beset by these negative internal states even though under considerable objective demand, whereas others experience intense stress at low objective levels of hardship. The extent to which objective conditions translate into subjective stressors, then, plays a major role in accounting for variation in the impact of providing care upon caregivers.

In sum, the objective conditions of caregiving influence the process of stress proliferation along two fronts. One is the progression of the dementia itself, especially the rate at which cognitive abilities are deteriorating and personality is fading. The other is the expansion of responsibilities for attending to the care recipient's needs and for supervising his or her behavior. Characteristics of the illness and the ways in which caregivers respond to them contribute to both the genesis and intensification of subjective primary stressors, which, in turn, influence emotional well-being.

The Impact of Secondary Stressors

The results of this investigation demonstrate that caregiving cannot be understood in isolation from the social context within which the role is enacted. The lives of caregivers necessarily entail connection to and participation in other social institutions, even though some caregivers feel quite isolated from society. The multiple institutional ties of caregivers are evidenced by their occupancy of other social roles and by the emergence of strain within these roles, especially strain that emanates from enactment of the role of caregiver. Caregivers differ from one another with regard to the configuration of their attachments to such social institutions as occupation and family. Moreover, it cannot be assumed that role strain flows inevitably from role occupancy because some caregivers experience little conflict between caregiving and their other social roles, whereas others grapple with seemingly irreconcilable demands among their multiple roles.

We have demonstrated that the lives of caregivers do indeed extend beyond the confines of caregiving, that there is considerable variation among caregivers with regard to the extent of their attachments to various social institutions, and, perhaps most importantly, that these attachments sometimes serve as additional sources of stress. The key point is not simply that caregivers encounter stress from social roles other than caregiving, but rather that caregiving is the origin of stress in these other social roles.

Clearly, caregiving is not the source of all stress: these social roles are quite capable of exerting stress in their own right. For example, workers who are not caregivers certainly encounter problematic conditions in their occupational lives. Employed caregivers, however, are exposed to strains that have no presence in the experience of other workers; namely, conflict between working and caregiving. Such strains are unique to caregivers. A distinctive contribution of this investigation, therefore, is the identification of specific types of secondary stressors, and, perhaps more importantly, the demonstration that caregivers differ from one another in their exposure to these secondary stressors.

Our differentiation of primary and secondary stressors, therefore, is essential to understanding why caregiving has more deleterious effects among some caregivers than others. The total burden of care encompasses both components: difficulties encountered in the actual provision of care, and problems encountered in other areas of life as a consequence of being a caregiver. As reported in chapter 6, increases in primary stressors are accompanied by increments in certain role strains and by an erosion of personal identity and other self-concepts, secondary stressors with depressive consequences. Secondary stressors, therefore, serve both as a conduit through which the tasks of providing care affect emotional well-being and, once they are established, as sources of stress in their own right.

Although primary and secondary sources of stress tend to accompany one another, it is also true that some highly stressful care situations are tightly contained, whereas some less demanding circumstances may disrupt virtually all aspects of life. The spread of stress from one domain of life to another is not determined solely by the course of the dementia; if this were the case, then caregivers would appear more homogeneous than they are with respect to their exposure to secondary stressors. Instead, we have seen that caregivers differ widely from one another in the extent to which caregiving is accompanied by difficulties within the family, in regard to employment, and in respect to finances.

For some considerations, the relationship between primary and secondary stressors is of less import than their combined impact upon the caregiver. Each tells only half of the story. Unfortunately, it is not possible to enumerate exhaustively all of the stressors potentially impinging upon caregivers because this universe is infinite. Consequently, it is necessary to sample this universe and to sample it in a manner that surveys the entire area encompassed by its boundaries. Measuring caregiving stress solely in terms of difficulties encountered in the provision of care is problematic because this strategy omits a substantial component of this universe, and, most importantly, because the omitted component is conceptually distinct. Primary stressors cannot be thought of as proxies for secondary stressors. Hence, primary stressors are not adequate measures of the entire spectrum of care-related stressors.

This issue is critical to the explanation of variation in outcomes among caregivers. The most straightforward explanation attributes differences in these outcomes to corresponding differences in exposure to care-related stressors (i.e., some people are more harmed by caregiving than others because they encounter more severe care-related stressors). If exposure is measured exclusively in terms of primary stressors, however, only the variation attributable to this component is taken into consideration. As we have seen, this component is quite distinctive from that of secondary stressors. Estimates of the impact of differential exposure based upon primary stressors, therefore, are poor proxies for the contribution of differential exposure to secondary stressors or to care-related stressors in toto.

If the secondary stressors contributing to variation in outcomes are ignored, the variation is likely to be attributed erroneously to other factors, especially factors that covary with exposure. The issue, then, is not that each and every stressor to which a caregiver might be exposed needs to be taken into account; it is, rather, that those stressors stemming from the caregiver's integration into the larger social system should not be overlooked because these kinds of stressors contribute importantly to the psychological costs of caregiving. As we have seen, caregivers are not uniformly at risk for secondary stressors; instead, the chances of such exposure are related to the social, personal, and economic circumstances within which care is provided. For example, low income, low education, and running out of money each month exacerbate anticipatory worries about the institutionalization of the dementia patient.

In sum, caregivers do not respond uniformly to being a caregiver. Some of these differences in outcomes are due to parallel differences in exposure to care-related stressors. Exposure, in turn, must be gauged in relation to two conceptually distinct types of stressors, one anchored directly in providing care to the impaired relative and the second anchored in other activities and self-knowledge. It is understandable that the constellations of stressors surrounding caregivers may be composed of a richly mixed array of hardships.

Psychosocial Resources and Stress Containment

The psychosocial resources people possess potentially have an explanatory function within the stress process framework similar to that of secondary stressors. We emphasized that people alike in their exposure to primary stressors can be quite different with regard to the secondary stressors to which they are exposed, and the assessment of such differences can help to explain variations in outcome. Now we consider those who may be similar in their exposure to stressors, primary or secondary, but still differ in the outcomes they manifest. One reason for such variation, we submit, is that people differ in their access to and use of resources having the capacity to constrain the effects of care-related stressors. Thus, both differences in the mix of primary and secondary stressors and differences in the possession of constraining resources can help make sense of the outcomes being observed.

There are at least three ways in which resources may constrain the stress process. First, they may mediate the impact of the stressors, a case where stressors exert an impact on outcomes through their effects on the resources. Next, they may moderate or buffer the impact of the stressor on the outcome. In this instance, the resource combines with the stressor such that those exposed to the most intense stressors benefit most from the resource. Finally, resources may affect the outcomes independently of the stressors, exerting a direct influence on the outcomes, effects that are referred to as main or additive effects. Each of these approaches was empirically tested but the only constraining effects revealed by our analyses were those that were independent. Thus, to the extent that the resources matter to the ultimate emotional well-being of caregivers, they matter in ways other than the transformation of the relationship between the stressors and indicators of well-being.

Our analysis of the independent effects of psychosocial resources illustrates vividly the complex intertwining of resources with the various junctures of the stress process. Generally, the analysis revealed a picture involving some specialization between the type of resource and the nature of the outcome it was constraining. In particular, informal instrumental support, especially where it provides hands-on help with patient care, is effective in constraining the levels of two subjective primary stressors over a period of a year, role captivity and role overload. However, the same type of support does not directly constrain any of the secondary stressors. By contrast, socioemotional support has a direct constraining effect on only one subjective primary stressor, the loss of intimate exchange, but does reduce family conflict and elevate caregivers' assessments of their competence and gains from being a caregiver. Still different in its effect is mastery, which constrains each of the three subjective primary stressors as well as work strain.

This picture of the specialized constraining effects of resources, especially on the intermediate outcomes of the stress process, strongly indicates that research in this area should adopt a more advanced conceptual orientation. Concretely, our findings suggest that it is necessary to ask a more detailed question than usually raised about resources and their effects: what kind of resource, in relation to what kind of stressor, has what kind of effect, on what kind of outcome, over what period of time. This is not a question that can be answered with ease, but the more closely we approximate an answer, the closer we shall come to understanding the naturalistic interventions that occur at the various points of the stress process, interventions that undoubtedly help most caregivers continue in the role over the long haul.

An additional aspect of our findings with regard to social support deserves emphasis, namely that caregivers as a group do not receive sufficient support. The overall level of instrumental social support is deficient. This conclusion pertains to both informal and formal sources of support: Caregivers do not receive sufficient assistance from their families and friends and this deficiency is not offset by the receipt of health and social services. Moreover, whether or not informal instrumental support is received is largely independent of the conditions of caregiving (i.e., need is unrelated to assistance).

This observation invites speculation that instrumental support does not appear to be as important as we had anticipated simply because the amount of assistance received, relative to need, is not sufficient to make a difference. Our failure to detect buffering or mediating effects may be due to the weak association observed between need and the receipt of instrumental social support. Although some primary stressors are related to the amount of support received, these effects are neither strong nor widespread. For example, having formal support, an in-home attendant, depends upon the level of cognitive impairment of the dementia patient and the rate at which cognitive abilities are declining. However, other dimensions of primary stress, most notably the subjective stressors of role overload and role captivity, which capture the impact of caregiving demands on the caregiver, do not exert independent effects on whether there is an attendant assisting with patient care. Under these circumstances, it is hardly surprising that formal support neither mediates nor moderates the impact of stress on the caregiver's emotional well-being. Thus, psychosocial resources are pervasively beneficial, but those who need these resources most are not especially likely to have them. Consequently, these resources do little to alleviate the pernicious effects of care-related stress.

Whereas the effects of stressors are generally negative, those of resources are generally in a positive direction. Thus resources contribute to the variability in the responses of caregivers to seemingly similar stressors by counterbalancing or offsetting the pernicious effects of the stressors. Some of the caregivers exposed to intense stressors fare better than others because they receive more support from friends and family and feel a greater sense of self-efficacy. Exposure to stress remains harmful, but its damage is compensated for by these assets. Furthermore, these resources affect subsequent exposure to care-related stressors. Among caregivers who face similar initial conditions, those who have adequate psychosocial resources are likely subsequently to encounter improved circumstances, whereas those who lack social and personal resources are likely to face deteriorating conditions. The conclusion we wish to emphasize is that psychosocial resources influence not only the ultimate outcome of care-related stress, such as emotional distress or the risk of nursing home admission, but rather the entire process of stress proliferation.

Interpreting Variation in the Impact of Stressors

A theme recurring throughout this volume concerns variation in reactions to caregiving, specifically the question of why some caregivers seem impervious to hardships that severely damage others. Variations in outcomes, such as depression, are often equated with individual differences in vulnerability, that is, the idea that some caregivers are more susceptible to the deleterious effects of stress. Individual differences in stress reactivity may exist, of course: some people seem to be especially resilient or to cope extremely well. This investigation, however, has provided evidence supporting three alternative explanations that should be considered before resorting to vulnerability, which, we submit, should be viewed as the explanation of last resort (i.e., the residual explanation).

First, differential stress reactivity may be illusory, the result of mistakenly attributing unmeasured differences in exposure to vulnerability. We have demonstrated that caregivers who are similar with regard to the primary stressors of caregiving often face dissimilar secondary stressors. Under conditions of stress proliferation, the total level of exposure to care-related stressors is heightened. Variation in outcomes, therefore, can be attributed to parallel variation in exposure. From this perspective, caregivers are not reacting differently to the same level of exposure, their exposure differs. Thus, it is necessary to conduct a comprehensive assessment of exposure to both primary and secondary stressors to accurately identify the components of outcomes that are attributable to exposure versus vulnerability.

The second explanation focuses upon the notion that stress is not solely an attribute of demand, but of resources as well: specifically, that stress arises when demands exceed resources. The results pertaining to stress containment (chapter 7) clearly indicate that differential access to psychosocial resources is responsible for some of the variation in outcomes observed among caregivers. In this regard, it is necessary to emphasize that resources exert independent effects on outcomes as distinct from altering the impact of stressors; the latter would be more consistent with a stress-reactivity explanation. Thus, some caregivers appear more damaged by exposure to care-related stressors because they also lack psychosocial resources and because this deficit itself is damaging.

Third, some caregivers only appear to be unaffected when they are indeed damaged by care-related stressors. Most assessments of the impact of caregiving focus on single outcomes (e.g., depression) and implicitly count those who do not manifest that outcome (e.g., those who are not depressed) as unaffected by exposure. At least some of these persons are in fact affected but manifest it as other outcomes (e.g., premature institutionalization). The absence of one type of negative outcome, therefore, should not be confused with the absence of any stress-induced harm.

In large part, this investigation has been dedicated to describing the multiple outcomes of care-related stress, such as the emergence of secondary stressors, premature institutionalization, adaptation to institutionalization, grief, and social readjustment. In the absence of this type of comprehensive assessment, the impact of caregiving inevitably is underestimated. Equally important, focusing on a single outcome runs the risk of attributing variation in that outcome to individual differences in vulnerability, whereas it may be due to systematic differences in the form of reaction. Thus, the calculation of the consequences of caregiving, especially variation in the magnitude of these consequences, requires that a comprehensive and inclusive approach be taken to identify potential outcomes or costs.

The Impact of Social Standing

It is compellingly evident, then, that exposure to care-related stressors is not a uniform occurrence, nor is its distribution happenstance. Instead, variability in the types and intensity of stressors depend, at least in part, upon circumstances *external* to caregiving. Caregiving does not go on in a vacuum, separated either from one's social and experiential past or present. On the contrary, caregiving is likely to be but one facet of people's lives, a component integrated into the overall arrangement of their multiple roles and selves. Although caregiving has an imperialistic quality, typically constricting involvements in other social activities, it usually does not stand as the sole activity or relationship in which one is involved. Instead, the circumstances and experiences of caregiving are influenced by the caregiver's engagement in other domains of his or her life, and conversely, the quality of experience within these domains is influenced by caregiving. In essence, the experience of care-related stress is organized by the overarching structure implicit in the lives of caregivers.

This conclusion is not immediately apparent from empirical results that seem to place the characteristics of caregivers at the periphery of stress proliferation. Specifically, sociodemographic and economic attributes do not emerge as potent independent influences on various outcomes, especially when these outcomes are examined over time. Most surprising in this regard is the relative insignificance of the kin relationship of caregivers and patients (i.e., the similarities observed among wives, husbands, daughters and sons are far more numerous than the observed differences). However, it would be erroneous to interpret these kinds of results as evidence that the impact of caregiving is universal, not dependent upon the caregiver's characteristics or locations in the social system. Such a conclusion is not justified.

Instead, it is likely that the impact of background characteristics is exerted almost immediately with the initiation of caregiving and, therefore, is captured in the baseline levels of care-related stressors. This early influence of background factors on stressors is then transmitted over time via the stability of these stressors (i.e., in the marked tendency for caregivers to maintain their relative standing to one another over time). In cross-sectional analysis of these rankings, kin relationship and income emerge as key correlates of exposure to both primary and secondary stressors. The main exception to this generalization is severity of the dementia patient's cognitive impairment, which is virtually independent of the socioeconomic background characteristics of caregivers, testimony to the democratic nature of dementia.

For kin relationship, it is not simply the case that combinations of gender and generation result in more or less exposure to stress. For example, adult children, on average, encounter a heavier burden of primary stressors, but husbands are most laden with ADL dependencies, and wives are most keenly troubled by their affectional detachment from the patient. Consequently, spouses and offspring, husbands and wives, appear to differ most in which stressors they are apt to encounter as distinct from simple differences in the quantity or overall level of the stressors.

The results for income confirm our hypothesis that socioeconomic resources enable caregivers to contain the extent to which the patient's condition becomes burdensome. When income matters to exposure, the pattern is consistently negative in sign: exposure declines as income increases. The exception, again, is the level of cognitive impairment, which is independent of income or other indicators of social standing. Thus, at similar levels of patient disability, those with the least economic resources are most likely to be providing extensive help to the patient, help that is experienced as overwhelming and that interferes with the enactment of other social roles. Thus, caregiving should not be viewed as a closed system the components of which are influenced only by other components of the system. Instead, caregiving is embedded within the context of the caregiver's life course and his or her contemporaneous social standing.

In Retrospect

It is in the very nature of scientific inquiry that new knowledge is built on the shoulders of what is already known. We believe that the work reported here realizes this ideal, at least to some modest degree. Certainly, we are the beneficiaries of many committed researchers who preceded us and whose work laid much of the foundation for this inquiry. To the extent that we have succeeded in advancing our understanding of a population whose ranks can only grow in the future, it should be taken as a tribute to others who have also dedicated themselves to rigorous research into stress and caregiving. And we await with pleasure those who are undoubtedly at this time preparing to go beyond this work. However, it would not be an exaggeration to assert that the theoretical perspectives guiding this investigation and the scope and richness of the data gathered over the years have resulted in what is probably the most comprehensive inquiry yet undertaken into long-term caregiving and its stresses. We cannot assert, however, that the work is without its share of shortcomings. We briefly point to three of these areas because they are especially relevant to the design of future research.

One concerns the composition of our sample. It will be recalled that for the most part the sample was gathered from the rolls of the San Francisco Bay Area and Los Angeles chapters of the ADRDA. We are not concerned that this method of recruitment cannot result in a representative sample. For the most part, the social and economic diversity of our sample, although probably not representative of the universe of caregivers, is sufficient to satisfy the analytic goals and strategies of the study. However, we have a pair of regrets about the composition of the sample. First, we suspect that there are caregivers who "go it alone" in the community, providing care without benefit of ties to voluntary associations or other organizations, including care facilities. If there are such independent and invisible caregivers in any appreciable numbers, their experiences could be highly instructive. In particular, they could help to reveal the kinds of conditions that lend themselves to self-sufficient caregiving, such as family organization, personal and social resources, and so on. Next, although the sample contains a fairly sizable number of ethnic and racial minority group members, there are too few in each group to permit comparative analyses. Future research should seek to specify the cultural factors that undoubtedly influence the career trajectories and stressful experiences of caregivers.

Second, our sample predominantly is caring for someone with AD, which precludes an assessment of whether disease makes a unique contribution to the caregiving career. Thus, we do not have a sufficient number of cases of other specific forms of dementia to determine whether the underlying disease matters to the evolution of this social role. More generally, at this point, we cannot ascertain which components are shared across different forms of impairment, for example, dementia versus cancer. Thus, it is important that future research be designed in such a way as to permit the identification of both the unique features associated with specific impairments and those that are shared in common across all caregiving contexts. For practical reasons, it may not be feasible to study multiple disorders in a single study. However, coordination of research strategies across studies would facilitate this type of metacomparison.

Finally, we can also observe that our treatment of the care recipient is considerably more limited than that of the caregiver, a deficiency future research should correct. By and large, this study does not take sufficient account of dementia patients as actors in the caregiving process. We have, of course, assessed the range of their functional dependencies, their cognitive status, and their behavioral symptoms, but we know little of their modes of interaction with and emotional responses to the caregiver. This does not mean that we should necessarily know the care recipient as well as we know the caregiver or that attention to each party should be balanced. It is reasonable and legitimate to place the caregiver at the forefront of our interests, just as other types of inquiries principally concern the dementia patient. What we would argue, however, is that our vision of the trials and triumphs of caregivers might come into sharper focus by taking greater account in future research of caregiving as an interactive system.

Closing Commentary

None of the collaborators in this research is or has been a long-term caregiver to a relative or friend. It is understandable, then, that initially we viewed our participants across some distance; much as one would regard any alien group, we thought of caregivers as "they" or "them." This was particularly the case, of course, with those of us having no prior professional contact with caregivers. This distance quickly began to close when the interviewing process began; although early in the work it remained difficult to appreciate fully what it is like to be a caregiver, the very first interviews provided ample opportunity to acquire a large measure of compassion and sympathy for caregivers. As our knowledge of caregiving accumulated in the course of trying to make sense out of the data we were collecting, it gradually became apparent that caregivers' careers, although unique in some respects, share some elements in common with the careers of others. With this awareness, we began to understand that the fates of caregivers are bound up, however indirectly, with those of others who, like ourselves, are not caregivers.

The fun side of me is back.

The sense of unity that emerged over the course of the inquiry fundamentally stems from the recognition that all of us are influenced by and struggling to make our way through many of the same institutions. Whether we are caregivers or not, most of us are members of larger family systems in which there are passionate loyalties; we must reconcile our engagement in occupational systems with our participation in other activities just as employed caregivers do; economic resources affect the choices we can make, no less then as in the case of caregivers; our networks support us as do those of caregivers, and so on. The point is not that groups are identical in their interests and the demands they face; far from it. It is rather, that everyone has a stake in seeing the surrounding social institutions of which we are all a part function effectively for everyone. If these institutions fail some segments of society in efforts to attain legitimate goals, then surely they fail us all.

References

Abel, E. K. (1987). *Love is not enough. Family care of the frail elderly*. Washington, DC: American Public Health Association.

Afifi, A. A., & Clark, V. (1984). Canonical correlation analysis: Examining linear relationships between two sets of variables. In *Computer-aided multivariate analysis* (pp. 361–378). Belmont, CA: Lifetime Learning.

American Psychiatric Association. (1994). *Diagnostic and statistical manual of mental disorders* (4th ed.). Washington, DC: Author.

Aneshensel, C. S. (1992). Social stress: Theory and research. *Annual Review of Sociology, 18*, 15–38.

Aneshensel, C. S. (in press). Consequences of psychosocial stress. In H. B. Kaplan (Ed.), *Psychosocial stress*. San Diego, CA: Academic Press.

Aneshensel, C. S., Pearlin, L. I., & Schuler, R. H. (1993). Stress, role captivity, and the cessation of caregiving. *Journal of Health and Social Behavior, 34*, 54–70.

Anthony, J. C., & Aboraya, A. (1992). The epidemiology of selected mental disorders in later life. In J. E. Birren, R. B. Sloane, & G. D. Cohen (Eds.), *Handbook of mental health and aging* (2nd ed., pp. 27–72). San Diego, CA: Academic Press.

Arthur, M. B., Hall, D. T., & Lawrence, B. S. (1989). Generating new directions in career theory: The case for a transdisciplinary approach. In M. B. Arthur, D. T. Hall, & B. S. Lawrence (Eds.), *Handbook of career theory* (pp. 7–25). Cambridge, UK: Cambridge University Press.

Barley, S. R. (1989). Careers, identities, and institutions: The legacy of the Chicago School of Sociology. In M. B. Arthur, D. T. Hall, & B. S. Lawrence (Eds.), *Handbook of career theory* (pp. 41–65). Cambridge, UK: Cambridge University Press.

Bass, D. M., & Bowman, K. (1990). The transition from caregiving to bereavement: The relationship of care-related strain and adjustment to death. *Gerontologist, 30*, 35–44.

Baumgarten, M. (1989). The health of persons giving care to the demented elderly: A critical review of the literature. *Journal of Clinical Epidemiology, 42*, 1137–1148.

Beck, A. T., Rush, D., Shaw, D., & Emery, G. (1979). *Cognitive therapy of depression*. New York: Guilford Press.

Becker, H. S. (1953). Becoming a marihuana user. *American Journal of Sociology, 59*, 235–242.

Belloni-Sonzogni, A., Tissot, A., Tettamanti, M., Frattura, L., & Spagnoli, A. (1989). Mortality of demented patients in a geriatric institution. *Archives of Gerontology and Geriatrics, 9*, 193–197.

Belsley, D. A. (1984). Demeaning conditioning diagnostics through centering. *American Statistician, 38*, 73–93.

Berg, S., Nilsson, L., & Svanborg, A. (1988). Behavioral and clinical aspects: Longitudinal studies. In J. P. Wattis & I. Hindmarch (Eds.), *Psychological assessment of the elderly* (pp. 47–60). London: Churchill-Livingstone.

Bernstein, G. M., & Offenbartl, S. K. (1991). Adverse surgical outcomes among patients with cognitive impairments. *American Surgeon, 57*, 682–690.

Berry, G. L., Zarit, S. H., & Rabatin, V. X. (1991). Caregiver activity on respite and nonrespite days: A comparison of two service approaches. *Gerontologist, 31*, 830–835.

Binstock, R. H., & Post, S. G. (1991). Old age and the rationing of health care. In R. H. Binstock & S. G. Post (Eds.), *Too old for health care? Controversies in medicine, law, economics, and ethics* (pp. 1–12). Baltimore: Johns Hopkins University Press.

Bodnar, J. C., & Kiecolt-Glaser, J. K. (1994). Caregiver depression after bereavement: Chronic stress isn't over when it's over. *Psychology and Aging, 9,* 372–380.

Bowlby, J. (1980). *Attachment and loss* (Vol. 3). New York: Basic Books.

Branch, L. G., & Jette, A. M. (1982). A prospective study of long-term care institutionalization among the aged. *American Journal of Public Health, 72,* 1373–1379.

Brauer, E., Mackeprang, B., & Bentzon, M. W. (1978). Prognosis of survival in a geriatric population. *Scandinavian Journal of Social Medicine, 6,* 17–24.

Brody, E. M. (1985). Parent care as a normative family stress. *Gerontologist, 25,* 19–29.

Callahan, D. (1987). *Setting limits: Medical goals in an aging society.* New York: Simon & Schuster.

Callahan, J. J., Jr. (1989b). Case management for the elderly: A panacea? *Journal of Aging and Social Policy, 1,* 181–195.

Callahan, J. J., Jr. (1989a). Play it again Sam: There is no impact. *Gerontologist, 29,* 5–6.

Cantor, M. H. (1983). Strain among caregivers: A study of experience in the United States. *Gerontologist, 23,* 597–604.

Carcagno, G. J., & Kemper, P. (1988). The evaluation of the national long-term care demonstration: An overview of the Channeling demonstration and its evaluation. *HSR: Health Services Research, 23,* 1–22.

Caserta, M. S., Lund, D. A., Wright, S. D., & Redburn, D. E. (1987). Caregivers to dementia patients: The utilization of community services. *Gerontologist, 27,* 209–214.

Chenoweth, B., & Spencer, B. (1986). Dementia: The experience of family caregivers. *Gerontologist, 26,* 267–272.

Cobb, S. (1976). Social support as a moderator of life stress. *Psychosomatic Medicine, 38,* 300–314.

Cohen, M. A., Tell, E. J., & Wallack, S. S. (1986). Client-related risk factors of nursing home entry among elderly adults. *Journal of Gerontology, 41,* 785–792.

Cohler, B. J. (1983). Autonomy and interdependence in the family of adulthood: A psychological perspective. *Gerontologist, 23,* 33–39.

Cohler, B. J., Groves, L., Borden, W., & Lazarus, L. (1989). Caring for family members with Alzheimer's disease. In E. Light & B. D. Lebowitz (Eds.), *Alzheimer's disease treatment and family stress: Directions for research* (pp. 50–105). Rockville, MD: U.S. Department of Health and Human Services.

Cressey, P. G. (1932). *The taxi-dance hall: A sociological study in commercialized recreation and city life.* Chicago: University of Chicago Press.

Cummings, J. L. (1987). Dementia syndromes: Neurobehavioral and neuropsychiatric features. *Journal of Clinical Psychiatry, 48,* 3–8.

Cummings, J. L., & Benson, D. F. (1992). *Dementia: A clinical approach* (2nd ed.). Stoneham, MA: Butterworth-Heinemann.

Day, A. T. (1985). Who cares? Demographic trends challenge family care for the elderly. *Population Trends and Public Policy, 9,* 1–17.

Diamond, E. E. (1987). Theories of career development and the reality of women at work. In B. A. Gutek & L. Larwood (Eds.), *Women's career development* (pp. 15–27). Newbury Park, CA: Sage.

Diesfeldt, H. F. A., van Houte, L. R., & Moerkens, R. M. (1986). Duration of survival in senile dementia. *Acta Psychiatrica Scandinavica, 73,* 366–371.

Dolinsky, A. L., & Rosenwaike, I. (1988). The role of demographic factors in the institutionalization of the elderly. *Research on Aging, 10,* 235–257.

Doty, P. (1986). Family care of the elderly: The role of public policy. *Milbank Quarterly, 64,* 34–75.

Doty, P. (1990). Dispelling some myths: A comparison on long-term-care financing in the United States and other countries. *Generations, 14,* 10–14.

Dwyer, J. W., & Coward, R. C. (1992). Gender, family, and long-term care of the elderly. In J. W. Dwyer & R. C. Coward (Eds.), *Gender, families, and elder care* (pp. 3–15). Newbury Park, CA: Sage.

Eckert, J. K., Namazi, K. H., & Kahana, E. (1987). Unlicensed board and care homes: An extra-familial living arrangement for the elderly. *Journal of Cross-Cultural Gerontology, 2,* 377–393.

Engström, M., Greene, R., & O'Connor, M. C. (1993). Adult day care for persons with dementia: A viable community option. *Generations, 17*, 75–76.

Ensel, W. M., & Lin, N. (1991). The life stress paradigm and psychological distress. *Journal of Health and Social Behavior, 32*, 321–341.

Evans, D. A., Funkenstein, H., Albert, M. S., Scherr, P. A., Cook, N. R., Chown, M. J., Hebert, L. E., Hennekens, C. H., & Taylor, J. O. (1989). Prevalence of Alzheimer's disease in a community population of older persons. *JAMA, Journal of the American Medical Association, 262*, 2551–2556.

Folstein, M. F., Folstein, S. E., & McHugh, P. R. (1975). "Mini-mental state": A practical method for grading the mental state of patients for the clinician. *Journal of Psychiatric Research, 12*, 189–198.

Fox, P. (1989). From senility to Alzheimer's disease: The rise of the Alzheimer's disease movement. *Milbank Quarterly, 67*, 58–102.

Friss, L. (1990). A model state-level approach to family survival for caregivers of brain-impaired adults. *Gerontologist, 30*, 121–125.

Funkenstein, H. H. (1988). Cerebrovascular disorders. In M. S. Albert & M. B. Moss (Eds.), *Geriatric neuropsychology* (pp. 179–210). New York: Guilford Press.

Gallagher, D. E., Breckenridge, J. N., Thompson, L. W., & Peterson, J. A. (1983). Effects of bereavement on indicators of mental health in elderly widows. *Journal of Gerontology, 38*, 565–571.

Gallagher-Thompson, D. (1994). Direct services and interventions for caregivers: A review of extant programs and a look to the future. In M. H. Cantor (Ed.), *Family caregiving: Agenda for the future* (pp. 102–122). San Francisco: American Society for Aging.

George, L. K., & Gwyther, L. P. (1986). Caregiver well-being: A multidimensional examination of family caregivers of demented adults. *Gerontologist, 26*, 253–259.

Gerhardt, U. (1990). Patient careers in end-stage renal failure. *Social Science and Medicine, 30*, 1211–1224.

Given, B. A., & Given, C. W. (1991). Family caregiving for the elderly. *Annual Review of Nursing Research, 9*, 77–101.

Goffman, E. (1961). *Asylums.* New York: Anchor.

Goldfarb, A. I. (1969). Predicting mortality in the institutionalized aged: A seven-year follow-up. *Archives of General Psychiatry, 21*, 172–177.

Gove, W. R., & Geerken, M. R. (1977). The effect of children and employment on the mental health of married men and women. *Social Forces, 56*, 66–76.

Gove, W. R., & Tudor, J. F. (1973). Adult sex roles and mental illness. *American Journal of Sociology, 78*, 812–835.

Greenberg, J. N., & Ginn, A. (1979). A multivariate analysis of the predictors of long-term care placement. *Home Health Care Services Quarterly, 1*, 75–99.

Greene, V. L., & Ondrich, J. I. (1990). Risk factors for nursing home admissions and exits: A discrete-time hazard function approach. *Journal of Gerontology: Social Sciences, 45*, S250-S258.

Haley, W. E., Brown, S. L., & Levine, E. G. (1987). Experimental evaluation of the effectiveness of group intervention for dementia caregivers. *Gerontologist, 27*, 376–382.

Haley, W. E., & Pardo, K. M. (1989). Relationship of severity of dementia to caregiving stressors. *Psychology and Aging, 4*, 389–392.

Harkness, G. A., Bentley, D. W., & Roghmann, K. J. (1990). Risk factors for nosocomial pneumonia in the elderly. *American Journal of Medicine, 89*, 457–463.

Heagerty, B., & Eskenazi, L. (1994). A practice and program perspective on family caregiving: Focus on solutions. In M. H. Cantor (Ed.), *Family caregiving: Agenda for the future* (pp. 35–48). San Francisco: American Society for Aging.

Hill, C. D., Thompson, L. W., & Gallagher, D. (1988). The role of anticipatory bereavement in older women's adjustment to widowhood. *Gerontologist, 28*, 792–796.

Horowitz, A. (1985a). Family caregiving to the frail elderly. *Annual Review of Gerontology and Geriatrics, 5*, 194–246.

Horowitz, A. (1985b). Sons and daughters as caregivers to older parents: Differences in role performance and consequences. *Gerontologist, 25*, 612–617.

House, J. S., & Kahn, R. L. (1985). Measures and concepts of social support. In S. Cohen & S. L. Syme (Eds.), *Social support and health* (pp. 83–108). Orlando, FL: Academic Press.

Humphry, D. (1984). *Let me die before I wake*. New York: Grove Press.

Jahnigen, D. W., & Binstock, R. H. (1991). Economic and clinical realities: Health care for elderly people. In R. H. Binstock & S. G. Post (Eds.), *Too old for health care? Controversies in medicine, law, economics, and ethics* (pp. 13–43). Baltimore: Johns Hopkins University Press.

Johansson, B., Zarit, S. H., & Berg, S. (1992). Changes in cognitive functioning of the oldest old. *Journal of Gerontology: Psychological Sciences, 47*, 75–80.

Johnson, C. L., & Catalano, D. J. (1983). A longitudinal study of family supports to impaired elderly. *Gerontologist, 23*, 612–618.

Jorm, A. F., Kortem, A. E., & Henderson, A. S. (1987). The prevalence of dementia: A quantitative integration of the literature. *Acta Psychiatrica Scandinavica, 76*, 465–479.

Kay, D. W. K., & Bergmann, K. (1980). Epidemiology of mental disorders among the aged in the community. In J. E. Birren & R. B. Sloane (Eds.), *Handbook of mental health and aging* (pp. 34–56). Englewood Cliffs, NJ: Prentice-Hall.

Kelman, H. R., & Thomas, C. (1990). Transitions between community and nursing home residence in an urban elderly population. *Journal of Community Health, 15*, 105–122.

Knopman, D. S., Kitto, J., Deinard, S., & Heiring, J. (1988). Longitudinal study of death and institutionalization in patients with primary degenerative dementia. *Journal of the American Geriatrics Society, 36*, 108–112.

Kokmen, E., Beard, C. M., Offord, K. P., & Kurkland, L. T. (1989). Prevalence of medically diagnosed dementia in a defined United States population: Rochester, Minnesota, January 1, 1975. *Neurology, 39*, 773–776.

Kunkel, S. R., & Applebaum, R. A. (1992). Estimating the prevalence of long-term disability for an aging society. *Journal of Gerontology, 47*, S253-S260.

Larwood, L., & Gutek, B. A. (1987). Working toward a theory of women's career development. In B. A. Gutek & L. Larwood (Eds.), *Women's career development* (pp. 170–184). Newbury Park, CA: Sage.

Lawton, M. P., Brody, E. M., & Saperstein, A. R. (1989). A controlled study of respite services for caregivers of Alzheimer's patients. *Gerontologist, 29*, 8–16.

Lazarus, R. S. (1966). *Psychological stress and the coping process*. New York: McGraw-Hill.

Lewis, J. (1987). *Daughters caring for mothers*. Technical report to the Rockefeller Foundation, London School of Economics.

Liang, J., & Tu, E. J. (1986). Estimating lifetime risk of nursing home residency: A further note. *Gerontologist, 26*, 560–563.

Litwak, E. (1985). *Helping the elderly: The complementary role of informal and formal systems*. New York: Guilford Press.

Lopata, H. Z. (1987). Women's family roles in life course perspective. In B. B. Hess & M. M. Ferree (Eds.), *Analyzing gender* (pp. 381–407). Newbury Park, CA: Sage.

Lund, D. A., Caserta, M. S., & Dimond, M. F. (1993). The course of spousal bereavement in later life. In M. S. Stroebe, W. Stroebe, & R. O. Hanson (Eds.), *Handbook of bereavement: Theory, research and intervention* (pp. 240–254). New York: Cambridge University Press.

Mace, N. L., & Rabins, P. (1991). *The 36-hour day: A family guide to caring for persons with Alzheimer's disease, related dementing illnesses, and memory loss in later life* (rev. ed.). Baltimore: Johns Hopkins University Press.

Malmberg, B., & Zarit, S. H. (1993). Group homes for people with dementia. *Gerontologist, 31*, 682–686.

MaloneBeach, E. E., Zarit, S. H., & Spore, D. L. (1992). Caregivers' perceptions of case management and community-based services: Barriers to service use. *Journal of Applied Gerontology, 11*, 146–159.

Manton, K. G. (1989). Epidemiological, demographic, and social correlates of disability among the elderly. *Milbank Quarterly, 67*, 13–58.

Marris, P. (1974). *Loss and change*. New York: Pantheon.

Martin, D. C., Miller, J. K., Kapoor, W., Arena, V. C., & Boller, F. (1987). A controlled study of survival with dementia. *Archives of Neurology (Chicago), 44*, 1122–1126.

Matthews, S. H., & Rosner, T. T. (1988). Shared filial responsibility: The family as the primary caregiver. *Journal of Marriage and Family, 50,* 185–195.

McConnell, S., & Riggs, J. A. (1994). A public policy agenda: Supporting family caregiving. In M. H. Cantor (Ed.), *Family caregiving: Agenda for the future* (pp. 25–34). San Francisco: American Society for Aging.

McCoy, J. L., & Edwards, B. E. (1981). Contextual and sociodemographic antecedents of institution·alization among aged welfare recipients. *Medical Care, 19,* 907–921.

Menaghan, E. G. (1983). Individual coping efforts: Moderators of the relationship between life stress and mental health outcomes. In H. B. Kaplan (Ed.), *Psychosocial stress: Trends in theory and research* (pp. 157–191). New York: Academic Press.

Miller, B., & McFall, S. (1991). The effect of caregiver's burden on change in frail older persons' use of formal helpers. *Journal of Health and Social Behavior, 32,* 165–179.

Mirowsky, J. (1985). Depression and marital power: An equity model. *American Journal of Sociology, 91,* 557–592.

Mirowsky, J., & Ross, C. E. (1984). Mexican culture and its emotional contradictions. *Journal of Health and Social Behavior, 25,* 2–13.

Moen, P., Robison, J., & Fields, V. (1994). Women's work and caregiving roles: A life course approach. *Journal of Gerontology: Social Sciences, 49,* S176-S186.

Mölsä, P. K., Marttila, R. J., & Rinne, U. K. (1986). Survival and cause of death in Alzheimer's disease and multi-infarct dementia. *Acta Neurologica Scandinavica, 74,* 103–107.

Montgomery, R. J. V. (1992). Gender differences in patterns of child-parent caregiving relationships. In J. W. Dwyer & R. C. Coward (Eds.), *Gender, families, and elder care* (pp. 65–83). Newbury Park, CA: Sage.

Morris, J. N., Sherwood, S., & Gutkin, C. E. (1988). Inst-Risk II: An approach to forecasting relative risk of future institutional placement. *HSR: Health Services Research, 23,* 511–536.

Mortimer, J. A. (1988). Epidemiology of dementia: International comparisons. In J. Brody & G. Maddox (Eds.), *Epidemiology and aging* (pp. 151–164). New York: Springer.

Mortimer, J. A., & Hutton, J. T. (1985). Epidemiology and etiology of Alzheimer's disease. In J. T. Hutton & A. D. Kenney (Eds.), *Senile dementia of the Alzheimer type* (pp. 177–196). New York: Alan R. Liss.

Moss, M. S., & Moss, S. Z. (1989). Death of the very old. In K. Doka (Ed.), *Disenfranchised grief: recognizing hidden sorrow* (pp. 213–227). Lexington, MA: Lexington Books.

Mowry, B. J., & Burvill, P. W. (1988). A study of mild dementia in the community using a wide range of diagnostic criteria. *British Journal of Psychiatry, 153,* 328–334.

Mullan, J. T. (1992). The bereaved caregiver: A prospective study of changes in well-being. *Gerontologist, 32,* 673–683.

Mullan, J. T. (1993). Barriers to the use of formal services among Alzheimer's caregivers. In S. H. Zarit, L. I. Pearlin, & K. W. Schaie (Eds.), *Caregiving systems: Formal and informal helpers* (pp. 241–259). Hillsdale, NJ: Erlbaum.

Mullan, J. T., Pearlin, L. I., & Skaff, M. M. (1995). The bereavement process: Loss, grief, recovery. In I. B. Corless, B. B. Germino, & M. A. Pittman (Eds.), *A challenge for living: Dying, death and bereavement* (pp. 221–240). Boston: Jones & Bartlett.

Nilsson, L. V., & Persson, G. (1984). Prevalence of mental disorders in an urban sample examined at 70, 75, and 79 years of age. *Acta Psychiatrica Scandinavica, 69,* 519–527.

Noelker, L. S., & Bass, D. M. (1989). Home care for elderly persons: Linkages between formal and informal caregivers. *Journal of Gerontology, 44,* 563–570.

Norris, F. H., & Murrell, S. A. (1987). Older adult family stress and adaptation before and after bereavement. *Journal of Gerontology, 42,* 606–612.

Osterweis, M., Solomon, F., & Green, M. (Eds.). (1984). *Bereavement: Reactions, consequences, and care.* Washington, DC: National Academy Press.

Parkes, C. M. (1987). *Bereavement: Studies of grief in adult life.* Madison, CT: International Universities Press.

Pearlin, L. I. (1983). Role strains and personal stress. In H. B. Kaplan (Ed.), *Psychosocial stress: Trends in theory and research* (pp. 3–32). New York: Academic Press.

Pearlin, L. I. (1989). The sociological study of stress. *Journal of Health and Social Behavior, 30,* 241–256.

Pearlin, L. I. (1992). The careers of caregivers. *Gerontologist, 32,* 647.

Pearlin, L. I., & Aneshensel, C. S. (1986). Coping and social supports: Their functions and applications. In L. H. Aiken & D. Mechanic (Eds.), *Application of social science to clinical medicine and health policy.* New Brunswick, NJ: Rutgers University Press.

Pearlin, L. I., & Aneshensel, C. S. (1994). Caregiving: The unexpected career. *Social Justice Research, 7,* 373–390.

Pearlin, L. I., Lieberman, M. A., Menaghan, E., & Mullan, J. T. (1981). The stress process. *Journal of Health and Social Behavior, 22,* 337–356.

Pearlin, L. I., Mullan, J. T., Semple, S. J., & Skaff, M. M. (1990). Caregiving and the stress process: An overview of concepts and their measures. *Gerontologist, 30,* 583–594.

Pearlin, L. I., & Schooler, C. (1978). The structure of coping. *Journal of Health and Social Behavior, 19,* 2–21.

Pearlin, L. I., & Turner, H. A. (1987). The family as a context of the stress process. In S. V. Kasl & C. L. Cooper (Eds.), *Stress and health: Issues in research methodology* (pp. 143–164). New York: Wiley.

Pearson, J., Verma, S., & Nellett, C. (1988). Elderly psychiatric patient status and caregiver perceptions as predictors of caregiver burden. *Gerontologist, 28,* 79–83.

Pillemer, K., & Suiter, J. J. (1994). Violence in caregiving relationships: Risk factors and interventions. In E. Light, G. Niederehe, & B. D. Lebowitz (Eds.), *Stress effects on family caregivers of Alzheimer's patients* (pp. 205–221). New York: Springer.

Pratt, C., Schmall, V., Wright, S., & Hare, J. (1987). The forgotten client: Family caregivers to institutionalized dementia patients. In T. H. Brubaker (Ed.), *Aging, health, and family: Long-term care* (pp. 197–213). Beverly Hills, CA: Sage.

Pruchno, R. A., Michaels, E. J., & Potashnik, S. L. (1990). Predictors of institutionalization among Alzheimer disease victims with caregiving spouses. *Journal of Gerontology: Social Sciences, 45,* S259-S266.

Pruchno, R. A., & Resch, N. L. (1989). Aberrant behaviors and Alzheimer's disease: Mental health effects on spouse caregivers. *Journal of Gerontology, 44,* 177–182.

Rando, T. A. (1986). A comprehensive analysis of anticipatory grief: Perspectives, processes, promises, and problems. In T. A. Rando (Ed.), *Loss and anticipatory grief* (pp. 3–37). Lexington, MA: D. C. Heath.

Raphael, B. (1983). *The anatomy of bereavement.* New York: Basic Books.

Regier, D. A., Boyd, J. H., Burke, J. D., Jr., Rae, D. S., Myers, J. K., Kraemer, M., Robins, L. N., George, L. K., Karno, M., & Locke, B. Z. (1988). One-month prevalence of mental disorders in the United States. *Archives of General Psychiatry, 45,* 977–986.

Roach, M. J., & Kitson, G. C. (1989). Impact of forewarning on adjustment to widowhood and divorce. In D. A. Lund (Ed.), *Older bereaved spouses: Research with practical applications* (pp. 167–184). New York: Hemisphere.

Rogers, R. G., Rogers, A., & Bélanger, A. (1989). Active life among the elderly in the United States: Multistate life-table estimates and population projections. *Milbank Quarterly, 67,* 370–411.

Rosenthal, C. J., & Dawson, P. (1991). Wives of institutionalized elderly men: The first stage of the transition to quasi-widowhood. *Journal of Aging and Health, 3,* 315–334.

Rosenthal, C. J., & Dawson, P. (1992). Families and the institutionalized elderly. In G. M. M. Jones & B. M. L. Miessen (Eds.), *Care-giving in dementia: Research and applications* (pp. 398–418). New York: Tavistock/Routledge.

Rosenthal, C. J., Sulman, J., & Marshall, V. W. (1993). Depressive symptoms in family caregivers of long-stay patients. *Gerontologist, 33,* 249–257.

Sanders, C. M. (1994). Risk factors in bereavement outcome. In M. S. Stroebe, W. Stroebe, & R. O. Hansson (Eds.), *Handbook of bereavement: Theory, research, and intervention* (pp. 255–267). New York: Cambridge University Press.

Scharlach, A. E., & Boyd, S. L. (1989). Caregiving and employment: Results of an employee survey. *Gerontologist, 29,* 382–387.

Schoenberg, B. S., Okazaki, H., & Kokmen, E. (1981). Reduced survival in patients with dementia: A population study. *Transactions of the American Neurological Association, 106,* 306–308.

Schulz, R., Visintainer, P., & Williamson, G. M. (1990). Psychiatric and physical morbidity effects of caregiving. *Journal of Gerontology: Psychological Sciences, 45,* P181-P191.

Shafritz, J. M. (1980). *Dictionary of personnel management and labor relations.* Oak Park, IL: Moore.

Shah, K. V., Banks, G. D., & Merskey, H. (1969). Survival in atherosclerotic and senile dementia. *British Journal of Psychiatry, 115,* 1283–1286.

Shanas, E. (1979). The family as a support system in old age. *Gerontologist, 19,* 169–174.

Shapiro, E., & Tate, R. B. (1985). Predictors of long term care facility use among the elderly. *Canadian Journal on Aging, 4,* 11–19.

Shuchter, S. R., & Zisook, S. (1993). The course of normal grief. In M. S. Stroebe, W. Stroebe, & R. O. Hansson (Eds.), *Handbook of bereavement: Theory, research and Intervention* (pp. 23–43). New York: Cambridge University Press.

Singer, J. D., & Willett, J. B. (1991). Modeling the days of our lives: Using survival analysis when designing and analyzing longitudinal studies of duration and the timing of events. *Psychological Bulletin, 110,* 268–290.

Skaff, M. M., & Pearlin, L. I. (1992). Caregiving: Role engulfment and the loss of self. *Gerontologist, 32,* 656–664.

Sloane, P. D., & Mathew, L. J. (1991). *Dementia units in long-term care.* Baltimore: Johns Hopkins University Press.

Smith, K., & Bergston, V. (1979). Positive consequences of institutionalization: Solidarity between elderly parents and their middle-aged children. *Gerontologist, 19,* 438–447.

Stoller, E. P. (1990). Males as helpers: The role of sons, relatives, and friends. *Gerontologist, 30,* 228–235.

Stoller, E. P. (1989). Formal services and informal helping: The myth of service substitution. *Journal of Applied Geronotology, 8,* 37–52.

Stroebe, M. S., Stroebe, W., & Hansson, R. O. (Eds.). (1993). *Handbook of bereavement: Theory, research and intervention.* New York: Cambridge University Press.

Stroebe, W., & Stroebe, M. S. (1987). *Bereavement and health: The psychological and physical consequences of partner loss.* New York: Cambridge University Press.

Stylianos, S. K., & Vachon, M. L. S. (1993). The role of social support in bereavement. In M. S. Stroebe, W. Stroebe, & R. O. Hansson (Eds.), *Handbook of bereavement: Theory, research and intervention* (pp. 397–410). New York: Cambridge University Press.

Sulkava, R., Wikström, J., Aromaa, A., Raitasalo, R., Lehtinen, V., LicPh, K. L., & Palo, J. (1985). Prevalence of severe dementia in Finland. *Neurology, 35,* 1025–1029.

Sutherland, E. H. (1937). *The professional thief: By a professional thief.* Chicago: University of Chicago Press.

Thoits, P. A. (1982). Life stress, social support, and psychological vulnerability: Epidemiological considerations. *Journal of Community Psychology, 10,* 341–362.

Thoits, P. A. (1987). Gender and marital status differences in control and distress: Common stress versus unique stress explanations. *Journal of Health and Social Behavior, 28,* 7–22.

Thomas, D. R., Bennett, R. G., Laughon, B. E., Greenough, W. G., III, & Bartlett, J. G. (1990). Postantibiotic colonization with *clostridium difficile* in nursing home patients. *Journal of the Medical Geriatrics Society, 38,* 415–420.

Thorslund, M. (1991). The increasing number of very old people will change the Swedish model of the welfare state. *Social Science and Medicine, 32,* 455–464.

Townsend, A. L., & Noelker, L. S. (1987). The impact of family relationships on perceived caregiving effectiveness. In T. H. Brubaker (Ed.), *Aging, health, and family: Long-term care* (pp. 80–99). Beverly Hills, CA: Sage.

U.S. Bureau of the Census. (1990). *The need for personal assistance with everyday activities: Recipients and caregivers* (Current Population Reports, Series P-70, No. 19). Washington, DC: U.S. Government Printing Office.

U.S. Bureau of the Census. (1992). *Population projections of the United States, by age, race, sex, and*

Hispanic origin: 1992 to 2050 (Current Population Reports, Series P-25, No. 1092). Washington, DC: U.S. Government Printing Office.

U.S. Department of Health and Human Services. (1992). *Social security area population projections 1991* (Publication No. 11–11553). Washington, DC: U.S. Government Printing Office.

van Dijk, P. T. M., Dippel, D. W. J., & Habbema, J. D. F. (1991). Survival of patients with dementia. *Journal of the American Gerontological Society, 39*, 603–610.

van Dijk, P. T. M., van de Sande, H. J., Dippel, D. W. J., & Habbema, J. D. F. (1992). The nature of excess mortality. *Journal of Gerontology: Medical Sciences, 47*, M28-M34.

Varsamis, J., Zuchowski, T., & Maini, K. K. (1972). Survival rates and causes of death in geriatric psychiatric patients: A six-year follow-up study. *Canadian Psychiatric Association Journal, 17*, 17–22.

Vicente, L., Wiley, J. A., & Carrington, R. A. (1979). The risk of institutionalization before death. *Gerontologist, 19*, 361–367.

Vitaliano, P. P., Peck, A., Johnson, D. A., Prinz, P. N., & Eisdorfer, C. (1981). Dementia and other competing risks for mortality in the institutionalized aged. *Journal of the American Geriatrics Society, 29*, 513–519.

Walker, A. J. (1992). Conceptual perspectives on gender and family caregiving. In J. W. Dwyer & R. C. Coward (Eds.), *Gender, families, and elder care* (pp. 34–46). Newbury Park, CA: Sage.

Walsh, J. S., Welch, H. G., & Larson, E. B. (1990). Survival of outpatients with Alzheimer-type dementia. *Annals of Internal Medicine, 113*, 429–434.

Wheaton, B. (1980). The sociogenesis of psychological disorder: An attributional theory. *Journal of Health and Social Behavior, 21*, 100–124.

Wheaton, B. (1985). Models for the stress buffering functions of coping resources. *Journal of Health and Social Behavior, 26*, 352–364.

Whitlatch, C. J., Zarit, S. H., & von Eye, A. (1991). Efficacy of interventions with caregivers: Reanalysis. *Gerontologist, 31*, 9–14.

Wiener, J. M., Hanley, R. J., Spence, D. A., & Murray, S. E. (1989). We can run but we can't hide: Toward reforming long-term care. *Journal of Aging and Social Policy, 1*, 87–102.

Wilensky, H. L. (1961). Orderly careers and social participation: The impact of work history on social integration in the middle mass. *American Sociological Review, 26*, 521–539.

Wilson, H. S. (1989). Family caregiving for a relative with Alzheimer's dementia: Coping with negative choices. *Nursing Research, 38*, 94–98.

Wolinsky, F. D., Callahan, C. M., Fitzgerld, J. F., & Johnson, R. J. (1992). The risk of nursing home placement and subsequent death among older adults. *Journal of Gerontology: Social Sciences, 47*, S173-S182.

Wortman, C. B., & Silver, R. C. (1989). The myths of coping with loss. *Journal of Consulting and Clinical Psychology, 57*, 349–357.

Wortman, C. B., Silver, R. C., & Kessler, R. C. (1993). The meaning of loss and adjustment to bereavement. In M. S. Stroebe, W. Stroebe, & R. O. Hansson (Eds.), *Handbook of bereavement: Theory, research and intervention* (pp. 349–366). New York: Cambridge University Press.

Wright, L. K., Clipp, E. C., & George, L. K. (1993). Health consequences of caregiver stress. *Medicine, Exercise, Nutrition, and Health, 2*, 181–195.

Yale, R. (1991). *A guide to facilitating support groups for newly diagnosed Alzheimer's patients.* San Francisco: Alzheimer's Association Greater San Francisco Bay Area Chapter.

Zarit, S. H. (1989). Interventions with frail elders and their families: Are they effective and why? In M. A. P. Stephens, J. H. Crowther, S. E. Hobfoll, & D. L. Tennenbaum (Eds.), *Stress and coping in later-life families* (pp. 241–265). New York: Hemisphere.

Zarit, S. H., Orr, N. K., & Zarit, J. M. (1985). *The hidden victims of Alzheimer's disease: Families under stress.* New York: New York University Press.

Zarit, S. H., & Teri, L. (1991). Interventions and services for family caregivers. *Annual Review of Gerontology and Geriatrics, 11*, 287–310.

Zarit, S. H., Todd, P. A., & Zarit, J. M. (1986). Subjective burden of husbands and wives as caregivers: A longitudinal study. *Gerontologist, 26*, 260–266.

Zarit, S. H., & Whitlatch, C. J. (1992). Institutional placement: Phases of the transition. *Gerontologist, 32*, 665–672.

Zedlewski, S. R., Barnes, R. O., Burt, M. R., McBride, T. D., & Meyer, J. A. (1990). *The needs of the elderly in the 21st century*. Washington, DC: Urban Institute Press.

Zisook, S., & Shuchter, S. R. (1986). The first four years of widowhood. *Psychiatric Annals, 16*, 288–294.

Index